Celiac Disease and Gluten

Multidisciplinary Challenges and Opportunities

Celiac Disease and Gluten

Multidisciplinary Challenges and Opportunities

Herbert Wieser
Scientific advisor at Deutsche Forschungsanstalt für Lebensmittelchemie, Leibniz Institut

Peter Koehler
Vice director of Deutsche Forschungsanstalt für Lebensmittelchemie, Leibniz Institut
And
Professor for Food Chemistry at Technische Universität München

Katharina Konitzer
Research scientist at Deutsche Forschungsanstalt für Lebensmittelchemie, Leibniz Institut

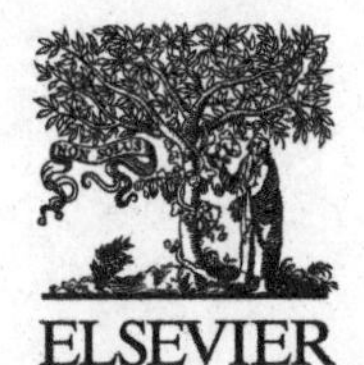

AMSTERDAM • BOSTON • HEIDELBERG • LONDON
NEW YORK • OXFORD • PARIS • SAN DIEGO
SAN FRANCISCO • SINGAPORE • SYDNEY • TOKYO

Academic Press is an imprint of Elsevier

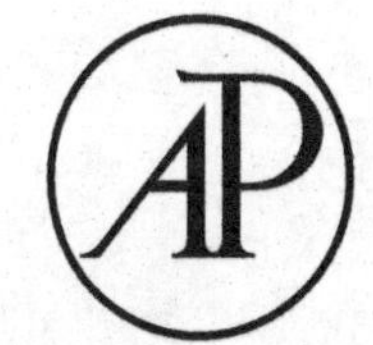

Academic Press is an imprint of Elsevier
32 Jamestown Road, London NW1 7BY, UK
225 Wyman Street, Waltham, MA 02451, USA
525 B Street, Suite 1800, San Diego, CA 92101-4495, USA

British Library Cataloguing-in-Publication Data
A catalogue record for this book is available from the British Library

Library of Congress Cataloging-in-Publication Data
A catalog record for this book is available from the Library of Congress

ISBN : 978-0-12-420220-7

For information on all Academic Press publications
visit our website at elsevierdirect.com

Typeset by TNQ Books and Journals Pvt Ltd.
www.tnq.co.in

Printed and bound in United States of America

14 15 16 17 10 9 8 7 6 5 4 3 2 1

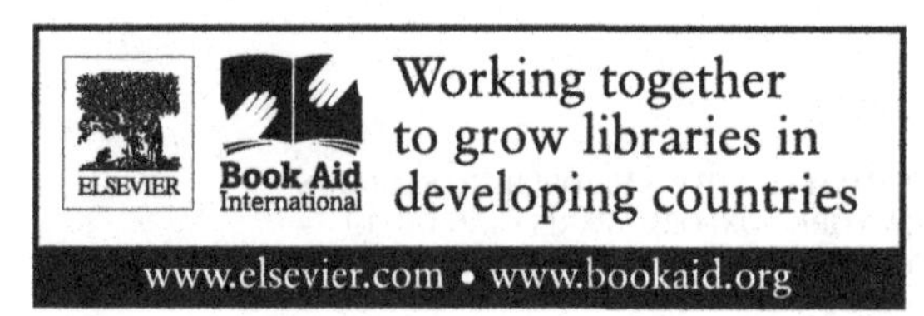

Contents

Preface

Research on celiac disease (CD) has progressed enormously over the last two decades with an explosion of new information. Evidence for this tremendous increase is provided by a literature search using the electronic databases MEDLINE and CAplus and "c(o)eliac disease" as MeSH terms, which yielded 260 references in 1990 and 1045 in 2012. In addition to more widespread awareness and improved diagnostic tools leading to earlier and more accurate recognition of CD, a rise of gluten-related disorders has contributed to this surge of research activity in multiple disciplines. Not only are physicians, pediatricians, pathologists, immunologists, gastroenterologists, neurologists, dermatologists, gynecologists, and pharmacists involved from the medical side, but also are analytical and food chemists, food technologists, cereal breeders, and genetic engineers from the cereal side and lawyers from the legal side. Due to the complexity of CD and the exceptionally high number of publications, experts in one discipline may find it difficult to keep track of recent developments in other disciplines.

To fill this gap, the aim of this book is to provide a unique, comprehensive overview on the multidisciplinary approaches to all essential aspects related to CD. History, epidemiology, genetics, clinical features, diagnosis, and pathomechanism of CD are covered as well as in-depth insights into cereal proteins. Legislation concerning gluten-free foods, novel treatment strategies, analytical methods for gluten quantitation, and concepts for future research complete the picture. Based on several hundred systematic reviews and original articles, the book reports up-to-date scientific findings and provides extensive opportunities for profound further reading. Thanks to the complete coverage of all scientific topics regarding CD, experts in one field may benefit from additional resources in their own field and broaden their knowledge of other fields. Over 60 illustrations and tables help the reader understand complex features like the pathomechanism of CD and the structure of cereal proteins. Careful cross-referencing, indexing, and a compilation of frequent abbreviations ensure easy navigation through the book.

This book will be a useful resource for medical practitioners and scientists, nutritionists, dietitians, producers of gluten-free foods, manufacturers of kits for clinical diagnostics and gluten detection, analytical and protein chemists, food technologists, and, of course, CD patients. It will also be interesting for hospitals, universities, research centers, analytical laboratories, and celiac societies worldwide.

We wish to express our thanks to Mrs Irmgard Bauer for ordering countless papers that were not available online, to Mrs Sabine Bijewitz for designing the illustrations, and to Mrs Anneliese Stoiber for all her work with the preparation of the manuscript. We would also like to thank the authors, editors, and publishers who have allowed reproduction of some of the illustrations included in this book.

Finally, we want to take the opportunity to thank the editorial and production team at Elsevier for their time, effort, expertise, and advice. We hope that this book will serve as a valuable basis of knowledge and as a comprehensive reference for all people involved in the fields of CD and gluten research.

Freising, December 2013.
Dr. Herbert Wieser, Prof. Dr. Peter Koehler, Katharina Konitzer.

Biography

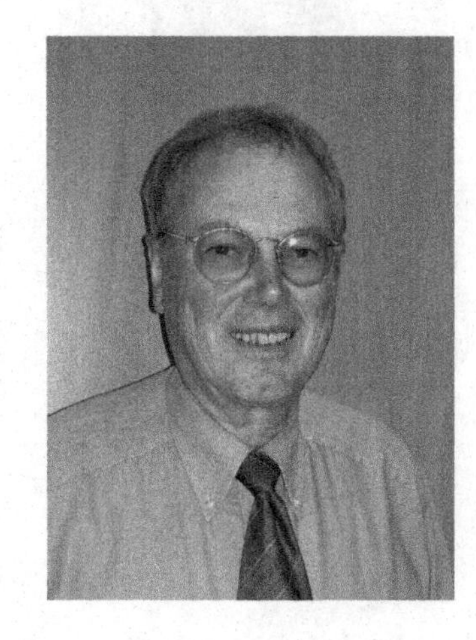

Herbert Wieser is one of the pioneers in celiac disease research. In 1984, he was the first to isolate a peptide from wheat gliadin with in vivo toxicity in celiac disease. In his career, Wieser has published more than 300 scientific papers. More than 100 articles are devoted to celiac disease research, mainly in cooperation with the most important clinical centers for this disease in Western Europe, the United States, and Israel. Herbert Wieser was a member of the Working Group on Prolamin Analysis and Toxicity (Prolamin Working Group, PWG) and scientific advisor of the German Celiac Society for more than 20 years. Currently, he works as a scientific advisor at the Deutsche Forschungsanstalt für Lebensmittelchemie, Leibniz Institut, in Freising, near Munich, Germany. He was awarded the Max-Rubner Award of the German Nutrition Society in 1984, the Osborne Medal of the AACC International in 2007, and the Neumann Medal of the German Association of Cereal Research in 2009.

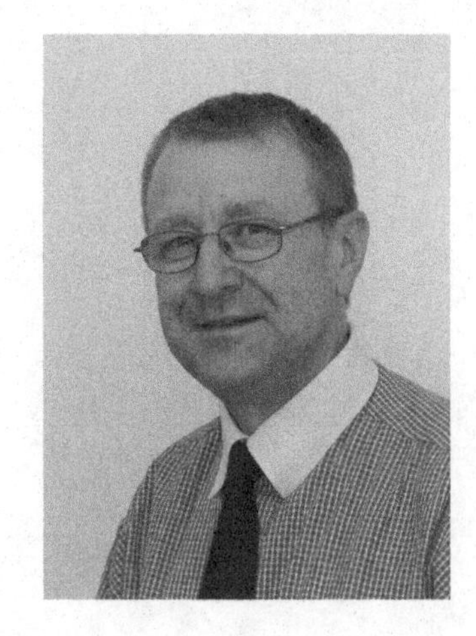

Peter Koehler is vice-director of the Deutsche Forschungsanstalt für Lebensmittelchemie, Leibniz Institut, professor for Food Chemistry at Technische Universität München, and vice-director of the Hans-Dieter-Belitz-Institute for Cereal Grain Research in Freising, near Munich, Germany. Currently, he is the chairman of the Working Group on Prolamin Analysis and Toxicity (Prolamin Working Group, PWG) and scientific advisor of the German Celiac Society. His research on celiac disease is focused on gluten analysis and gluten detoxification by means of enzymes. He developed a novel reference material for competitive ELISAs for gluten quantitation and coordinated collaborative studies on the validation of ELISA kits. Koehler is in charge of the PWG-gliadin reference material of the Working Group on Prolamin Analysis and Toxicity. He was awarded the Scientific Award of the German Bread Industry in 1994, Fellow of the ICC (International Association for Cereal Science and Technology) Academy in 2013, and "Bread Senator" of the German Association of Industrial Bakers in 2013.

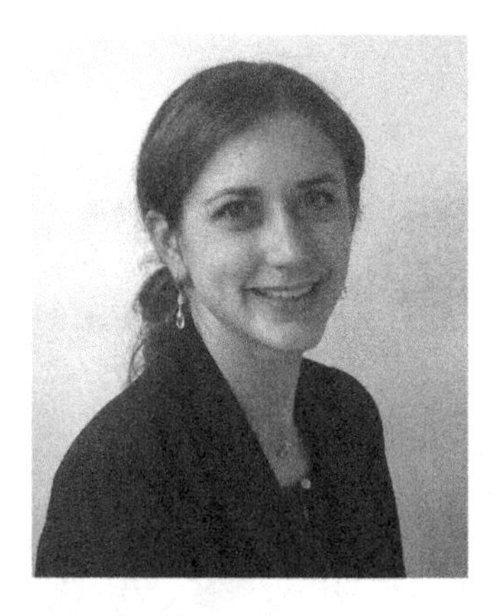

Katharina Konitzer studied food science at the Technische Universität München (TUM) and did research on new methods for the analysis of *Alternaria* mycotoxins via LC-MS/MS as a graduate student. She continued with her Ph.D. on "Studies on saltiness perception in bread and texture model systems—A contribution to salt reduction in foods" at the Chair of Food Chemistry and Molecular Sensory Science of the TUM. Currently, she works as a research scientist at the Deutsche Forschungsanstalt für Lebensmittelchemie, Leibniz Institut, in Freising, near Munich, Germany. Her present research deals with analytical and biochemical aspects of celiac disease, including the development of nonimmunochemical methods for gluten quantitation. She was awarded third prize at the Best Student Research Paper Competition of the AACC International in 2012 and won the Best Oral Student Paper Award at the Cereals and Europe Spring Meeting in 2013.

Frequent Abbreviations

2-D	Two-dimensional
AGA	Anti-gliadin antibody
Amino acid codes	see Table 2.1 (Chapter 2, Section 2.1)
AN	*Aspergillus niger*
APC	Antigen-presenting cell
ATI	Amylase trypsin inhibitor
CD	Celiac disease
DGPA	Deamidated gliadin peptide antibody
DNA	Deoxyribonucleic acid
ELISA	Enzyme-linked immunosorbent assay
EMA	Anti-endomysium antibody
ESPGHAN	European Society for Pediatric Gastroenterology, Hepatology and Nutrition
GFD	Gluten-free diet
GP	Gel permeation
GS	Glutenin subunit
HLA	Human leukocyte antigen
HMW	High-molecular-weight
HPLC	High-performance liquid chromatography
IBS	Irritable bowel syndrome
IEL	Intraepithelial lymphocyte
IFN	Interferon
Ig	Immunoglobulin
IL	Interleukin
LMW	Low-molecular-weight
LOD	Limit of detection
LOQ	Limit of quantitation
mAb	Monoclonal antibody
MALDI-TOF	Matrix-assisted laser desorption/ionization time-of-flight
MHC	Major histocompatibility complex
MS	Mass spectrometry
NCGS	Non-celiac gluten sensitivity
pAb	Polyclonal antibody
PAGE	Polyacrylamide gel electrophoresis
PBMC	Peripheral blood mononuclear cell
PCR	Polymerase chain reaction
PEP	Prolyl endopeptidase
POC	Point-of-care
PT	Peptic-tryptic
PWG	Prolamin Working Group
RCD	Refractory celiac disease
RNA	Ribonucleic acid
RP	Reversed-phase
SDS	Sodium dodecylsulfate

TCR	T-cell receptor
TG	Transglutaminase
TGA	Anti-transglutaminase antibody
Th	T-helper
TJ	Tight junction
TNF	Tumor necrosis factor
Treg	Regulatory T cell
VCE	Video capsule endoscopy
ZO	Zonulin

Introduction

Celiac disease (CD) is an immune-mediated inflammatory disease of the upper small intestine in genetically susceptible individuals triggered by the ingestion of the storage proteins (gluten) from wheat, rye, barley, and possibly oats. Intestinal symptoms similar to the clinical picture of CD nowadays were already described in the Roman Empire in the second century AD, and the idea that the disorder may be associated with food ingestion was discovered in the nineteenth century. Yet it was not until the 1950s that gluten was identified as the precipitating factor of CD, and a gluten-free diet was successfully introduced as treatment. For a long time, CD was considered to be a rare childhood enteropathy. Thanks to modern diagnostic techniques and increased awareness, epidemiological studies of the past decade revealed that CD is one of the most frequent food intolerances in many parts of the world, affecting about 1% of the population. While CD is typically characterized by a flat intestinal mucosa with villous atrophy resulting in a generalized malabsorption of nutrients, the spectrum of clinical manifestations is very complex, including silent and atypical presentations as well as numerous extraintestinal symptoms and nonspecific findings. This is why many cases remain undiagnosed and entail the risk of long-term complications such as osteoporosis, anemia, or malignancy in addition to a substantial burden of illness. Strategies like raising awareness and screening in at-risk groups have been successful in identifying previously undiagnosed patients, but the risks and benefits of screening the general population for CD remain controversial.

In addition to medical sciences like pediatrics, pathology, immunology, gastroenterology, neurology, and dermatology, other sciences like pharmaceutics, analytical and food chemistry, food technology, cereal breeding, genetic engineering, and law are involved in CD and gluten research. These multidisciplinary challenges and opportunities are highlighted in this book.

Starting with definitions and a historical perspective on previous milestones of CD investigations, recent epidemiological studies on CD prevalence worldwide are presented in the first chapter. Over the past few decades tremendous progress has been made in elucidating the complex pathomechanism of CD, which involves an intricate interplay of gluten, other environmental factors, genetics, and immunity. The strong association between HLA-DQ2/8 alleles and CD development has been proven conclusively, but the relative contributions of other unknown genetic risk factors and environmental factors such as infections, timing of gluten introduction into the infants' diet, and standards of hygiene have yet to be evaluated. Beside CD, other related disorders like dermatitis herpetiformis, gluten ataxia, wheat allergy, irritable bowel syndrome, and non-celiac gluten sensitivity are included as well as associated genetic and autoimmune diseases. The onset of CD may occur at any age, and the majority of patients nowadays present with predominantly extraintestinal complaints. This diagnostic challenge has been met with improved serological tests and HLA-DQ genotyping, but small intestinal biopsy is still considered the gold standard. Recent advances have been made in understanding the steps in the pathomechanism of CD, beginning with gluten intake and digestion followed by epithelial passage and induction of the adaptive and innate immune responses. With each advance in understanding within the single steps, new questions have arisen that will need to be investigated. As probably the only autoimmune disease in which the triggering environmental factor (gluten) is known, CD may serve as a unique model of autoimmunity that may be transferred to other immune-mediated diseases.

The second chapter gives an overview on cereals and provides an in-depth description of cereal proteins. The storage proteins of all cereals have a very intricate composition with hundreds of single proteins. When comparing the amino acid sequences, there are distinct differences between the CD-toxic storage proteins from wheat, rye, barley, and oats and the CD-safe storage proteins from corn, rice, sorghum, and millet. Advances in DNA and RNA sequencing have contributed to an increased knowledge of protein structures, which helps identify CD-toxic epitopes. Testing for CD toxicity may be done in vivo or in vitro using cereal flours or extracts, protein fractions, protein types, single proteins, or peptides. Whereas prolamins from wheat with an emphasis on α-gliadins and avenins have been studied most thoroughly regarding their CD toxicity, little is known about prolamins from rye and barley and all glutelins. CD epitopes are derived from all protein types from wheat, rye, barley, and oats, and further research on these proteins will help identify more relevant structures and allow an assessment of toxicity levels.

The treatment of CD, including both conventional and alternative therapies, is discussed in the third chapter. The conventional treatment, a strict, lifelong gluten-free diet, is currently the only safe option available. Patients adhering to a gluten-free diet need to be followed-up for an assessment of improvement of symptoms and recovery of normal intestinal architecture, not least because of the risk of refractory CD. Compliance to the gluten-free diet is essential not only to prevent a recurrence of symptoms, but also to reduce the risk of complications. An assessment of nutritional status is recommended at regular intervals, and monitoring the health-related quality of life of CD patients may help identify factors for its improvement. Alternative therapeutic options such as oral enzyme therapy, permeability inhibitors, inhibition of transglutaminase 2, HLA-DQ blocking, modulation of inflammation, and vaccination are in various stages of development and may become promising strategies. As more and more steps in the pathomechanism of CD are unraveled, further interesting approaches for alternative treatments will arise.

The fourth chapter deals with gluten-free products, legislation, and gluten analysis. While the production of gluten-free foods was a niche market only a few years ago, annual sales continue to experience a double-digit growth rate and are estimated to be worth more than (US) $6.2 billion worldwide by 2018. Only a small portion of this growth can be traced back to improved diagnosis of CD patients, and the larger portion can be attributed to an increasing number of gluten-sensitive individuals or of persons who seem to feel better on a gluten-free diet. Improving textural and flavor attributes, especially of breads and beer, is still a challenge for food technologists, but many acceptable products are already available not only in natural food stores but also in supermarkets and online. A variety of gluten-free symbols is used to distinguish these products, which have to comply with national and international legislation concerning foods for special dietary use for persons intolerant to gluten. To guarantee the safety of products for CD patients, several analytical methods for gluten quantitation have been developed, which are used in support of food labeling legislation. After an appropriate extraction of gluten proteins from the food matrix, enzyme-linked immunosorbent assays based on specific antibodies are most widely used for quantitation of gluten. Nonimmunochemical methods like mass spectrometry of gluten peptides as specific markers are promising alternatives. Despite major efforts, an accurate quantitation of gluten in a variety of food matrices still represents a considerable challenge owing to the great variability and complexity of gluten as the target analyte.

The last section includes a list of relevant research papers and reviews for readers wishing to delve deeper into the topic. Further on, it is dedicated to an overview on unresolved issues in the multidisciplinary fields of CD and gluten research, which deserve special attention and need to be addressed in future studies. Providing answers to these open questions will deepen our understanding not only of CD but also of other autoimmune and inflammatory disorders, which may open up exciting new concepts for the prevention and treatment of these diseases.

Definitions and Terms

CELIAC DISEASE

The relevant scientific literature suffers from a lack of consensus on the use of terms related to celiac disease (CD). Therefore, a multidisciplinary task force of 16 physicians from seven countries reviewed the literature for CD-related terms up to January 2011 and recommended definitions for each term (the so-called "Oslo definitions") [1]. Historically, different names (e.g. nontropical sprue, idiopathic steatorrhea, Heubner-Herter disease, celiac sprue, gluten-sensitive enteropathy, gluten intolerance, gluten sensitivity) were equivalently used for CD. The Oslo definitions suggest the term "celiac disease" (American English) or "coeliac disease" (British English) and define CD as "a chronic small intestinal immune-mediated enteropathy precipitated by exposure to dietary gluten in genetically predisposed individuals". The relevant scientific literature perceives CD, in part, as a food hypersensitivity disorder (gluten is the responsible food antigen) and, in part, as an autoimmune condition (presence of autoantibodies against tissue transglutaminase).

In addition, the authors of the Oslo definitions recommend terms for the different forms of CD and gluten-related disorders, and some terms were abandoned. The terms "classical" and "typical" CD have traditionally been similar concepts defining the presence of a gluten-induced enteropathy with diarrhea, malnutrition, and malabsorption syndromes. The word "typical" implies that this form is the most frequently encountered form of CD. However, many current patients have symptoms such as anemia, fatigue, and abdominal pain, which is why the use of the term "typical" CD has been discouraged. "Symptomatic" CD is characterized by clinically evident gastrointestinal and/or extraintestinal symptoms attributable to gluten intake. What was previously called "overt" CD should be part of "symptomatic" CD. "Nonclassical" CD presents itself without signs and symptoms of malabsorption. Similarly, "asymptomatic" CD does not show any symptoms commonly associated with CD. "Subclinical" CD is below the threshold of clinical detection without signs or symptoms sufficient to trigger CD testing in routine practice. The term "gluten intolerance" has been used as a synonym for CD and to indicate that a patient experiences a clinical improvement after starting a gluten-free diet. However, this term is nonspecific and has weaknesses and contradictions, and should not be used. "Gluten-related disorders" is the "umbrella" term for all diseases triggered by gluten. These may include disorders such as dermatitis herpetiformis, gluten ataxia, and non-celiac gluten sensitivity beside CD (see Chapter 1, Section 4.5). "Gluten sensitivity" has been used either as a synonym for CD or as an umbrella term for all disorders triggered by gluten. Most recently, the term was used for non-celiac gluten sensitivity. Due to these inconsistencies, it has been recommended that the term "gluten sensitivity" should no longer be used.

According to the guidelines of the European Society for Pediatric Gastroenterology, Hepatology and Nutrition (ESPGHAN) for the diagnosis of CD, "silent" CD is defined as "the presence of positive CD-specific antibodies and human leukocyte antigens (HLAs), and small-bowel biopsy findings that are comparable with CD but without sufficient symptoms and signs to warrant clinical suspicion of CD" [2]. "Latent CD" is defined by "the presence of compatible HLA but without enteropathy in a patient who has had a gluten-dependent enteropathy at some point in his or her life. The patient may or may not have symptoms and may or may not have CD-specific antibodies". "Potential CD" is defined by "the presence of CD-specific antibodies and compatible HLA but without histological abnormalities in duodenal biopsies. The patient may or may not have symptoms and signs and may or may not develop a gluten-dependent enteropathy later".

Considering that the terms "potential CD" and "latent CD" have often been used interchangeably, resulting in confusion, the authors of the Oslo definitions discouraged the use of the term "latent CD" [1]. The term "potential CD" should be used for people with normal small intestinal mucosa who are at increased risk of developing CD as indicated by positive CD serology.

GLUTEN

Primarily, "gluten" (from Latin for "glue") has been defined as "the rubber-like proteinaceous mass that remains, when wheat dough is washed with water or salt solution to remove soluble constituents and starch granules". The procedure of wheat gluten preparation was first described by Beccari in 1745 [3] and is nowadays widely used for the industrial isolation of "vital gluten", a byproduct of wheat starch production (see Chapter 2, Section 2.3). The starch industry expanded the meaning of gluten by the introduction of the term "corn gluten" as the proteinaceous byproduct of corn starch production. In the field of CD and according to the Codex Alimentarius, gluten is defined as "a protein fraction from wheat, rye, barley, oats or their crossbred varieties and derivatives thereof, to which some persons are intolerant and that is insoluble in water and 0.5 mol/l NaCl" [4] (see Chapter 4, Section 3.1). This protein fraction comprises hundreds of different components and corresponds to the storage proteins exclusively present in the starchy endosperm of the grains. Following the classical definition of Osborne, cereal storage proteins soluble in aqueous alcohols without reduction of disulfide bonds are designated as "prolamins" and the insoluble proteins as "glutelins" [5]. Shewry and coworkers used the term "prolamins" for all storage proteins (including glutelins) [6]. To prevent confusion, however, the classical definitions of prolamins and glutelins according to Osborne are used in this book.

REFERENCES

[1] Ludvigsson JF, Leffler DA, Bai JC, Biagi F, Fasano A, Green PHR, et al. The Oslo definitions for coeliac disease and related terms. Gut 2013;62:43–52.

[2] Husby S, Koletzko S, Korponay-Szabo IR, Mearin ML, Phillips A, Shamir R, et al. European Society for Pediatric Gastroenterology, Hepatology, and Nutrition guidelines for the diagnosis of coeliac disease. J Pediatr Gastroenterol Nutr 2012;54:136–60.

[3] Bailey CH. A translation of Beccari's lecture "concerning grain" (1728). Cereal Chem 1941;18:555–61.

[4] ALINORM 08/31/26, Appendix III, Codex Alimentarius Commission. Rome: WHO; 2008.

[5] Osborne TB. The vegetable proteins. 2nd ed. London: Longmans, Green; 1924.

[6] Shewry PR, Miflin BJ, Kasarda DD. The structural and evolutionary relationships of the prolamin storage proteins of barley, rye and wheat. Philos Trans R Soc Lond B Biol Sci 1984;304:297–308.

Chapter 1

Celiac Disease—A Complex Disorder

CHAPTER OUTLINE

Celiac Disease and Gluten. http://dx.doi.org/10.1016/B978-0-12-420220-7.00001-8

1. HISTORY

Until the Neolithic age, humans were not exposed to gluten for hundreds of thousands of years. Only about 10,000 years ago, cereal farming started in the Middle East, including the Tigris, Euphrates, and Upper Nile regions, and gradually spread across Europe with wheat and barley as prominent crops. The process of breadmaking was developed in Egypt about 5000 years ago and transferred via Greece to the Romans and then to other European regions. Wheat and rye bread became a staple food for Western populations; consequently, gluten consumption increased enormously. It appears that many individuals did not adapt to this "new" food item and did not develop an immunological tolerance [1].

Aretaeus of Cappadocia, a Greek physician practicing in Rome and Alexandria in the first and second centuries AD, was the first to describe an intestinal disorder similar to the picture of celiac disease (CD) nowadays. It was a general report on patients with chronic diarrhea, but some passages suggest that CD patients were among them. He wrote: "If diarrhea does not proceed from a slight cause of only one or two days duration, and if, in addition, the general system be debilitated by atrophy of the body, the celiac sprue of chronic nature is formed." He called these patients "koiliakos" according to the Greek term "koilia", which simply means abdomen. He believed the disease to be caused by partial indigestion of food, which should be treated by relieving the bowel of stress by rest and fasting. The case of a first century AD young woman, found in the archaeological site of Cosa, impressively demonstrated that a CD-like disorder existed in antiquity [2,3]. She was characterized by clinical signs of malnutrition, such as short height, osteoporosis, dental enamel hypoplasia, and indirect signs of anemia, which are all strongly suggestive for CD. Deoxyribonucleic acid (DNA) from bone and tooth followed by human leukocyte antigen (HLA)-typing displayed HLA-DQ2.5, the haplotype associated with the highest risk of CD (see Section 3.1).

It was not until the year 1888 that Samuel Gee, an English physician and pediatrician, presented the first accurate description of the clinical syndrome of CD. He used the term "celiac affection" and defined the disease as "a kind of chronic indigestion, which is met within persons of all ages, yet especially occurs in children between one and five years old." He recommended a dietary treatment without knowing the precipitating factor: "To regulate the food is the main part of the treatment" and "If the patient can be cured at all, it must be by means of the diet" [4]. Thereupon, different dietary therapies were recommended during the subsequent decades. For example, in 1908, Christian Herter stated that fats are better tolerated than carbohydrates. In 1918, George F. Still drew attention to the poor tolerance of bread; in 1921, John Howland recognized intolerance to carbohydrates; and in 1924, Sidney V. Haas recommended that all sources of carbohydrates (bread, cereals, potatoes) except bananas have to be excluded [5]. Nevertheless, most CD patients were branded by serious clinical features and 15–20% of the children died of the so-called celiac crisis characterized by acute diarrhea, metabolic and electrolyte abnormalities, and weight loss.

The Dutch pediatrician Willem K. Dicke (Figure 1.1) observed a decline of CD in The Netherlands, when there was a scarcity of cereals and bread during World War II. In his thesis, Dicke described that CD children benefited dramatically when wheat, rye, and oat flours were excluded from the diet [6]. Afterwards, the deleterious effect of wheat was clearly demonstrated by gastrointestinal studies [7,8]. The fractionation of wheat dough into

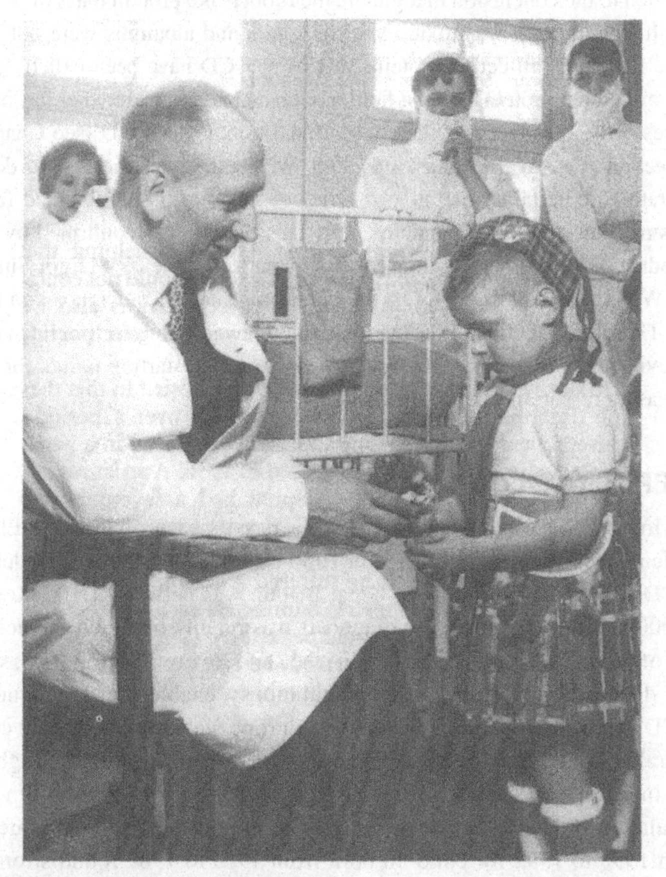

FIGURE 1.1 Willem Karel Dicke (1905–1962).

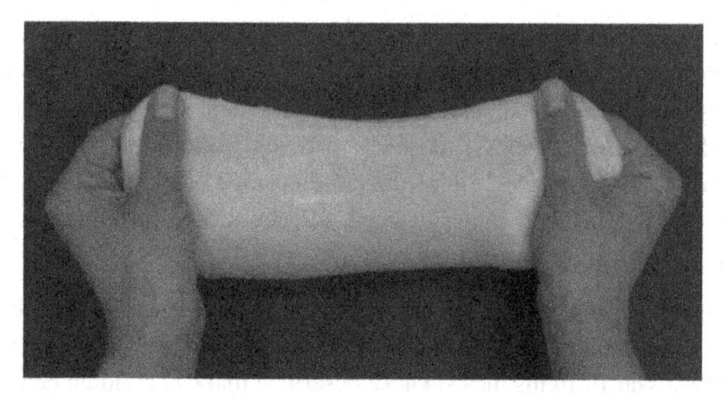

■ **FIGURE 1.2** Wheat gluten, the first cereal constituent detected to trigger celiac disease.

water-soluble albumins, gluten, and starch and in vivo testing of these fractions led to the conclusion that gluten, the rubber-like protein mass of wheat dough (Figure 1.2), was toxic, whereas starch and albumins were not [9]. Since that time, all cereal proteins that trigger CD have been called "gluten" or "gluten proteins" in the field of CD, and a gluten-free diet has been successfully introduced as the conventional treatment of CD (see Chapter 3, Section 1.1). At the same time, John W. Paulley was the first to demonstrate with certainty the abnormalities of mucosal tissue obtained from the small intestine of CD patients [10]. This finding was confirmed by the introduction of the peroral biopsy of the small intestine by Margot Shiner and William H. Crosby [11,12], the criterion standard of diagnosis to this day. Thus, the detection of the environmental precipitating factor gluten and the evidence of intestinal mucosal atrophy were the starting points for the increasing research activities in CD.

2. EPIDEMIOLOGY

Previously, CD was considered to be a rare disease of infancy. Early epidemiologic studies published in 1950 established that the prevalence of CD-like sprue syndrome in Great Britain was between 1:10,000 and 1:5000 [13]. At that time, the diagnosis was mainly based on the detection of typical symptoms, such as diarrhea and steatorrhea. Later on, specific diagnostic tools, such as intestinal biopsy, enabled better diagnosis of CD. In the 1970s, the prevalence in Europe was estimated to be considerably higher than before, from around 1:500 to 1:1000. The highest rate in Europe was found in Ireland, from 1:300 to 1:450 in the general population of the Galway region [14]. A multicenter study conducted from 1990 to 1992 for children born from 1975 to 1989 found strongly variable rates in different European areas, from 1:3200 (Copenhagen,

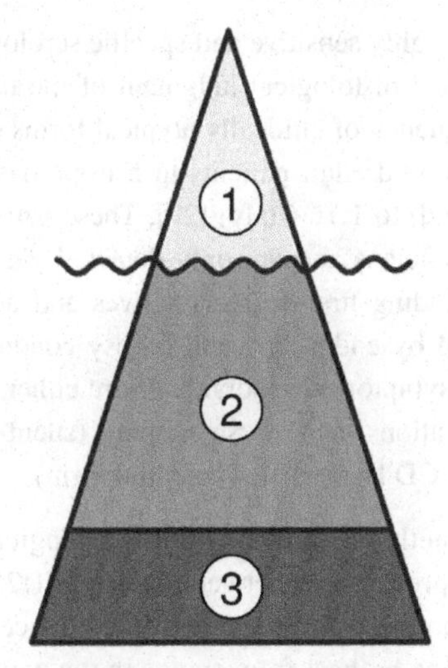

FIGURE 1.3 The iceberg model of celiac disease (CD). 1 = diagnosed patients; 2 = patients with undiagnosed silent CD; 3 = patients with undiagnosed potential CD. *Adapted from Ref. [17].*

Denmark) to 1:239 (Norrkoeping, Sweden) [15]. Outside Europe, CD awareness and diagnostic possibilities were less than in Europe, and the disease was thought to be rare. However, during the last decades the perception of CD has changed from a rather uncommon enteropathy to a common multiorgan disease.

In 1992, Logan published his frequently cited model of a "celiac iceberg", with the intention to demonstrate that CD patients with classical symptoms (symptomatic CD) are only a small minority compared with asymptomatic patients [16]. Since that time, different iceberg models with three, four, or five compartments have been suggested, including varying definitions of the compartments. Figure 1.3 shows the simplest three-section model [17]. Accordingly, the tip of the iceberg is formed by patients who have been diagnosed by biopsy, live gluten-free now, and show a normal mucosa. Below the water line, there are two big groups of asymptomatic cases that are not diagnosed due to atypical, minimal, or even missing complaints. These individuals either have a flat mucosa ("silent"; central part of the iceberg) or have immunological abnormalities (increased intraepithelial lymphocytes [IELs] or antitransglutaminase serum antibodies [TGAs]), but a normal mucosa ("potential"; lower part of the iceberg). Potential CD is not a rare form of CD. A retrospective study revealed a 18.3% prevalence among all celiac patients evaluated [18], and 62 children with normal villous morphology (19%) were identified among 320 children with positive serology by another study [19].

The development of highly sensitive and specific serological tests followed by mucosal biopsy and histological judgment of the tissue resulted in an unexpected high frequency of clinically atypical forms of CD. The ratio of diagnosed to undiagnosed adult patients in Europe has been estimated to be around 1:3 (Finland) to 1:16 (Italy) [20]. These patients usually remain unrecognized by physicians and are only detected via screening of high-risk individuals, including first-degree relatives and autoimmune disease patients, or identified by endoscopy and biopsy conducted for other reasons. Undiagnosed asymptomatic individuals are either exposed to the risk of long-term complications such as osteoporosis (silent form) or are at risk of developing typical CD later in life (potential form).

Modern diagnostic methods, including both serological tests and intestinal biopsy, revealed prevalences between 1:70 and 1:200 in most Western populations, corresponding to an average prevalence of approximately 1% [20,21]. One of the highest frequencies in the world, reaching 5.6%, has been reported among the Saharawi refugees of Berber-Arabic origin in North Africa [22]. CD is not reported in black African people. Exact figures on the worldwide prevalence vary according to population, age, year of measurement, and how CD is defined. Even though there is incomplete knowledge of the worldwide prevalence of CD, there appear to be differences among ethnic groups: the disease is obviously particularly common among Caucasians. A significant increase has been proposed during the last decades [23]. This may partly be attributed to an increase in awareness and to improved diagnostic techniques, but increased wheat and gluten consumption and changes in the environment have also been considered a major cause [24]. Moreover, modern wheat breeding may also have contributed to an increased prevalence [25]. However, a survey of data from the twentieth and twenty-first centuries for the United States did not support the likelihood that wheat breeding has increased the protein content proportionally to the gluten content [26].

In contrast, the statistical evaluation of more than 500 relevant papers published between 1995 and 2010 revealed that the average prevalence of CD in the general population remained constant (≈1:160). It seems to have been stable over the last decades and does not vary significantly in different geographical regions [27]. Thus, the prevalence of CD in the general population appears to be overestimated in recent years, and this is mainly due to the use of serological tests as the only diagnostic tool [27]. Nevertheless, CD is one of the most frequent food intolerances. It is not only a childhood disease anymore and can develop at any age. More than half of the new cases occur in individuals above the age of 50 [28].

Similar to most autoimmune disorders, the disease is more common in women than in men (ratio between 2:1 and 3:1), possibly because the necessary HLA-DQ2/8 alleles are more frequent in female than male patients [29]. The prevalence among first-degree relatives has been reported to be strongly elevated (≈10–20%), and the rate in monozygotic twins is approximately 75–80%, showing the strong genetic influence in CD (see Section 3.1). The prevalence of CD is significantly increased in autoimmune diseases, such as type 1 diabetes or autoimmune thyroid disease, and some genetically associated diseases such as Down's syndrome (see Section 4.6). Previously, CD was thought to be prevalent only in Europe and in countries to which Europeans have emigrated, including Australia, North America, and South America. Nowadays, the disease is increasingly found in areas of the developing world such as North Africa, the Middle East, and India, whereas only sporadic cases have been found in the Far East and sub-Saharan countries. In traditional rice-eating Asian countries, wheat is becoming a preferred staple. Due to these alimentary trends, an increased prevalence of CD in the Asian population can be anticipated in the near future.

Considering the key roles of the environmental (gluten) and genetic (HLA-DQ2/8) factors (see Section 3), Abadie and coworkers compiled the prevalence of CD, the levels of wheat consumption, and the frequencies of HLA-DQ2/8 alleles for different regions of the globe [30]. Surprisingly, a significant correlation between these three parameters was not observed. However, after outlier countries (Algeria, Finland, Mexico, North India, and Tunisia) were eliminated, the prevalence of CD was significantly correlated with wheat consumption, the frequencies of HLA-DQ2/8, and the combination of both risk factors. The existence of clear outliers and the fact that correlation coefficients were rather low suggest that other environmental and genetic factors must contribute to CD development.

3. GENETICS AND ENVIRONMENTAL FACTORS

CD is a multifactorial disorder and its development is controlled by a combination of genetic and environmental risk factors. The genetic predisposition to CD is complex and includes HLA-DQ2/8 genes as major factors. These are estimated to explain approximately 40% of the genetic susceptibility to CD. The other 60% are shared between an unknown number of non-HLA genes, each of which is estimated to contribute only a small risk effect. Genetic susceptibility and dietary gluten are necessary but not sufficient for the disease to develop. Thus, environmental factors beside gluten intake contribute to disease onset. For example, infections, microbiota, age of gluten introduction, initial dose of gluten, and breastfeeding have been considered to be important.

3.1 Genetics

Each complex disease, such as CD, has a unique genetic architecture. The main genetic factors in CD known today are HLA genes. The first insight into the links of CD to HLA alleles was presented in 1973 [31,32]. Since that time, it became obvious that CD has a stronger genetic component than many other common complex diseases. The pronounced genetic predisposition to CD is apparent because the concordance between monozygotic twins is 75–80% and between first-degree relatives it is approximately 10%. The latter is about 10 times greater than in the general population (see Section 2). The HLA class II alleles HLA-DQ2 and HLA-DQ8 at the major histocompatibility complex (MHC) on chromosome locus 6p21 have the strongest association with CD. Indeed, almost all CD patients express at least one of these HLA molecules. HLA-DQ proteins are heterodimers with α- and β-chains, both responsible for the CD-specific binding of gluten peptides by antigen-presenting cells (APCs) (see Section 6.3.1). The large majority of CD patients (≈90–95%) are DQ2 positive; the remainder are DQ8 positive. Two common DQ2 isoforms, DQ2.5 and DQ2.2, have been found. Most DQ2 patients have the DQ2.5 isoform, which is encoded by DQ A1*05 (α-chain) and DQ B1*02 (β-chain), either in *cis* position when these two genes (DQ A1*0501, DQ B1*0201) are located on the same DR3-DQ2 haplotype (on one parental chromosome) or in *trans* position, where the α-chain (DQ A1*0505) is encoded on the DR5-DQ7 haplotype on one chromosome and the β-chain (DQ B1*0202) on the DR7-DQ2 haplotype on the other chromosome (on one chromosome of each parent) [30] (Figure 1.4). The DQ2.2 heterodimer is encoded by the DQ A1*0201 and DQ B1*0202 alleles on the DR7-DQ2 haplotype. The DQ8 heterodimer is formed by α- and β-chains encoded by DQ A1*03 and DQ B1*0302, respectively, on the DR4-DQ8 haplotype. A minor subset of patients carries both DQ2 and DQ8 alleles. As a result, these patients may express two types of mixed DQ2/8 transdimers (encoded by DQ A1*05/DQ B1*03 and DQ A1*03/DQ B1*02) in addition to DQ2 and DQ8 [33]. A few remaining CD patients, who are neither DQ2 nor DQ8 positive (≈6%) [34], carry either the α-chain or the β-chain of the DQ2 heterodimer.

The HLA-DQ2.5 genotype is associated with a very high risk for CD, followed by DQ8 (high) and DQ2.2 (low) [30]. This disease susceptibility has been explained by the different dosage effects of the heterodimers [35] (see Section 6.3.1). Further, the increased risk of DQ2.5 over DQ2.2 correlates with a different ability of the two HLA molecules to form stable complexes with many gluten peptides [36]. In addition, Fabris and colleagues described an increased risk of developing CD in HLA-DQ2 positive individuals who carry an HLA-GI allele [37].

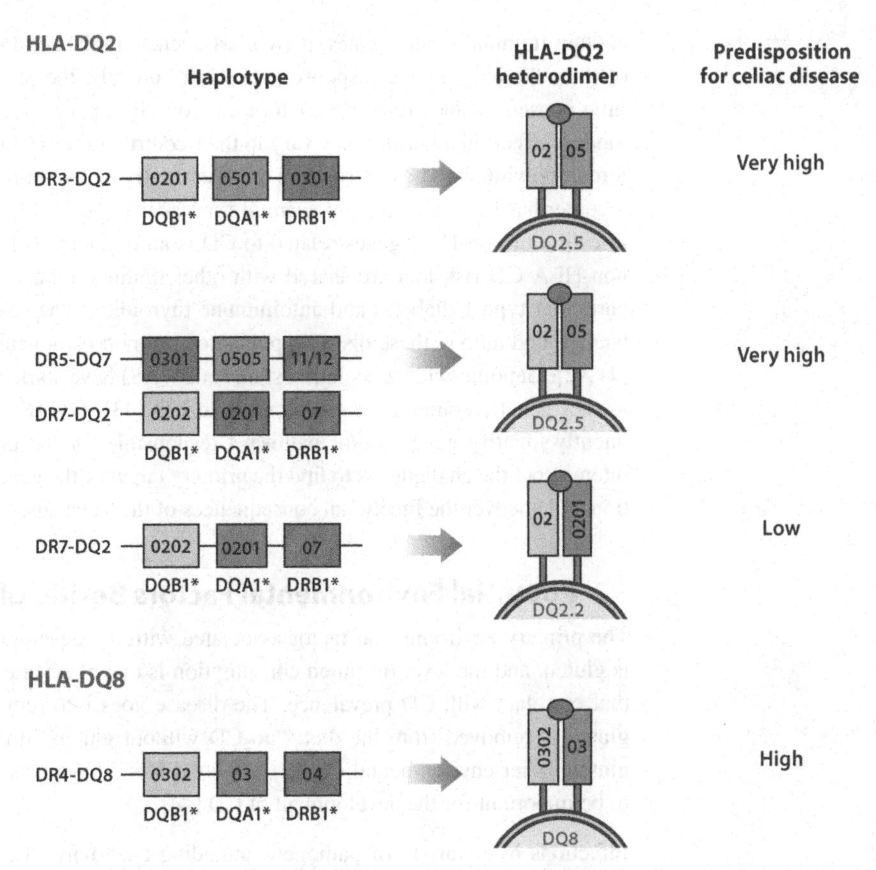

■ **FIGURE 1.4** Human leukocyte antigen (HLA) associations in celiac disease (CD). The great majority of CD patients express the HLA-DQ2.5 heterodimer, which is more strongly associated with CD than are the DQ8 and DQ2.2 heterodimers. *From Abadie et al. [30], with permission.* (Please see color plate at the back of the book.)

While approximately 97% of CD patients have HLA-DQ markers, these alleles are also common in approximately 30% of the general population; consequently, most individuals who express DQ2 or DQ8 never develop CD. Therefore, HLA-DQ2 or -DQ8 is thought to be necessary, but not sufficient, for the development of CD. The absence of these genes, however, is a reliable negative predictor of CD: if individuals do not have DQ2/8 alleles, they are unlikely to have CD. Due to the fact that HLA-DQ alleles are considered to account for only approximately 40–50% of the genetic susceptibility to CD, further genome research to identify risk factors, mainly focused on non-HLA genes, has been performed. A number of new loci (e.g., 2q33, 5q31–33, 19p13.1), including many immunological candidates, have been identified [38–40]. To date, around 40 such genomic regions harboring more than 60 candidate genes have been described. Most of these loci contain immune-related genes, particularly genes implicated in the control of the adaptive immune response [41]. Unfortunately, the results indicate little consensus and show that each of the non-HLA genes has a relatively modest effect; in addition, they vary in their contribution to CD among different individuals. The contribution of all currently known non-HLA genes together has been estimated to account for less than 10% [40]. Thus, identification of non-HLA genes related to CD is an ongoing challenge. Many non-HLA CD risk loci are shared with other immune-related diseases, in particular type 1 diabetes and autoimmune thyroiditis. The shared genetic background among these diseases points to common pathogenic pathways [41,42]. Genome-wide association studies (GWAS) have started to uncover further genetic components contributing to CD [43]. GWAS findings frequently identify genes and/or pathways responsible for the phenotype of interest, but the challenge is to find the primary target of the genetic association and uncover the functional consequences of the true causal risk variant.

3.2 Potential Environmental Factors Beside Gluten

The primary environmental factor associated with the development of CD is gluten, and the level of gluten consumption is one of several parameters that correlate with CD prevalence. The disease goes into remission when gluten is removed from the diet: "no CD without gluten". In addition to gluten, other environmental triggers ("second hits") have been considered to be important for the development of CD [44].

Infections by a variety of pathogens including adenovirus 12 and hepatitis C virus have been associated with CD, and there are descriptions on the increased onset of CD following rotavirus infection, the most common cause of childhood gastroenteritis [45]. The increased risk of subsequent CD development is perhaps due to a disruption of the intestinal barrier and facilitation of gluten peptide penetration. Indeed, double-stranded ribonucleic acid (RNA) viruses are strong inducers of interferon-γ (IFN-γ) and interleukin (IL)-15, key players of CD pathogenesis [46]. Remarkably, predisposed individuals born in the summer were proposed to have a higher risk of getting CD than those born in winter, possibly because the introduction of gluten at around 6 months of age occurs in winter accompanied by the seasonal peak of infections [47]. Although a causal relationship between infections and CD has not been demonstrated, rotavirus and other intestinal pathogens may create a proinflammatory environment that initiates and enhances the immune response to dietary gluten. A nationwide study of more than 29,000 CD patients and more than 140,000 controls examined the association between summer birth (March–August) and later CD diagnosis [48]. The results indicated a small risk of summer birth for CD, and the risk factor was most prominent for children with CD before the age of 2 years. The authors concluded that seasonal exposures early in life, such as infectious diseases, are unlikely to be a major cause of CD. Another multicenter study proposed that the season of birth may be an environmental risk for CD, particularly in boys diagnosed before the age of 15 years [49].

Likewise, an imbalanced intestinal microbiota has been reported in CD patients compared to healthy individuals [50]. The intestinal microbiota comprises bacteria that promote regulatory immune responses and bacteria that promote inflammatory immune responses [51,52]. In CD patients, decreases in regulatory bacteria *Faecalibacterium prausnitzii* and representatives of the genus *Bifidobacterium* were reported [50,53], as well as an expansion of potentially pathogenetic bacterial populations, such as *Escherichia coli* and *Staphylococcus* spp [54]. Two probiotic strains, *Bifidobacterium longum* and *Bifidobacterium bifidum*, were shown to reverse the deleterious effects of the proinflammatory milieu of the disease [55]. These findings may hold future perspectives of interest in CD therapy. Neonatal bacterial colonization has been associated with a future risk of CD, but it was not confirmed in all studies [56]. Children born by cesarean section, having a modest increased risk of later CD, harbor flora resembling skin bacterial communities, whereas children born vaginally have microbiota that resemble their mothers' vaginal flora [57].

The so-called hygiene hypothesis, postulating that a high hygiene level in the industrialized world has led to increased allergic and autoimmune disorders, has been used to explain the drastically different prevalences of CD in Finland (1.0%) and the neighboring Russian Karelia (0.2%). Both populations have similar wheat consumption levels and comparable HLA haplotype frequency, but Karelia is characterized by lower standards of hygiene [58]. However, the low prevalence found in Germany (0.3–0.5%) [20] appears contradictory to this hypothesis.

A reduced risk of developing CD has been associated with both breastfeeding during gluten introduction and the amount and timing of gluten exposure [59–61]. Children that were breastfed at the first exposure to gluten, even with high amounts, showed a lower risk of developing CD than those who were formula-fed. The cause of this effect is unknown. The microbiota as well as nutritional and immune system supporting factors in breast milk may contribute to the reduced gastrointestinal illness, and this reduction in infection extends beyond the time of breastfeeding. The epidemic of CD among Swedish children observed in the mid-1980s suggests that the amount of gluten during weaning can play a pivotal role in the development of CD [62]. Later findings indicated that the amount of gluten introduced during weaning might affect the development of symptomatic CD, but it does not protect the children from being affected by subclinical or silent forms of CD [63].

The timing of gluten introduction also seems to be relevant: children younger than 4 months and older than 7 months at the first exposure to gluten have an increased risk of CD compared to children aged 4–7 months [64]. Therefore, the ESPGHAN Committee and the international project PREVENTCD recommend avoidance of both early (<4 months) and late (>7 months) introduction of gluten and gradual introduction of small amounts of gluten while the child is still breastfed [65,66]. However, it is not clear whether the onset of symptoms is delayed or a permanent protection against CD is provided. Studies on 9408 Swedish children, including parent-reported data on gluten introduction, breastfeeding duration, and infections, found no association between breastfeeding, age at gluten introduction, and future CD [67]. Infection at the time of gluten introduction was not a major risk factor for CD. Studies on 324 Norwegian children with CD in a cohort of 82,167 children showed an increased risk in children introduced to gluten after 6 months and a higher risk in children breastfed after 12 months of age [68].

Ongoing research will hopefully determine the optimum practice; in particular, the possible risk related to a late introduction of gluten (>7 months) deserves further confirmation. Several population studies are currently being carried out to look for new strategies for CD prevention during the first stages of life [69]. Important issues are to determine the following:

1. the long-term effects of breastfeeding and the molecular basis for the protective effect;
2. the role of timing and dose of gluten during introduction;
3. the role of probiotics and prebiotics.

3.3 Interplay Between Genetics and the Environment

Abadie and coworkers described the spectrum of CD susceptibility as a complex interplay between genes and environment [30]. On the one end, there are individuals with HLA-DQ2/8 alleles, a large number of non-HLA genes, and a limited need for environmental hits. This group of patients may get CD as soon as gluten is introduced into the diet. On the other end, there are individuals with a limited number of genetic risk factors (e.g., correct HLA genes but a limited number of non-HLA genes) who require multiple environmental hits to develop CD. This group may never develop CD or may develop it late in life. How gluten influences disease development can vary depending on the amount of gluten and when it is introduced into the diet, which further suggests a complex interplay between genetic risk factors and the environment.

4. CLINICAL FEATURES

CD was originally considered to be a pediatric disorder characterized by diarrhea and malabsorption. Subsequently, it was recognized that CD can also affect adults at any age. The clinical appearance of CD is highly variable and can range from asymptomatic to full-blown symptoms. CD predominantly affects the upper small intestine and is characterized by inflammation and damage of the small intestinal mucosa. Beside intraintestinal symptoms, CD includes a number of extraintestinal features involving endocrinological, cutaneous, and neurological manifestations. Gluten intake induces the production of CD-specific serum antibodies, which can act as markers of the untreated disease. As an immune-mediated disease with an autoimmune component, CD shares different genes with other autoimmune diseases and shows a strong association with these disorders.

4.1 Symptoms

Numerous symptoms are associated with CD. They can be divided into intestinal disorders and extraintestinal features mainly caused by malabsorption of essential nutrients. Patients with only extraintestinal manifestations have a major potential disadvantage: They are less likely to be diagnosed with CD as compared to patients with gastrointestinal symptoms. CD is a disease of all ages, but with a trend towards older age at diagnosis. Whether these patients have had CD since their childhood but only became symptomatic later on in life or whether they actually developed CD in adulthood is still under debate. Probably both scenarios exist [70]. The systemic manifestations of CD include a wide clinical spectrum involving endocrinological, cutaneous, and neurological manifestations, among others. The wide variety of presentations is addressed in the National Institute for Health and Care Excellence guidelines drawn up to improve recognition and diagnosis of CD [71]. The pattern of clinical signs has significantly shifted toward later presentation and more extraintestinal manifestations in recent decades.

In predisposed infants, symptoms of CD can be observed within weeks to months of starting introduction of gluten into the diet. Classical symptoms in infants are diarrhea, steatorrhea, abdominal distension (Figure 1.5), vomiting, failure to thrive, stunted growth, and apathy. Iron-deficiency anemia is one of the most common extraintestinal manifestations of CD. The so-called celiac crisis, frequently described previously and characterized by explosive watery diarrhea, marked abdominal distension, metabolic and electrolyte disturbances, and shock, is now observed rarely. These patients require hospitalization and parenteral nutrition, and most cases show a full response to a gluten-free diet. In older children and adolescents, the clinical

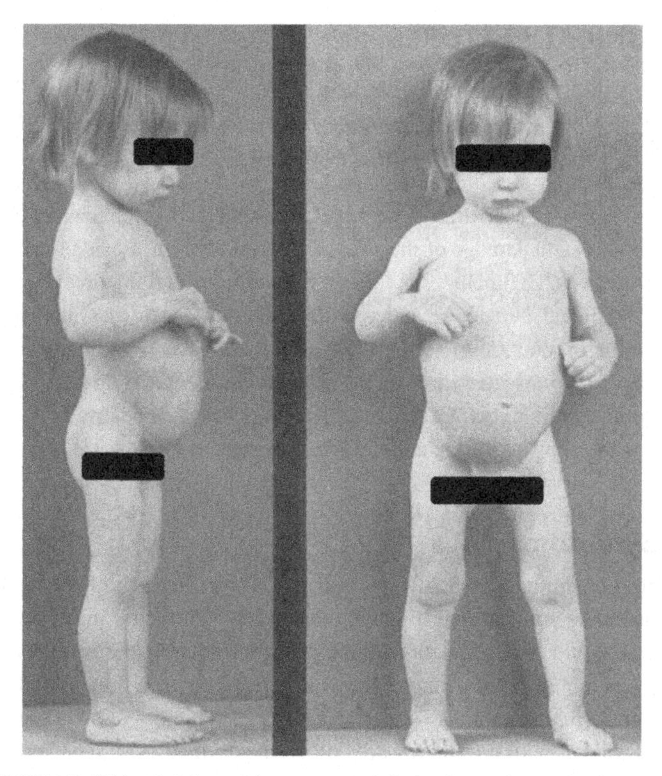

■ **FIGURE 1.5** Child with abdominal distension typical of celiac disease. *Reprinted with permission from the German Celiac Society.*

presentation of CD is usually less obvious, with diarrhea, loss of appetite, constant fatigue, anemia, and short stature predominating. CD is the most common cause of slow growth rate and is much more common than growth hormone deficiency. Delayed sexual maturation of adolescents is also a known complication of CD.

In addition to the classical symptoms, adults show increased effects of mineral and vitamin deficiencies, such as anemia, decreased bone mineral density, bone pain and fractures, osteoporosis, dental enamel defects, skin lesions, and night blindness. The presentation of CD both clinically and histologically is similar in young and elderly patients [72]. The nutrition status depends on the length of time the disease has been active and on the extent of intestinal damage. Malabsorption of fat-soluble vitamins (A, D, E, and K) as well as folic acid are frequently observed, whereas deficiencies of water-soluble vitamins are less common. The level of certain minerals including iron, magnesium, calcium, copper, zinc, and selenium can be low, depending on disease severity and dietary intake. Active CD is frequently accompanied by lactose intolerance due to the reduced activity of the enzyme lactase. Historically, weight loss has been a classical symptom of CD. Recent studies, however, suggest that untreated CD patients are more likely to be obese [73]. The traditional image of CD patients characterized by thin and diarrhetic individuals contrasts with the subsequent situation, as up to 30% of all patients are overweight and 50% suffer from constipation [74]. CD has been associated with several hepatic disorders, such as modest hypertransaminasemia. In rare cases, untreated CD may even lead to fulminant hepatitis and liver failure [75]. Treatment with a gluten-free diet may prevent progression to hepatic dysfunction, even in cases in which liver transplantation is considered.

Early studies showed contradictory results with regard to the co-occurrence of CD and psoriasis. However, a large study revealed the relationship between the two diseases to be unequivocally present [76]. Patients with psoriasis should be investigated for potential CD and should be followed-up [77]. In women, CD may have implications on menstrual and reproductive health (e.g., delayed menarche, early menopause, recurrent miscarriages) [78,79]. These women especially benefit from early diagnosis and treatment. CD has also been linked to infertility. However, two large cohort studies could not show an association between CD and infertility, before or after CD diagnosis [80,81]. Reproductive disorders associated with CD in men seem to be less frequent than in women, but reduced sperm motility, abnormal sperm morphology, impotence, and loss of libido have been reported in untreated CD patients [79].

A minor number of patients show neurological or psychiatric symptoms such as depression, anxiety, peripheral neuropathy, migraine, cerebellar ataxia, and epilepsy [82]. Patients with established CD referred for neurological opinion showed significant brain abnormality on 3T magnetic resonance imaging, such as less grey matter density and white matter abnormalities in some regions [83]. The precise mechanism of the association between CD and neurological manifestations is unknown and several hypotheses have been proposed [84]. CD is characterized by malabsorption, and some neurological complications may be secondary to deficiencies of vitamins and minerals. Some authors suggest that the antibodies associated with CD (anti-endomysium antibodies [EMAs], TGAs) may be neurotoxic themselves, or, alternatively, may be a marker for a neurotoxic immunological process.

Data on the prevalence of CD cases in people with epilepsy differ from 1% to 8% [84]. The clinical picture generally includes a specific triad of symptoms—occipital calcifications, seizures originating from a number of brain locations, and CD. Some studies have reported an improvement in patients with this triad after going on a gluten-free diet [82]. Sleep disorders, which are common in CD, have been shown to be strongly associated with psychological illness [85]. The association between autism, schizophrenia, and CD is still controversial. Several studies have shown an association between autism and CD [82,86]. Individuals with normal mucosa but a positive CD serologic test result were found to have a markedly increased risk of autism spectrum disorders [87]. A gluten- and casein-free diet turned out to be beneficial in subjects with autism. However, it is difficult to discern whether the removal of casein or gluten had the beneficial effects. Currently, there is insufficient evidence to support instituting a gluten-free diet as a treatment of autism [86]. There may be a subgroup of patients who might benefit from a gluten-free diet, but the symptoms or testing profile of these candidates remain unclear.

Schizophrenia may be the psychiatric disorder with the most robust relationship to CD (the so-called bread madness) [82]. Since 1953, cases of schizophrenia have been described where a gluten-free diet improved schizophrenic symptoms. The level of anti-gliadin antibodies (AGAs) in people with schizophrenia was found to be significantly higher than that observed in the general population. A study in more than 10,000 patients with schizophrenia showed that these patients were at an increased risk for CD as well as other autoimmune diseases [88].

Untreated CD has been associated with an increased risk of comorbidity, mortality, and malignancy, such as T-cell lymphoma. However, the strength of this association is conflicting among different studies [89,90]. With the exception of reduced bone health, older adults with undiagnosed CD were shown to have only limited comorbidity [91]. Population-based studies indicated that the overall risks of malignancy and mortality in unrecognized CD are not increased compared to the general population during a 20-year follow-up [92]. Another study confirmed that persistent villous atrophy is not associated with increased mortality [93]. However, certain malignancies, such as non-Hodgkin lymphoma and esophageal cancer, seem to be significantly associated with the undiagnosed conditions [94]. Refractory CD (RCD) is a very severe form of CD (see Section 4.4), and RCD type II imposes a serious risk of virtually lethal enteropathy-associated T-cell lymphoma. The 5-year survival rate varies from 44% to 58% [95].

4.2 Pathology

CD predominantly affects the mucosa of the upper small intestine (duodenum, proximal jejunum). However, capsule endoscopy has revealed that over a third of CD patients have microscopic mucosal changes extended beyond the duodenum, and other mucosal surfaces (such as oral, esophageal, gastric, ileal, and rectal) belonging to the digestive tract can also be involved [96]. CD is classically characterized by damage of the intestinal mucosa, including villous atrophy, crypt hyperplasia, and increased lymphocyte infiltration of the epithelium [97]. The characteristic histological appearance of the mucosa in untreated CD exhibits a loss of the normal villous architecture and a reduction in the ratio of villous height to crypt depth (normally between 5:1 and 3:1). There is a general flattening of the mucosa, which can vary from mild partial villous atrophy to a total absence of villi (Figure 1.6). The number of IELs in relation to the number of surface cell enterocytes is increased (≥30 IELs per 100 enterocytes). In full-blown atrophic mucosa, the uptake of nutrients is strongly reduced by a dramatic decrease of the luminal small intestinal surface (approximately from the area of a tennis court to a sheet of paper) and the loss of mucosal enzyme/carrier systems.

In 1992, Marsh introduced a grading scheme to classify the morphologic spectrum of the mucosa of untreated CD patients [98]. Oberhuber and coworkers [99] modified some of Marsh's parameters, and the so-called Marsh-Oberhuber classification is used by many pathologists to evaluate the mucosal lesions in CD patients. This classification describes five interrelated states of the mucosa (types 0–4) as follows [99] (Table 1.1):

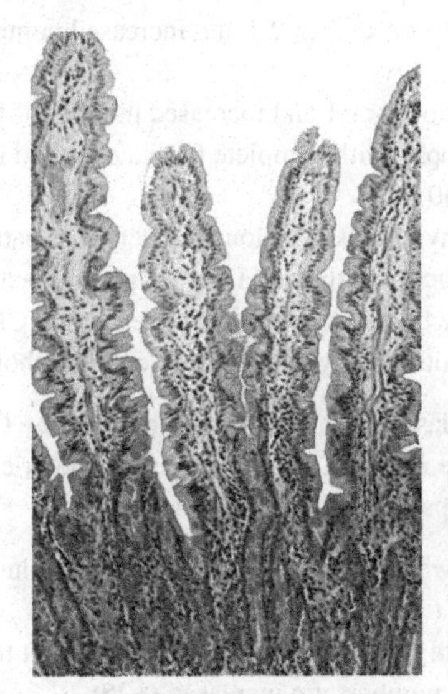
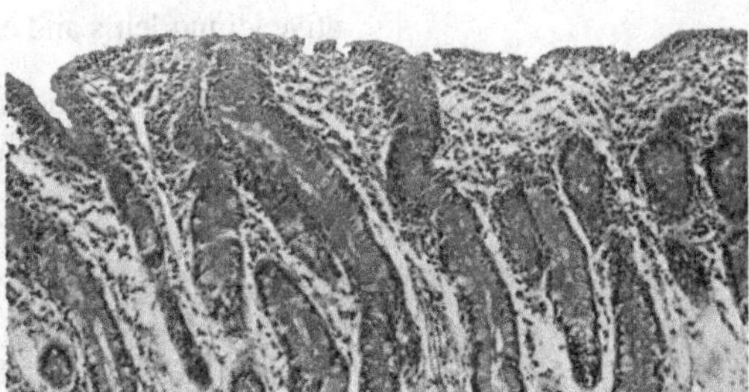

■ **FIGURE 1.6** Cross-section of normal (left) and celiac disease-damaged atrophical (right) intestinal mucosa. *Reprinted with permission from the German Celiac Society.* (Please see color plate at the back of the book.)

Table 1.1 Classification Schemes for the Pathologic Evaluation of CD[a]

Marsh [98]	Oberhuber et al. [99]	Corazza and Villanacci [100]	Ensari [101]
Type 1	Type 1	Grade A	Type 1
Type 2	Type 2	Grade A	Type 1
Type 3	Type 3A	Grade B1	Type 2
	Type 3B	Grade B1	Type 2
	Type 3C	Grade B2	Type 3
Type 4	Type 4	Obsolete	Obsolete

[a]*Adapted from Ensari [101].*

Type 0: preinfiltrate, normal small intestinal mucosa with less than 30 IELs per 100 enterocytes.
Type 1: infiltrative type, which is characterized by a normal villous to crypt ratio (>3:1) and an increased number of IELs (≥30).
Type 2: infiltrative-hyperplastic type, which is characterized by a normal villous architecture and crypt hyperplasia with an increased number of IELs (≥30). This stage is only very rarely encountered in CD patients and has mainly been observed in patients with dermatitis herpetiformis.
Type 3: destructive (flat mucosa) type of CD lesion. It has been divided into three different subgroups depending on the degree of villous atrophy:
3a: villous/crypt ratio of <3:1 or 2:1 and increased number of IELs (≥30).
3b: villous/crypt ratio of <1:1 and increased number of IELs (≥30).
3c: total villous atrophy with complete flat mucosa and increased number of IELs (≥30).
Type 4: atrophic type (hyperplastic lesion) is a very rare pattern, characterized by flat mucosa with only a few crypts and near-normal IEL counts. It is usually found in patients with refractory CD, ulcerative jejunoileitis and enteropathy-associated T-cell lymphoma.

An alternative histologic classification has been proposed by Corazza and Villanacci, who divided the mucosal lesions into two categories (A and B, the latter with two subgroups) as follows [100] (Table 1.1):

Grade A: nonatrophic, with normal villous and crypt architecture and increased IEL numbers (>25).
Grade B1: atrophic, with villous to crypt ratio of <3:1, but the villi are still detectable and IEL numbers are increased (>25).
Grade B2: atrophic and flat, where the villi are no longer detectable and IEL numbers are increased (>25).

A further updated version of the original Marsh classification was presented by Ensari in 2010 [101] (Table 1.1). The mucosal pathologic features are defined in three types, mainly depending on the degree of cellular and architectural abnormalities. Type 1 corresponds to type 1 of Marsh and Oberhuber and to grade A of Corazza–Villanacci. Type 2 corresponds to types 3A and 3B of Oberhuber and to grade B1 of Corazza–Villanacci. Type 3 corresponds to type 3 of Marsh, to type 3C of Oberhuber and to grade B of Corazza–Villanacci. This new classification has been proposed to be a simple and practical approach to improve clinical pathologic correlation in CD.

Most experts believe that a small-intestinal biopsy and the histopathologic judgment of the tissue are essential in the diagnosis of CD. Therefore, the pathology report is of great importance and should include information on site and number of biopsy specimens, architecture in terms of villous to crypt ratio, damage to surface epithelium, IELosis, and degree of inflammation [101]. Pathologists should communicate with the clinician and obtain serological and clinical data before making a definitive diagnosis (see Section 5.2).

Immunoelectron microscopic studies revealed heavy deposits of immunoglobulin (Ig) A TGAs in the intestinal mucosa of CD patients [102]. These deposits disappear during a gluten-free diet, but when gluten is reintroduced into the diet, the antibody deposition rapidly reappears. Interestingly, IgA deposits in intestinal biopsies of CD patients have the ability to bind external tissue transglutaminase (TG2) when added to the tissues [103]. Staining of intestinal IgA deposits, which are TG2-targeted autoantibodies, has extensively been used in the diagnostic workups of CD. Several studies demonstrated that all untreated CD patients, even seronegative ones, have these characteristic deposits in their intestinal mucosa [103,104]. These deposits appear early during disease development when the mucosa is still morphologically normal and before they are detectable in the periphery [105,106]. In IgA-deficient CD patients, these mucosal autoantibody deposits appear in the IgM-class instead [107].

4.3 Serology

CD is characterized by a disease-specific antibody response to gluten exposure. These antibodies belong to the Ig classes A and G and are produced by the anti-inflammatory T-helper (Th) 2 pathway in the lamina propria of the intestinal mucosa (see Section 6.3.1). CD patients with selective IgA deficiency are only positive for IgG antibodies. The antibodies bind to their specific antigen in the diseased intestinal mucosa and also appear in the blood. Antibody production starts early during the CD course and may precede the development of clinical symptoms and villous atrophy. CD-specific antibodies can act as markers of active disease and indicate an ongoing pathologic immune response to gluten. Successful treatment of CD with a gluten-free diet leads to the elimination of antibodies from both the tissue and the blood after a prolonged time. Testing of CD-specific antibodies from serum or plasma samples is currently the most important noninvasive diagnostic tool to recognize CD (see Section 5.1). However, it should be kept in mind that the prevalence of seronegative CD has been shown to be in a range of 6–9% of diagnosed cases [108].

The intake of gliadin, a main trigger of CD, causes the production of IgA and IgG AGAs. Both IgG and IgA types were shown to be largely specific for the amino acid sequence QPFXXQXPY (in which X can be various amino acids) [109]. The specificity of AGAs is fairly poor because they can be detected in non-CD enteropathies as well as in healthy individuals (2–8%). It has been shown that selective deamidation of gliadin peptides by TG2 specifically increases circulating antibody recognition in CD patients, and such serum antibodies against deamidated gliadin peptides (DGPA) have been proven to be highly accurate indicators of untreated CD [110] (see Section 5.1). In 1971, Seah and coworkers incubated CD patient sera with rodent liver and kidney sections; they observed binding of antibodies to these tissues and identified reticulin, a type of fiber in the connective tissue, as antigen [111]. Later on, Chorzelski and colleagues described the production of EMAs in patients with CD and dermatitis herpetiformis [112]. Endomysium is a connective tissue protein found in the collagenous matrix of human and monkey esophagus. In 1997, Dieterich and coworkers identified TG2 as the autoantigen of CD, a milestone in the history of CD [113]. Thereafter, it was shown that TG2 is also the CD-specific antigen in reticulin and endomysium. The formation of TGAs as well as its gluten dependence was absolutely unexpected, but since that time, it has been clear that the immune response in CD has an autoimmune component. The TGAs disappear if gluten is removed from the diet, and they reappear if a gluten-containing diet is reintroduced. The dependence of an autoimmune response on the exposure to an external protein (gluten) antigen makes CD unique among autoimmune disorders.

TGAs primarily interact with extracellular TG2. They are highly specific to TG2 and bind preferentially to the open, Ca^{2+}-activated enzyme conformation [114]. The IgA antibody response is focused on the active site of TG2 responsible for its transamidation and deamidation reactions, whereas the IgG antibody targets other regions of the enzyme [115]. TGAs are deposited in the small intestinal mucosa and also in extraintestinal sites, such as muscle and liver [116]. Furthermore, such deposits have been found around blood vessels of the brain in patients with gluten ataxia [117]. The question is how these CD-specific antibodies are linked with the pathogenesis of the disease. Koning and colleagues suggested that the antibodies are, in fact, specific indicators of CD, but they are not initiators of CD and are unlikely to cause disease symptoms [118]. Today, evidence is emerging in favor of their pathogenic potential. However, it remains to be determined how antibodies contribute to the progression of the disease at an intestinal and extraintestinal level [119,120]. It is a fact that TGAs increase the activity of TG2 and thereby accelerate the immune response in the mucosa [121]. The hypothesis that TGAs may affect TG2 functions is still controversial. If TGAs play an inhibitory role on TG2, they might also block the proposed role of TG2 in driving the immune response through deamidation and crosslinking. Dieterich and coworkers suggested that despite a partial inhibitory effect of TGAs, residual enzymatic activity of TG2 remains sufficiently high for deamidation and transamidation [122]. Experiments with cell cultures revealed that TGAs can have various biological effects: induction of epithelial proliferation, neuronal and trophoblast apoptosis, inhibition of epithelial differentiation and angiogenesis, increase in epithelial and vascular permeability, interference with gliadin uptake, and binding to placential tissue [119]. However, in vivo studies have so far not been able to confirm that TGAs play a pathogenic role in CD [123].

Only a few studies have assessed serum cytokine levels. A case-control study showed that patients with active CD and those on a gluten-free diet with positive TGAs have significantly higher levels of proinflammatory cytokines (e.g., IL-2, IL-18, IFN-γ, tumor necrosis factor-α [TNF-α]) compared with controls and patients on a gluten-free diet without antibodies [124]. A significant correlation between IgA TGA levels and levels of cytokines IL-1α, IL-1β, IL-4, IL-8, and IL-10 was observed. Most of these cytokines decrease when the patients commence a gluten-free diet. Thus, serum cytokines may be good markers of CD activity as well as indicators for adherence to a gluten-free diet. However, a few cytokines that have been implicated in tissue damage, such as IFN-γ, persist in the circulation despite a gluten-free diet. The variation of cytokine mean concentrations in CD patients from very high values to undetectable values makes the clinical diagnostic use of serum testing of cytokines very problematic [124].

4.4 Refractory Celiac Disease

A small percentage of CD patients (2–5%), especially among those diagnosed above the age of 50, develops a primary or secondary resistance to a strict gluten-free diet. This condition, called RCD, is characterized by persistence or recurrence of villous atrophy and elevated levels of IELs despite a strict diet for at least 6–12 months [125]. It has been suggested to be the link between CD and overt lymphoma [126]. Persistent diarrhea, abdominal pain, and involuntary weight loss are the most common symptoms in RCD. Most patients are negative for EMA and TGA at the time of RCD diagnosis, reflecting strict adherence to a gluten-free diet. Interestingly, many of the RCD patients are homozygous for HLA-DQ2 alleles [127], eliciting much stronger gluten-specific T-cell responses than in those heterozygous for HLA-DQ2 (see Section 6.3.1). Studies on the tight junctions (see Section 6.2) in RCD demonstrated that tightening claudin-4 and -5 are downregulated and the pore-forming claudin-2 is upregulated [128].

A combination of clinical and pathological findings is required for diagnosing RCD [125,129]. The diagnosis is made on the basis of strong evidence of CD supplemented with systematic exclusion of other causes of nonresponsiveness, such as trace gluten contamination of the gluten-free diet [130]. Tests for the detection of abnormal IELs in the intestine have facilitated the confirmation of RCD type II (see below). It is important to distinguish between true RCD patients and those who do not respond for other reasons [131]. True RCD carries a significant burden of morbidity and mortality, mainly from malnutrition and lymphoma. Early identification of RCD enables early intervention, which results in a reduction of morbidity and mortality. It is therefore imperative that clinicians are aware of how RCD is diagnosed and can be differentiated from related disorders. The management of RCD should be undertaken in specialist centers [132]. It requires initial intensive dietary supervision, strict gluten exclusion, and subsequent re-evaluation.

According to the immunophenotype of IELs, RCD can be classified into type I and type II. In type I, the majority of IELs have normal expression of surface markers, and the T-cell receptors are polyclonal. In type II, a far more serious condition, loss of IEL markers CD3 and CD8 and abnormal clonality of the γ/δ receptor of T cells occur. Type II imposes a serious risk of developing a virtually lethal enteropathy-associated T-cell lymphoma and small intestinal adenocarcinoma. Such patients require evaluation for potential small intestinal cancer. The diagnostic use of video capsule endoscopy may predict the type of RCD and allows for the early detection of overt lymphoma [133]. Early differentiation between the different types is necessary as the reported 5-year survival rate varies between 40% and 58% for type II and 93% for type I [134]. The main cause of death in type II RCD is progression to an enteropathy-associated T-cell lymphoma and progressive malnutrition. To discriminate between RCD I and RCD II, a clinically validated cutoff value of 20% aberrant IELs, determined by the analysis of small intestinal biopsy samples by flow cytometry, is used [135]. As flow cytometry is not available in all medical centers, immunohistochemistry for CD3 and CD8 would also be helpful.

RCD is a rare disease and, to date, there is no standard therapy. The latest insights into treatment options are summarized by Nijeboer and coworkers [129]. Corticosteroids may improve clinical symptoms in some patients, but the histological response to steroids is not consistent. Patients with RCD I can be treated effectively with prednisone with or without azathioprine or, in some cases, cyclosporine. However, the use of these medications is limited by systemic side effects. Therefore, the use of budesonide has been considered a breakthrough for patients with RCD I, as it produces rapid symptomatic improvement with fewer side effects compared with prednisone [136]. As long-term treatment with budesonide leads to traditional steroid side effects, small intestinal release mesalamine is recommended as a safe and efficacious treatment option in patients with RCD I, either as primary therapy or in patients with incomplete response to budesonide [137]. Recently, tioguanine was recommended as a convenient drug for the treatment of RCD I [138]. Patients with RCD II may respond to cladribine or to stem cell transplantation. The application of cladribine (a synthetic purine nucleoside analog) found excellent 2-year clinical and histological response rates of 81% and 47%, respectively [139]. Patients responsive to cladribine have been trialed with stem cell transplantation to replace the abnormal IEL population and the blocking of IL-15. Four-year survival rates were 60%, with 5 of 13 patients achieving complete histological remission.

4.5 Other Gluten-Related Disorders

The term "gluten-related disorders" is the commonly accepted umbrella term for describing all intolerances related to the ingestion of gluten-containing food. There are five main forms of gluten-related disorders besides CD: dermatitis herpetiformis, gluten ataxia, wheat allergy, non-celiac gluten sensitivity, and irritable bowel syndrome [140–142]. Although these gluten-related disorders and CD are treated similarly—by removal of gluten from the diet—they are not the same conditions. It is important for patients and health-care practitioners to be able to differentiate between these disorders [140]. Based on a combination of clinical, biological, genetic, and histological data, an algorithm for the differential diagnosis of gluten-related disorders was proposed by Sapone and coworkers [142]. Future studies should focus on the extraintestinal manifestations as they could provide more clues and ultimately hold the key to fully understand the pathogenesis of gluten-related disorders beside CD.

4.5.1 Dermatitis Herpetiformis

Dermatitis herpetiformis (DH), also known as Duhring disease, is the cutaneous counterpart of CD ("skin CD"). In both conditions, HLA-DQ2 and -DQ8 are associated, and immune reaction to dietary gluten is mediated by T-cell activation in the intestinal mucosa. The relationship between CD and DH has been impressively illustrated by a report of monozygotic twins, one of whom had DH and the other CD [143]. DH is characterized by intense itching and burning of the skin caused by herpetiform clusters of pruritic urticated papules and vesicles, especially on the elbows, upper forearms, buttocks, and knees but also on other parts of the body (Figure 1.7 [144]). Typically, granular IgA deposits are present in the skin, and inflammatory cells and cytokines are found in the lesions. Furthermore, antibodies to

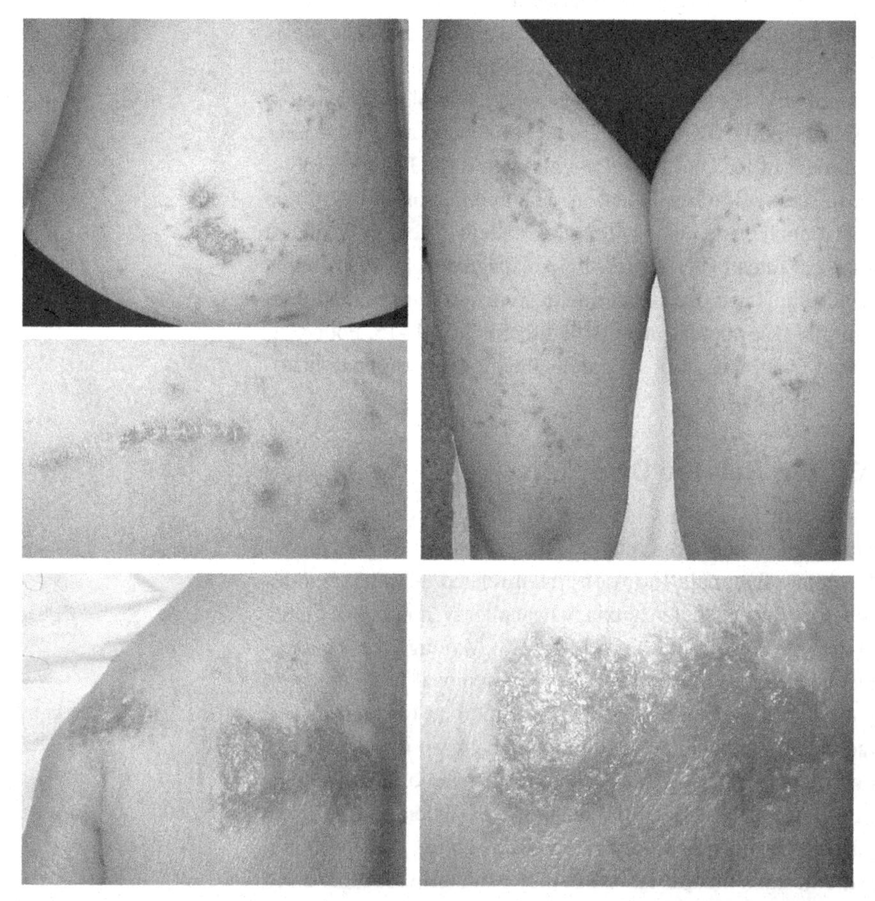

■ **FIGURE 1.7** Erythematous, papular, and vesiculous lesions in a patient with dermatitis herpetiformis. *From Caproni et al. [144].* (Please see color plate at the back of the book.)

epidermal transglutaminase (eTG), homologous to TG2 within the enzymatically active domain, occur in the serum. Serum IgA eTG antibody determination can effectively distinguish untreated DH from other dermatological itchy diseases and is highly sensitive to gluten-free diet [145]. Most patients with DH have the intestinal lesion of CD (Marsh type 2) but only a minority of patients have gastrointestinal symptoms, and these are usually mild. It is not known why only some patients with CD develop DH and what factors link the bowel and skin lesions.

The prevalence of DH is much lower than that of CD, ranging from around 1:2000 to 1:10,000. In contrast to CD, males have a higher prevalence of DH than females [145]. DH is most prevalent in patients of Northern European descent. The diagnosis of DH is based on immunofluorescent IgA determination in the skin and on serological tests, such as by IgA anti-eTG antibodies. When skin biopsy confirms the diagnosis, intestinal biopsies are not needed. After establishing the diagnosis, a gluten-free diet is recommended for treatment. Dapsone, an anti-inflammatory antibiotic, is the drug of choice to alleviate the acute pruritus. Often, a combined therapy of gluten-free diet and dapsone is needed to address acute cutaneous manifestations and provide long-term control, with gradual reduction in dose or complete withdrawal of dapsone over a few months [146]. Similar to CD, a wide range of autoimmune disorders are associated with DH; the most common is hypothyroidism [147]. Moreover, DH patients may have a higher risk of non-Hodgkin lymphoma as compared to the general population.

4.5.2 Gluten Ataxia

Gluten ataxia (GA) is one of a number of neurological manifestations attributed to CD and can be defined as idiopathic sporadic ataxia with positive serological markers (AGAs) for gluten sensitization, even in the absence of duodenal enteropathy. Serological tests revealed that around 20% of patients with sporadic ataxia have GA. All of these patients present gait ataxia, and the majority has limb ataxia and evidence of cerebellar atrophy [148]. Gaze-evoked nystagmus and other ocular signs of cerebellar dysfunction are seen in up to 80% of cases. IgA deposits seem to accumulate in the periphery of vessels, and antibodies against TG6, a primarily brain-expressed TG, have been found in the serum of GA patients [149]. Antibodies against TG6 are gluten-dependent and appear to be a sensitive and specific marker of GA [150]. The diagnosis of GA is not as straightforward as that of CD. The current recommendation is a serological screening for AGAs, TGAs, and anti-TG6 antibodies. Patients who are positive for any of these antibodies with no alternative cause for this ataxia should be offered a gluten-free diet. The response to this treatment depends on the duration of GA [151]. Loss of Purkinje cells in the cerebellum is irreversible, and prompt treatment is more likely to result in improvement or stabilization of the ataxia. Examples for other reported neurologic gluten-related disorders include inflammatory myopathy and sensory ganglion neuropathy.

4.5.3 Wheat Allergy

Wheat allergy (WA) is defined as an IgE-mediated immunological reaction to proteins of wheat and related cereals [152]. Baker's asthma is a well-characterized allergic reaction to the inhalation of wheat flour and dust. It is recognized as one of the most common types of occupational asthma. α-Amylase inhibitors have been identified as the most important allergens, but a number of other proteins present in wheat, including α- and β-amylases, germ agglutinin, and peroxidase, have also been shown to bind to IgE from patients with baker's asthma. Gluten-related allergic responses to the ingestion of wheat can be divided into two types—the clearly defined wheat-dependent exercise-induced anaphylaxis (WDEIA) and less understood immune reactions, including atopic dermatitis, urticaria, and anaphylaxis. WDEIA will be triggered neither by wheat ingestion nor exercise alone; the combination of food and increased physical activity is required [153]. Aspirin, in combination with wheat-containing food, is another well-known trigger for WDEIA and can induce anaphylaxis without apparent exercise [154]. Patients display a range of clinical symptoms from generalized urticaria to severe allergic reactions, including anaphylaxis. Skin prick tests and in vitro IgE assays are first-level diagnostics for WDEIA. However, the positive predictive value of these tests is less than 75%, and in many cases oral food (gluten) challenge in combination with exercise or aspirin intake is necessary for the final diagnosis. ω5-Gliadins (see Chapter 2, Section 2.2) were identified as the major allergens, and the following IgE binding epitopes were found to be dominant: QQIPQQQ, QQFPQQQ, QQSPEQQ, and QQSPQQQ. Further epitopes such as QQPGQ, QQPGQGQQ, and QQSGQG were detected in high-molecular-weight glutenin subunits (HMW-GS) [153]. It was hypothesized that exercise as well as aspirin may facilitate improperly digested allergen absorption from the gastrointestinal tract [155].

4.5.4 Non-Celiac Gluten Sensitivity

Non-celiac gluten sensitivity (NCGS), frequently termed gluten sensitivity, has most recently been described as gluten-meditated disorder. A double-blind randomized and placebo-controlled gluten challenge administered to 34 individuals without CD (DQ2/8 negative) revealed that NCGS exists [156]. NCGS prevalence is estimated to be much higher (≈6%) than CD's [142].

NCGS is characterized by gastrointestinal complaints including bloating, diarrhea, weight loss, and abdominal pain and may be the prime presentation [157]. Analogous to CD, extraintestinal symptoms (e.g., muscular disturbances, bone pain, tiredness, and neurological disorders) also have been described in patients with NCGS. Patients reported more abdominal and nonabdominal symptoms after a gluten challenge of 3 days than CD patients [158]. Removal of gluten from the diet results in symptomatic improvement. NCGS patients have neither CD nor WA; due to similar symptoms, both of these conditions must be ruled out before labeling a patient as NCGS positive. An overlap between irritable bowel syndrome (see below) and NCGS has been suspected, requiring even more stringent diagnostic criteria. The small intestine of NCGS patients is usually normal and serum TGAs and EMAs as well as wheat IgE are negative [159]. However, IgG AGAs may be positive in 40–50% of cases. Only around 50% of patients carry the HLA-DQ2 or -DQ8 haplotype [160]. In CD patients, mucosal IFN-γ levels were shown to be high both before and after in vivo gluten challenge, whereas the levels of TNF-α and IL-8 increased after challenge. In NCGS patients, however, only IFN-γ increased significantly [161]. Once CD has been excluded, the best available test for diagnosing NCGS is food sensitivity testing, such as a gluten-elimination diet for 2–3 months. If remission of symptoms is obtained, a definitive demonstration of NCGS can be counted if the symptoms reappear upon gluten reintroduction [160].

NCGS represents a unique condition with a potentially different mechanism and different manifestations than CD [82]. It appears that NCGS does not have a strong hereditary basis, is not associated with malabsorption or nutritional deficiencies, and is not associated with any increased risk for autoimmune disorders or intestinal malignancy. Studies proposed that, beside gluten, wheat amylase trypsin inhibitors (ATIs) [162] and fermentable, poorly absorbed, short-chain carbohydrates (FODMAP; fermentable oligo-, di- and monosaccharides, and polyols) [163] may contribute to symptoms of NCGS. Sapone and coworkers suggested an important role of the innate immune system without any involvement of the adaptive immune response [164]. Although NCGS gained medical credibility during recent years, many questions are not answered at this time. It is unclear which components of grains trigger symptoms in people with NCGS and whether some populations of patients with NCGS have subtle small intestinal morphological changes. There is currently no standard diagnostic approach to NCGS. Altogether, NCGS is currently an underrecognized and undertreated disorder. Future research is needed to generate more knowledge regarding NCGS, a condition that has a global acceptance but has only a few certainties and many unresolved issues [165].

4.5.5 Irritable Bowel Syndrome

The typical symptoms of irritable bowel syndrome (IBS) are similar to those of CD and NCGS, including abdominal pain, gas, bloating, and diarrhea with or without constipation [166]. Therefore, CD and NCGS have to be ruled out before making the diagnosis of IBS. Epidemiologic surveys suggest that IBS is a common condition with a prevalence between 5% and 30% [167,168]. Identification of patients with IBS is no longer considered to be based on the exclusion of other diseases, but on a positive diagnosis using symptom-based criteria. The so-called Rome III diagnostic criteria require recurrent abdominal pain or discomfort at least 3 days a month in the past 3 months associated with two or more of the following [169]:

1. improvement with defecation;
2. onset associated with a change in frequency of stool;
3. onset associated with a change in form (appearance) of stool.

The pathophysiologic mechanism of IBS is not completely understood but is thought to be due to intestinal bacterial overgrowth. Research suggests that some types of IBS may show symptomatic improvement on a gluten-free diet. For example, 60% of diarrhea-predominant IBS patients return to normal stool frequency and gastrointestinal symptom score. The patients who respond to the gluten-free diet are more likely to have positive AGAs and TGAs than those who do not respond. Several studies have shown increased gut permeability in IBS [170]. For example, intestinal biopsies of patients with IBS indicated increased paracellular permeability as compared to healthy subjects [171]. These findings might pave the way to identify novel biomarkers for IBS as well as new therapeutic targets.

4.6 **Associated Diseases**

CD is a disease with an autoimmune component (TG2) and shares important features with other autoimmune diseases: It is chronic, multifactorial, and shows a female-to-male ratio of roughly 2:1. CD puts patients at risk for other autoimmune conditions and vice versa. Screening studies have shown an increased prevalence of CD in individuals with Sjögren's syndrome (4–12%), type 1 diabetes mellitus (4–10%), autoimmune thyroid disease (4–5%), and primary biliary cirrhosis (3%) (Table 1.2) [121]. In total, about 30% of adult CD patients have one or more autoimmune disorders, compared with about 3% in the general population. In a study on subjects with CD and concurrent autoimmune diseases, roughly 75% of subjects were diagnosed first with another autoimmune disease and then with CD [172]. Type 1 diabetes is one of the most complicated associations with CD because it requires a lifelong adherence to two restrictive diets and lifestyles. Also, certain genetically determined syndromes (e.g., Down's syndrome, Turner syndrome, IgA deficiency) have a higher rate of CD than those of the general population.

The risks for CD-associated autoimmune disorders increase with the duration of gluten exposure. A multicenter national study revealed that the prevalence of autoimmune disorders in CD patients (n=909) was clearly dependent on the age of diagnosis of CD, ranging from 5.1% at the age of <2 years to 34.0% at the age of >20 years (Figure 1.8) [173]. These data strongly advocate the need for routine screening of patients with autoimmune diseases for CD, regardless of the presence or absence of symptoms [174].

Table 1.2 Conditions Associated with Celiac Disease (CD) [121]

Condition	Prevalence of CD (%)
Multiple autoimmune disorders	10
Sjögren's syndrome	4–12
Down's syndrome	5–10
Type 1 diabetes mellitus	4–10
Selective IgA deficiency	7
Addison's disease	5
Autoimmune thyroid disease	4–5
Autoimmune hepatitis	3–6

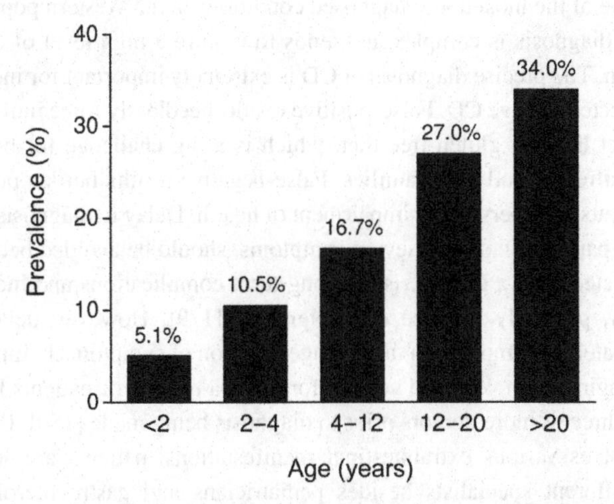

■ **FIGURE 1.8** Prevalence of autoimmune disorders related to age at diagnosis of celiac disease. *Adapted from Ref. [173].*

Different HLA and non-HLA genetic loci are shared in CD and autoimmune diseases, suggesting an overlap of the genetic mechanism involved in the development of such diseases [41]. The comparison of genetic pathways indicates that CD bears a stronger resemblance to T-cell-mediated organ-specific autoimmune diseases than to inflammatory diseases. For example, a large genetic study demonstrated that genetic susceptibility to both CD and type 1 diabetes shares at least seven common alleles [175]. Strikingly, individuals who carry the HLA haplotypes DR3-DQ2 and DR4-DQ8 have an increased risk of approximately 1 in 20 for a diagnosis of type 1 diabetes by the age of 15 years [176].

The relationship between the treatment of CD and the prevention of autoimmune diseases remains controversial [177]. Several studies have found that a gluten-free diet may prevent CD patients from contracting other autoimmune diseases, and that autoimmune diseases may improve on a gluten-free diet when concomitant CD is present. However, not all studies have supported the association of a gluten-free diet with a reduction in the risk of autoimmune diseases in CD patients. The association of CD with other autoimmune diseases would be an interesting area of future research. Using CD as an example, other exogenous factors might be identified as drivers of autoimmune processes, in particular when evidence for T cells with specificity for autoantigens driving the disease is lacking [178].

5. DIAGNOSIS

CD is one of the most underdiagnosed conditions in the Western population because diagnosis is complex and tends to require a high level of clinical suspicion. The precise diagnosis of CD is extremely important for individuals suspected to have CD. False-positive results needlessly force individuals to a strict lifelong gluten-free diet, which is a big challenge for both the persons affected and their families. False-negative results burden potential CD patients with permanent impairment of health. Delay in diagnosis, especially in patients who have severe symptoms, should be avoided because it is associated with a greater risk of long-term complications and increased mortality, primarily because of malignancy [179]. However, delays are unfortunately common, with the average duration of symptoms before diagnosis ranging from 4.5 to 11 years. Moreover, a quarter of patients have to consult three or more doctors prior to diagnosis being made [180]. Because CD involves various extraintestinal manifestations, patients are seen by many different specialists besides pediatricians and gastroenterologists, such as dermatologists, rheumatologists, dentists, endocrinologists, and neurologists.

Some of the CD-associated complications may be irreversible unless CD is treated in time. For example, growth retardation, osteoporosis, and abnormal dentition will remain permanent if not treated early. For these reasons, CD has been suggested as appropriate for mass screening. However, the role of widespread population screening remains controversial. Particularly, the benefit of screening for asymptomatic persons is still a subject of debate because it is not clear if the increase in health status will outweigh the burden of the adherence to the gluten-free diet. Arguments for and against mass screening have been summarized by Aggarwal and colleagues [177]. At present, screening is recommended for persons when first-degree family members or other close relatives have biopsy-confirmed CD. Individuals with autoimmune diseases known to be associated with CD (see Section 4.6) are also candidates for screening. Future studies should focus on the practical benefits of diagnosing CD in asymptomatic patients, with emphasis on measuring the quality of life before and after diagnosis and the introduction of a gluten-free diet [177]. An effective alternative to mass screening is active case finding by serological screening among individuals with only subtle or atypical symptoms and in risk groups. This approach, which involves education and increased awareness of health personnel, has led to the detection of a large number of CD patients in the general population in Finland [181].

Diagnostic approaches have changed during recent decades, owing to a better understanding of the pathomechanism of CD and the availability of more sensitive and specific serological tests. In summary, the diagnostic scheme consists of the following (Figure 1.9):

1. clinical history and symptomatology;
2. serological testing;
3. histological findings in small intestinal biopsies;
4. clinical and serological (optionally histological) response to a gluten-free diet.

Screening candidates should follow the same procedure. Genetic HLA testing is not indicated in the initial evaluation of CD but could be useful when CD diagnosis is controversial, for example, because of a discrepancy between symptomatology and serology or equivocal small intestinal biopsy.

The primary care doctor has a central role in the process of diagnosis. Well-known symptoms of CD should prompt the physician to initiate a serological test (see Section 5.1). Additionally, individuals with autoimmune diseases (see Section 4.6) and first-degree relatives of CD patients should be taken into consideration for serological testing. How to proceed with the

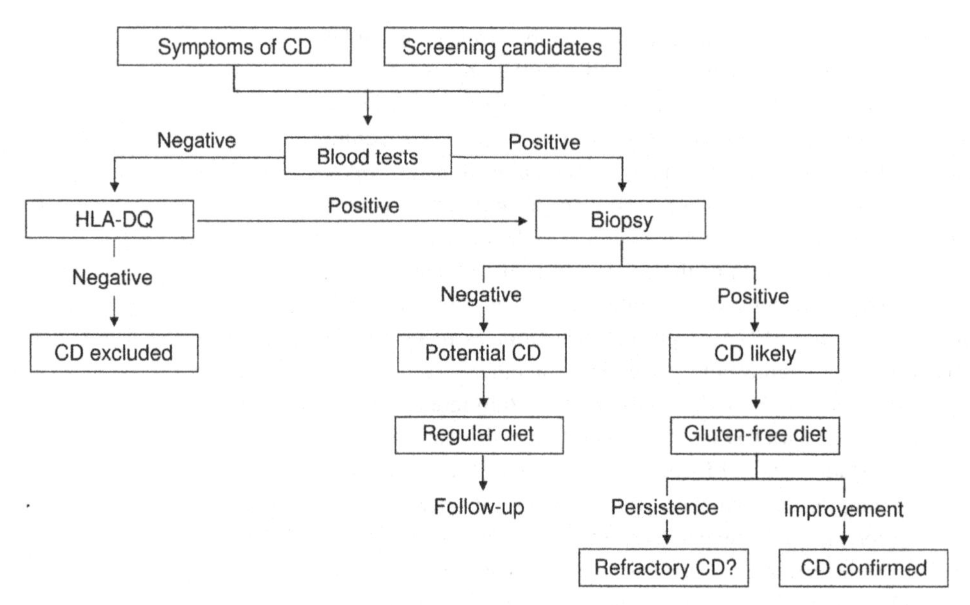

■ **FIGURE 1.9** Proposed algorithm to diagnose celiac disease (CD).

diagnostic procedure is differently assessed. The American Gastroenterological Association mandates an intestinal biopsy to confirm the diagnosis in people suspected of having CD. In contrast, in its consensus statement of 2004, the US National Institutes of Health recommends biopsies only after a positive serologic finding or when serologic results are nondiagnostic [101]. ESPGHAN previously recommended the following three steps:

1. biopsy→flat mucosa;
2. gluten-free diet, biopsy→mucosa in remission;
3. gluten challenge, biopsy→flat mucosa.

The challenge should be performed for 3–4 weeks with an average of three to four slices of wheat bread per day. The question of whether such patient-straining and time-consuming procedures, including three biopsies, are necessary has led to the suggestion of ESPGHAN in 1990 that a gluten challenge is not mandatory (except for children under 2 years of age), if a gluten-free diet has resulted in good improvement of the symptoms and morphology of the biopsy specimens [182].

In 2012, ESPGHAN presented another revision of the diagnostic guidelines [183]. The main conclusions are that the diagnosis of CD depends on

1. gluten-dependent symptoms;
2. CD-specific antibody levels;

3. the presence of HLA-DQ2 or HLA-DQ8 alleles;
4. histological changes (villous atrophy and crypt hyperplasia) in the duodenal biopsy.

In modification of the previous guidelines, the duodenal biopsy can be omitted if IgA TGA titers are high (>100 U/ml=>10 times the upper limit of normal). Particularly for children, omitting biopsies would avoid the burden of endoscopy with general anesthesia and the potential adverse effects of this procedure. It must be noted that the new ESPGHAN evidence-based guideline does not recommend skipping the biopsy in selected cases, but simply allows the physician to do so at her or his discretion. Studies by Klapp and colleagues supported the view that in selected children who are symptomatic and positive for TGAs, CD diagnosis could be established independent of histological findings [183]. Other studies, however, reported unexpectedly frequent cases of children with negative EMAs and TGAs, but a positive histology [184] and no cutoff TGA level was found to be associated with a positive CD-predictive value of 100% [185]. Thus, the need for a confirmatory intestinal biopsy may still be present. In every case, the recovery of the intestinal mucosa and a negative serological test after treatment with a gluten-free diet are important evidence for the diagnosis of CD.

If a biopsy is needed, at least five specimen samples should be collected, including one of the bulb, as this may be the only affected site (see Section 5.2). Villous atrophy according to Marsh 3 was previously required to set the diagnosis of CD, but the new ESPGHAN guidelines conclude that Marsh 2 is also sufficient for CD diagnosis [186]. When the diagnosis is established and a gluten-free diet is introduced, repeated serological tests are recommended for the follow-up and management of CD. In asymptomatic patients, a second biopsy under a gluten-free diet is advised to demonstrate the histologic recovery of the mucosa, which usually does not develop before 6 months.

The diagnosis of CD should be undertaken while patients are on a gluten-containing diet. Therefore, a normal gluten-containing diet has to be consumed until the end of the diagnostic process. This should be particularly emphasized to families that consume a gluten-free diet because a family member has been diagnosed with CD. Moreover, many patients initiate a gluten-free diet before appropriate diagnostic testing. In such cases, the effect of gluten withdrawal on the accuracy of diagnosis by serology or biopsy depends on duration and strictness of the gluten-free diet. In the case of unclear diagnostic results, gluten has to be reintroduced into the diet for a sufficient duration to reproduce the serological abnormality and the characteristic intestinal damage [187,188]. A gradual increase in gluten may be advised because a severe reaction to a gluten challenge may occur in some patients. Patients should be challenged for 3–4 weeks with three to four slices of wheat bread per day. If symptoms do not recur, antibody measurements may be used to guide the timing of intestinal biopsy. However, patients who have followed a gluten-free diet for prolonged periods may take several years to relapse in serology and mucosal histology after gluten is reintroduced.

Patients' reactions to the diagnosis of CD are different: The majority of patients having classical symptoms were satisfied at being diagnosed with CD and adapted to living with their condition [189]. However, screen-detected asymptomatic people and those with extraintestinal symptoms experienced the diagnosis more negatively than those having classical symptoms. A minority of patients diagnosed without classical symptoms regretted being diagnosed.

5.1 Serological Tests

CD is characterized by disease-specific antibodies, in response to gluten exposure, appearing both in the blood and the intestinal tissue (see Section 4.3). Tests for antibodies from serum or plasma samples are currently most often applied. These tests are important as a noninvasive diagnostic aid in symptomatic patients with a clinical suspicion of CD and to select patients for diagnostic small intestinal biopsy. Positive results strongly support the diagnosis of CD, whereas negative results can greatly help to distinguish the pathologic features from other conditions. Moreover, antibody tests are very useful for population screening and for follow-up of adherence to the gluten-free diet. Many disorders known to produce damage to the intestinal mucosa similar to that caused by CD do not give false-positive results with these tests. However, it should be mentioned that the prevalence of seronegative CD has been shown to account for up to 10% of all diagnosed cases [190]. Thus, it is important to keep in mind that seronegativity in individuals consuming gluten does not rule out the possibility of CD.

The terms *sensitivity* and *specificity* are used when evaluating the performance of serological tests. Sensitivity refers to the ability of the test to correctly identify those patients with the disease [191]. A test with 100% sensitivity correctly identifies all patients with the disease. A test with 80% sensitivity detects 80% of patients with the disease (true positive) but 20% with the disease go undetected (false negative). The specificity refers to the ability of the test to correctly identify those patients without the disease. A test with 100% specificity correctly identifies all patients without the disease. A test with 80% specificity correctly reports 80% of patients without the disease as test negative (true negatives) but 20% of patients without the

Table 1.3 Sensitivity and Specificity of Serologic Tests [194]

Antibody[a]	Sensitivity (Range) (%)	Specificity (Range) (%)
IgA AGA	85 (57–100)	90 (47–94)
IgG AGA	85 (42–100)	80 (50–94)
EMA	95 (86–100)	99 (97–100)
IgA TGA	98 (78–100)	98 (90–100)
IgG TGA	70 (45–95)	95 (94–100)
IgA DGPA	88 (74–100)	95 (90–99)
IgG DGPA	80 (63–95)	98 (90–99)

[a]AGA, anti-gliadin antibody; DGPA, antibody against deamidated gliadin peptides; EMA, endomysial antibody; TGA, TG2-antibody.

disease are incorrectly identified as test positive (false positive). Both sensitivity and specificity depend on the cutoff value of the test.

Initial serological tests were developed in the 1970s and 1980s using AGAs, first based on immunofluorescent staining and then on enzyme-linked immunosorbent assays (ELISAs) [192,193]. IgA class AGAs have been shown to have a similar to modestly higher sensitivity, but a significantly better specificity compared with IgG class AGAs. AGA tests initially seemed very promising, but they lost diagnostic significance because their sensitivities and specificities are fairly poor (Table 1.3); AGAs can also be detected in nonceliac enteropathies as well as in 5–10% of healthy individuals. Diagnostic guidelines have therefore recommended that AGA tests should be abandoned for routine diagnosis [195]. The testing of children younger than 2 years of age may be an exception because AGAs are considered to be the first to appear after exposure to a gluten-containing diet and remain positive, whereas other CD-specific antibodies may fluctuate [196]. More recent studies, however, showed that IgA and IgG AGA testing conferred no additional diagnostic benefit as compared to tests described below [197,198].

The problems with AGAs were overcome by the development of anti-reticulin antibody (ARA) and EMA tests. They are based on indirect immunofluorescence using rodent (ARA) or primate (EMA) tissues as antigens. In most studies, their sensitivities and specificities are both reported to be above 90%. In particular, EMA testing has been used for diagnostic and screening purposes for many years despite the difficulties inherent in immunofluorescence detection, which is a subjective semiquantitative method that is not easy to standardize. The test requires either monkey esophagus or human umbilical cord tissue as a substrate as well as individual reading of each sample under a microscope, which adds to the cost and leads to concerns about interobserver variability. For that reason, the specificities might not be so high in routine clinical settings as reported in research laboratories [199]. Reports on EMA results should contain the specification of investigated Ig class, cutoff dilution, interpretation (positive or negative), highest dilution still positive, and specification of the substrate tissue [186].

In 1997, TG2 was identified as CD-specific autoantigen [113], which allowed the development of ELISA-based TGA tests. Early assays used TG2 derived from guinea pig liver, leading to false-positive results due to impurities in these preparations. Afterwards, human recombinant TG2 was applied showing high sensitivity and specificity. The user-friendly test is now produced by a number of manufacturers and widely used as a first screening tool for CD. However, it is important to bear in mind that the performance of the commercial TG2 ELISA may vary depending on the quality of the TG2 antigen [119]. TGA laboratory test results should be communicated with the specification of the Ig class measured, the manufacturer, the cutoff value defined for the specific test kit and the level of antibody values [186].

Further studies evaluated whether the quantitative measurements of TGAs could be used to predict mucosal condition and disease severity. The results demonstrated that elevated IgA TGA levels (>30 U/ml) and IgG TGA levels (>15 U/ml) measured in 170 CD patients predicted a more severe intestinal atrophy, with a specificity of 99% for Marsh 3a–3c lesions [200]. The level of IgA TGAs was found to be highly correlated ($p<0.0001$) with the Marsh type in both children ($n=97$) and adults ($n=227$) [200]. CD patients with lesser degrees of villous atrophy are less likely to have positive serologic findings [201].

CD-specific antibody detection can also be done by means of fingersticks using rapid test kits in point-of-care (POC) tests, but only as semiquantitative tests for circulating antibodies [202–204]. There are currently several POC tests available for use by health professionals. The benefits of these tests include ease of interpretation (positive or negative), no need for laboratory processing, and availability of results within minutes. However, sensitivity and specificity are lower than with most ELISA-based assays and more studies are clearly needed. Detection of TGAs in human saliva is also possible and may be useful to monitor adherence to the gluten-free diet. Because the specificity of EMA has been proven to be higher than that of TGAs, the use of EMAs has been suggested as a confirmatory test after TGA testing [205]. Serial testing (TGA+EMA) may decrease the risk that a diagnosis of CD is falsely assigned to a truly healthy patient. EMA and TGA tests are usually based on IgA class antibodies, and only in the case of IgA deficiency (total serum IgA<0.2 g/l) are IgG class antibodies used. In 2004, a new test for detecting DGPAs recognizing the epitope QPEQPFP was introduced, which displays promising results according to sensitivity and specificity [110]. IgA TGA tests, however, perform significantly better and are less costly than IgA DGPA tests. Moreover, a recent meta-analysis indicates that IgA DGPA tests are less sensitive than IgA TGA tests [206].

Testing with IgA antibodies is not helpful in evaluating possible CD in patients with IgA deficiency. Selective IgA deficiency is found in about 10% of CD patients [190] (about 10 times higher than in the general population), which may cause false-negative results of IgA antibody testing. In this scenario, concurrent measurement of total IgA should be considered. Because sensitivity and specificity of IgG DGPA tests are higher than those of IgG TGA tests, they should be used for testing IgA-deficient individuals. Comparative test characteristics are presented in Table 1.3 [194]. As IgG EMA and IgG TGA tests seem to be less sensitive in children <2 years of age, the more sensitive IgG DGPA test is recommended for very young children [207]. DGPAs have been reported to appear earlier than TGAs in some cases and may even resolve sooner on a gluten-free diet, suggesting that they may be useful for monitoring dietary compliance. In summary, the combination of IgA TGA and IgG DGPA assays should be adapted as the best combination to screen for CD [160]. Duodenal biopsy may be avoided when high antibody titers are present [208].

The performance and diagnostic accuracy of 15 commercially available ELISA kits (IgA/IgG TGA and DGPA, IgG AGA) and an IgA EMA assay were compared by Rozenberg and colleagues [209]. The results demonstrated that the clinical demand for both maximal sensitivity and maximal specificity cannot be achieved with a single test. A combination of four tests (IgA DGPA, IgG DGPA, IgA TGA, IgA EMA) yielded positive and negative predictive values of 99% and 100%, respectively. However, if the intention is to avoid an intestinal biopsy for confirmation of CD, the accuracy of serological tests in clinical practice may require further study [210].

None of the tests described above show a high degree of responsiveness to modest changes in intestinal inflammation or limited duration of gluten exposure. A solution to this problem by measuring antibodies to the stabilized open (active) conformation of TG2 has been proposed [211]. This open conformation TG2 crosslinks with gluten peptides in the lamina propria, and the resulting conjugate triggers an additional immune response that produces antibodies to this conjugate. This test was shown to be more sensitive for the evaluation of the adherence to a gluten-free diet and may help in the diagnosis of patients with nonresponsive CD. With a combination of the three different antigens (conjugate, TG2, deamidated gliadin peptides), a new ELISA was developed as a screening test [212]. It seems to offer superior analytical sensitivity in identifying patients with subclinical or silent CD and may help explore the celiac iceberg.

In patients without overt gastrointestinal involvement, serum TGAs can be absent. Such patients typically have antibodies that react with different TG isoenzymes—TG3 (eTG) in dermatitis herpetiformis and TG6 in patients with neurological manifestations (see Section 4.5). Seronegative CD is a clinical challenge and requires integration of clinical, genetic, and histopathologic criteria because the individuals lack serum antibodies [190]. Biomarkers for CD that are present in the intestinal mucosa may be useful if the diagnosis via blood antibodies is not clear. For example, EMA assays in the intestinal culture medium have a higher sensitivity (98%) and specificity (99%) than serum EMAs [213]. Evaluation of the number and pattern of IELs at the villous tips and detecting increased intraepithelial γδ T cells in biopsy samples also helps in diagnosing cases of CD with mild inflammation, lacking serologic abnormalities [214].

All tests except POC tests require qualified personnel and laboratory facilities, and results are available only after a time delay. Several simple and rapid methods were therefore developed for the detection of serum or whole blood TGAs, which offer good sensitivity and specificity [215,216]. They can be performed with a drop of blood and allow visual reading after a few minutes. Balkenhohl and Lisdate developed impedimetric immunosensors for the detection of antibodies directed against gliadin and TG2 in human serum [217,218]. The immunosensors are based on the immobilization of the antigens onto disposable screen-printed gold electrodes, which are covered with a polyelectrolyte layer of poly(sodium 4-styrenesulfonic acid). Testing of the systems showed an acceptable sensitivity, whereas the specificity was lower compared to ELISA techniques. Overoxidized polypyrrole doped with gold-nanoparticles on a glassy carbon electrode was used as a platform to construct a novel label-free impedimetric immunosensor for TGAs [219]. Pividori and colleagues proposed an amperometric electrochemical immunosensor based on the physical absorption of the antigen (TG2) onto graphite-epoxy composite electrodes [220]. Testing of a small number of positive and negative serum samples (10 each) revealed a sensitivity of 70% and a specificity of 100%. More recently, a total number of 29 sera from CD patients and 19 negative control sera indicated a sensitivity of 100% and a specificity of 84% [221].

A magnetoelectrochemical immunosensor for CD diagnosis based on magnetic beads coated with TG2 antigen was applied for serum sample analysis [222]. Clinical sensitivity was 100%, clinical specificity was 98%, and the correlation with ELISA kit values was 0.943. An electrochemical system for the detection of TGAs using thiol-based surface chemistry was introduced by Dulay and colleagues [223]. The results showed an excellent degree of correlation with those of corresponding ELISA kits. A surface plasmon resonance biosensor based on the utilization of plastic optical fibers was developed to monitor the formation of the TG2/TGA complex [224]. The obtained results showed that the sensor is able to measure the complex in the range of concentrations between 30 and 3000 nmol/l. The simultaneous detection of IgA and IgG type AGAs and TGAs was achieved by means of an electrochemical dual immunosensor [225]. The results obtained indicated that the sensor can be a good alternative to traditional ELISA kits. The first electrochemical immunosensor for the detection of DGPAs was described by Neves and coworkers [226]. Real serum samples were successfully assessed, showing that the presented method is a promising analytical tool for CD diagnosis. In summary, electrochemical immunosensors appear as a promising alternative to conventional ELISA techniques because they are simple, cost-effective, and point-of-care analytical methods. However, some limitations still remain, such as long-term stability and surface effects, and future studies are necessary for a critical assessment of electrochemical immunosensors in comparison to established ELISA methods.

Beside serum antibodies, serum T cells can be used for diagnostic purposes. Fleur du Pré and coworkers identified a new subset of peripheral blood T cells that enables better detection of gluten-sensitive T cells, which in turn have better specificity for intestinal mucosa antigens [227]. This study may have important consequences for identifying subtypes of CD and provide a noninvasive method of evaluating therapeutic responsiveness.

5.2 Small Intestinal Biopsy

The histological judgment of small intestinal mucosa is commonly regarded as the criterion standard for CD diagnosis, despite the diagnostic advances afforded by the availability of serologic testing. The biopsy can be undertaken either with a small intestinal capsule or endoscopically. Capsule biopsies are taken by means of a capsule with a suction-guillotine-mechanism (e.g., Watson capsule) under fluoroscopic control. Tissue pieces are usually bigger and easier to orientate, but swallowing the capsule is uncomfortable for the patient and is more labor-intensive and time-consuming for the physician [101]. Thus, endoscopical biopsies using standard fiberoptic instruments have almost entirely replaced capsule biopsies. Video capsule endoscopy (VCE) was introduced into clinical practice for the diagnosis of gastrointestinal diseases several years ago. To evaluate current indications for the use of VCE in CD patients in everyday clinical practice, VCE was carried out in a number of CD patients at different European centers [228]. The results demonstrated that VCE may have a definitive impact on the management of RCD, but it plays a more limited role in the remaining patients. Kurien and coworkers advocate the use of VCE in equivocal cases, particularly in patients with antibody-negative villous atrophy [229]. VCE may also be performed in patients who are unable or unwilling to undergo conventional endoscopy—those with positive serology and normal duodenal biopsies and those who develop alarming symptoms [230].

Although CD is the most common cause of duodenal villous atrophy, nonceliac enteropathy is not rare and may easily be mistaken for CD [231]. For example, tropical sprue, autoimmune enteropathy, common variable immunodeficiency, collagenous sprue, bacterial overgrowth, inflammatory bowel disease, and drug-induced mucosal injury can cause villous atrophy and should be excluded by differential diagnosis [232]. Most of these disorders are characterized by a normal TGA level, a lack of intraepithelial lymphocytosis on biopsy, and a lack of histological response to a gluten-free diet. Nonceliac enteropathy can often be confirmed by negative HLA-DQ2/8 testing, and targeted investigations can ascertain a definitive etiology in most cases.

Historically, biopsies were taken from the jejunum. Later on, biopsies from the second part of the duodenum have been considered to be sufficient without loss of sensitivity and specificity. Biopsies from the duodenal bulb should be interpreted with caution because this area is exposed to gastric acid and is prone to peptic injury. However, the duodenal bulb is the most sensitive site to detect mucosal damage induced by gluten, and duodenal bulb biopsies can increase the accuracy of the histologic diagnosis [233]. For example, Tanpowpong and colleagues demonstrated that 6 out of 103 CD children had a Marsh 3 biopsy only in the duodenal bulb [234]. Hence, in practice, it seems reasonable to suggest that at least four to six endoscopic specimens be taken from the second part of the duodenum and two samples from the bulb region [232,235]. Given that patients with CD are frequently deficient in vitamin K, a coagulation study should be performed before the biopsy.

The biopsy pieces should be well orientated and should contain at least three to four consecutive villous-crypt units visualized in their entirety and arranged parallel to each other. The biopsies should be immediately fixed in buffered formalin, embedded on edge in paraffin, and stained with hematoxylin-eosin and Giemsa. Histopathologic evaluation should be performed by experienced pathologists who are blinded to the indication for endoscopy. Ideally, a pathologist with experience in gastrointestinal diseases should examine the biopsy slides to differentiate CD from other enteropathies, such as tropical sprue, peptic duodenitis, and graft-versus-host disease. Microscopic evaluation of the biopsies should consider the following targets: luminal surface (e.g., check for infection agents), enterocytes (e.g., loss of brushborder, villous and crypt architecture, crypt hyperplasia), number of IELs per enterocyte, basement membrane (e.g., thickening), and lamina propria (e.g., type and extent of inflammation). Villous and crypt architecture and number of IELs allow the judgment of the grade of mucosal damage from mild to marked and total villous atrophy (see Section 4.2). Nevertheless, false-positive and false-negative diagnosis may occur as a consequence of interobserver variability, patchy mucosal damage, low-grade histopathological abnormalities, and technical limitations [236].

Villous atrophy (Marsh 3) was previously required to set the diagnosis of CD. However, the new ESPGHAN guidelines have concluded that Marsh 2 is also sufficient to establish the diagnosis, as it has been proven that these patients actually suffer from CD. By contrast, a Marsh 1 lesion is still considered insufficient for the diagnosis of CD because this nonspecific lesion can also be associated with other diseases. To avoid variability in the reporting of villous atrophy and the diagnosis of CD, uniformity in small intestine histopathology reporting among pathologists is recommended [235]. In the case of equivocal serology and histology, biopsy tissues can be utilized further for measuring EMAs and TGAs [104,237–240]. The levels of these antibodies correlated with clinical symptoms, and after the introduction of a gluten-free diet, both the mucosal antibodies and symptoms resolved. The measurement of intestinal TGAs is also useful in identifying potential CD [239]. The analysis of IgM TGAs in the intestinal tissue may help to diagnose patients with IgA deficiency.

The increase in IELs is one of the hallmarks of CD and may be a more sensitive parameter of CD than the changes in villous structure as they are found earlier in the course of disease and disappear earlier in remission. However, intraepithelial lymphocytosis is not a CD-exclusive feature and, therefore, its diagnostic evidence can only be evaluated in a broader clinical context. IELs should be best immunostained with monoclonal anti-CD3 antibodies. This significantly increases the accuracy of IEL count, which is particularly important in the evaluation of biopsies with a normal villous/crypt ratio in the identification of Marsh 1 lesions, especially in patients with raised serum TGAs [241]. IELs isolated from intestinal biopsies can be measured by flow cytometry, a technique widely used for the study on solid tissues [242]. Counts between 25 and 29 IELs per 100 epithelial cells are considered a borderline increase, while a count of 30 or more represents a definite increase in IELs [232]. The increase in IELs can be a helpful diagnostic biomarker in cases of CD with mild inflammation lacking serologic abnormalities and in the differential diagnosis of CD versus other immune-mediated enteropathies. If histology shows lesions that are consistent with Marsh 2–3 (see Section 4.2), then the diagnosis of CD is confirmed. If histology is normal

(Marsh 0) or shows only increased IEL counts (Marsh 1), then further testing should be performed before establishing the diagnosis [186].

5.3 HLA-DQ Tests

Except for the CD-specific HLA-DQ2/8 alleles, no convincing disease association has been found for other genetic tests or the test did not find its way from the research field to clinical practice. It is estimated that more than 95% of CD patients are positive for HLA-DQ2/8. However, positive DQ2/DQ8 cannot be used to confirm a diagnosis of CD, because DQ2/DQ8 alleles are very common in the white population (more than 25%) and only approximately 1% develop CD. For instance, DQ2/DQ8 testing was shown to have a positive predictive value for CD of only 6% among 463 people [243]. CD risk prediction may be improved by adding non-HLA-susceptible variants to common HLA testing in the future [244]. Above all, HLA tests should be used to rule out the existence of CD because they have high negative predictive values (≈97%) [245]. HLA-DQ typing is a cost-saving first-line screening step in high-risk groups, including first-degree relatives of patients with a confirmed case and patients with autoimmune and non-autoimmune conditions known to be associated with CD, such as type 1 diabetes mellitus, Down's syndrome, and Turner's syndrome. Moreover, it can be a useful adjunct in an exclusionary sense when the diagnosis based on other tests is not clear [246]. In such cases, if a patient is negative for HLA-DQ2/8, CD can be excluded lifelong and no further investigations and follow-up are needed.

Commercial DNA tests based on polymerase chain reaction (PCR) are now available, allowing the determination of the alleles of HLA-DQ2/8. Even if HLA-DQ2.2 is rare, it should be included into testing beside DQ2.5 and DQ8 [247]. DNA is extracted from cells in a cheek swab or blood sample and then analyzed by PCR. New techniques, such as using tag single nucleotide polymorphisms, semiautomated sequence-specific primer PCR, and real-time PCR preceded by melting curve analysis, will make HLA typing simpler and faster at a relatively low cost [186]. Using capillary electrophoresis for directed HLA typing may reduce the reagent expenses and technical time [248]. A so-called HLA-DQ2-gliadin tetramer test was developed for the diagnosis of CD in patients already adhering to a gluten-free diet [249]. Biotinylated recombinant DQ2.5 heterodimers are complexed with gluten epitope peptides. These tetramers are multimerized with fluorescence-conjugated streptavidin and used to detect epitope-specific $CD4^+$ T cells in blood of potential CD patients challenged with four slices of white bread daily for 3 days. The number of tetramer-binding T cells is measured by flow cytometry on day 0 and day 6 after gluten challenge. This method offers an accurate alternative for detecting CD in individuals who have already established themselves on a gluten-free diet.

6. PATHOMECHANISM

The human gastrointestinal tract is constantly subjected to a high antigenic load and therefore has developed numerous strategies to maintain tolerance to ingested food. Under normal conditions, the mucosal immune system has developed a strict tolerance to these antigens by a combination of anergy and apoptosis of antigen-specific T cells and the active suppression of these cells by regulatory T cells (Tregs) [250]. These Tregs share a number of inhibitory mechanisms that involve production of the anti-inflammatory cytokine IL-10 and transforming growth factor-β, among others. Studies on suppressive activities have shown that the number of Tregs (subset FoxP3$^+$) is significantly increased in the mucosa of active CD and correlates with the histological severity [251,252]. However, the beneficial suppressor capacity of Tregs might be impaired by IL-15 [252], which is upregulated in the intestinal mucosa of CD (see Section 6.3).

The acquisition of oral tolerance is a complex process and is far from being fully understood. Intolerance to gluten may potentially be the result of two different phenomena: The first could be that, for unknown reasons, tolerance to gluten never developed in certain individuals; the second is that prior tolerance is lost at some point in life [253]. It has been hypothesized that molecular mimicry between pathogens and gluten could trigger the loss of gluten tolerance. For example, it was observed that the E1b protein of human adenovirus type 12 shares a sequence homology with an α-gliadin fragment [254], and the hyphal wall protein 1 from *Candida albicans* shares a sequence homology with α- and γ-gliadins [255]. However, no direct evidence and experimental findings have supported this hypothesis.

6.1 Gluten Intake and Digestion

Wheat, rye, barley, and oat products are staple foods in many parts of the world. In these countries, daily gluten intake is high, between 15 and 20 g on average, with segments of the general population consuming as much as 50 g and more. Gluten intake has apparently increased during the last decades, and it has been suggested that the higher gluten consumption is related to the increase in the prevalence of CD [24]. In fact, the worldwide production of wheat grains increased from 583 million metric tons per year during 2000–2002 to 676 million metric tons per year during 2010–2012 [256]. Because wheat is mainly used for human consumption, wheat gluten consumption may have increased accordingly. In contrast to IgE-mediated allergens, small amounts of gluten are tolerated by most CD patients. The important question on the maximum level of daily gluten intake not harmful to CD patients was addressed in only a few studies. The difficulties are obvious: Patients differ in the tolerable level of gluten, the time necessary to develop evidence of toxicity is variable and may be very long, and challenged volunteers have to be biopsied at least twice (before and after challenge). Nevertheless, some remarkable results have been obtained [257,258], which are described here.

A significant relapse of CD at the clinical, laboratory, and histological levels was observed in both children and adults, when 1–5 g of gluten, a moderate amount compared with the normal daily intake of 15–20 g, was given [259]. Four lower daily doses of gliadins were tested in a single patient: 10 mg produced no change, 100 mg produced a very slight measureable change, 500 mg produced a moderate change, and 1 g caused extensive damage of the small intestinal morphology [260]. In another study, the ingestion of 2.4–4.8 mg of gluten per day caused no change in the jejunal biopsy, neither after 1 nor 6 weeks of challenge [261]. Similarly, 4–16 mg gliadins [262] and 20–36 mg gluten [263,264] did not affect the intestinal mucosa of CD patients in remission. In contrast, a 4-week challenge with 100 mg gliadins per day caused deterioration of the small intestinal architecture, which was even more pronounced in patients challenged with 500 mg gliadins (corresponding to occasional dietary lapses) [265]. The most extensive study was published in 2007 describing a prospective, double-blind, placebo-controlled multicenter trial with 39 patients in remission [266]. They were assigned to ingest a capsule containing either 0, 10, or 50 mg of gluten daily and for a duration of 90 days. Despite a wide individual variability, it was demonstrated that 50 mg of daily gluten for 3 months are sufficient to cause significant damage of the intestinal mucosa. The kinetics of the histological, serological, and symptomatic responses to gluten intake were studied by Leffler and coworkers [188]. Twenty adult CD patients on a gluten-free diet were challenged with 3.0 or 7.5 g gluten per day for 14 days. Duodenal biopsies were taken at the beginning and at days 3 and 14 of challenge. TGAs and DGPAs, lactulose to mannitol ratio, and symptoms were assessed more frequently. A significant reduction in the ratio of villous height to crypt depth and increase in IELs were seen from the baseline to day 14. Antibody titers increased slightly from baseline to day 14, but markedly by day 28. The lactulose to mannitol ratio did not change significantly. Gastrointestinal symptoms increased significantly by day 3 and returned to baseline by day 28. No differences were seen between the two gluten doses.

Usually, food proteins are broken down into amino acids, dipeptides, and tripeptides by gastric, pancreatic, and intestinal brushborder enzymes (step 1 in Figure 1.10). The earliest theory on CD pathogenesis was based on the

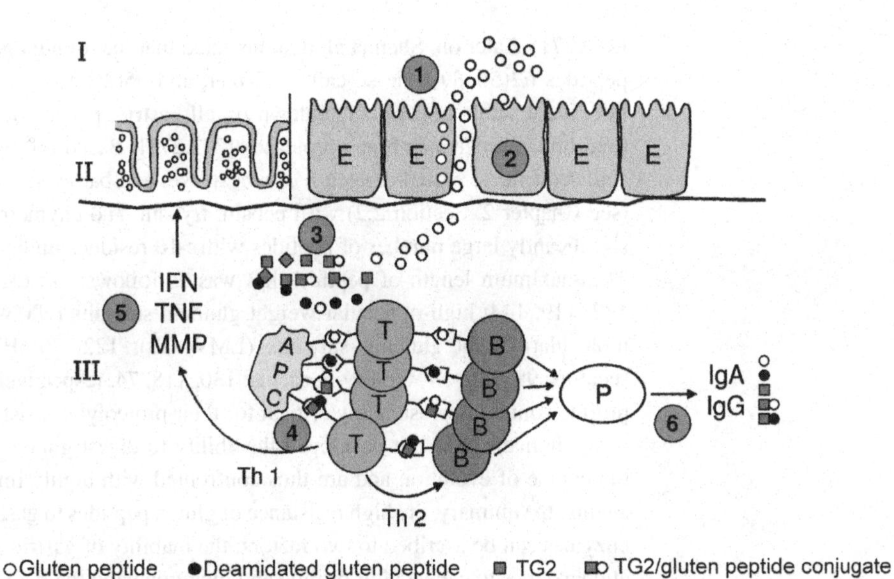

■ **FIGURE 1.10** Schematical representation of the adaptive immune response in the intestinal lymphatic tissue and destruction of enterocytes in the pathogenesis of celiac disease. I = intestinal lumen; II = epithelium; III = lamina propria; APC = antigen-presenting cell; B = B cell; E = enterocyte; IFN = interferon-γ; Ig = immunoglobulin; MMP = matrix metalloproteinase; P = plasma cell; T = CD4+ T cell; TG2 = tissue transglutaminase; Th = T helper; TNF = tumor necrosis factor. For steps 1–6, see text. (Please see color plate at the back of the book.)

"missing peptidase hypothesis" [267]. The basic effect was considered to be a deficiency of an enzyme in the small intestine, which is required for the digestion of CD-active peptides. Later on, however, other authors showed that peptidase activities are normal in the mucosa of CD patients on a gluten-free diet [268]. Therefore, impaired gluten digestion by jejunal mucosa from patients with active disease was viewed as a consequence, not a cause, of the disease [269]. Today, it is commonly accepted that the high frequency of proline in gluten proteins combined with the absence of prolyl endopeptidase activity in the human gastrointestinal tract makes these proteins resistant to digestion even in healthy individuals, so that long-chain peptides reach the intestinal mucosa. Nonetheless, the relatively poor digestion of gluten proteins alone is not sufficient to cause CD, and there is no known difference between healthy individuals and CD patients in their (non)ability to digest these proteins.

In the 1980s, studies on the CD toxicity of peptides isolated from enzymatic digests of gliadins revealed first insights into the partially poor digestibility of gluten proteins. Accordingly, peptides derived from the proline-rich amino acid sequences of α-gliadins (see Chapter 2, Section 2.2) with a length of up to 30 residues were resistant to pepsin, trypsin, chymotrypsin, and pancreatin

[270,271]. Later on, Shan et al. demonstrated that the immunogenic gliadin peptides α2(56–89), the so-called 33-mer, and γ5(26–51), a 26-mer peptide, were stable towards breakdown by all gastric, pancreatic, and intestinal brushborder membrane proteases [272,273]. Based on known amino acid sequences, virtual digestion of wheat, rye, and barley storage proteins (see Chapter 2, Section 2.2) with pepsin, trypsin, and chymotrypsin left a significantly large number of peptides with >10 residues undigested [274]. The maximum length of peptides left was as follows: ω-, α-, γ-gliadins: 132, 119, 144; high-molecular-weight glutenin subunits (HMW-GS), low-molecular-weight glutenin subunits (LMW-GS): 122, 70; HMW-, ω/γ-secalins: 99, 339; D-, C-, B/γ-hordeins: 130, 118, 74, respectively. The high proline content is presumably critical for their proteolytic resistance. Obviously, humans have not developed the ability to digest gluten well during the course of evolution and are thus confronted with highly immunogenic agents. In summary, the high resistance of gluten peptides to gastrointestinal enzymes can be ascribed to two factors: the inability of gastric and pancreatic enzymes to cleave after proline and glutamine and the inability of aminopeptidase N, dipeptidyl peptidase IV, and dipeptidyl carboxypeptidase I in the brushborder membrane to digest long-chain peptides.

As demonstrated below, the deamidation of glutamine side chains increases the damaging immune response. Several authors postulated that glutamine-containing gluten proteins and peptides may be partially deamidated in the acidic milieu of the stomach—however, without any proof. For clarification, the model peptide PQL, occurring in immunogenic epitopes of α-gliadins, was treated with 0.01 mol/l HCl (pH 2.0) at 37 °C for 240 min in order to study possible deamidation reactions [275]. The subsequent chemical analysis revealed that not even traces of the possible deamidation product PEL were generated. In conclusion, deamidation of glutamine-containing gluten peptides does not take place unspecifically in the stomach but specifically in the lamina propria catalyzed by TG2 (see Section 6.3.1).

To mimic human digestion for in vitro research studies, several systems have been employed [276]. For example, gluten digestion experiments were performed in beakers or tubes, where temperature, enzyme composition and levels, and duration had been adapted to physiological conditions. This simple in vitro system was used for the identification of the 33-mer peptide as a stable product of gluten digestion [272]. A dynamic gastrointestinal model developed by TNO (Wageningen, NL) is more sophisticated. The so-called TIM 1 system comprises four compartments mimicking the stomach, duodenum, jejunum, and ileum [277]. Peristaltic intestinal mixing is simulated by manipulating the jacket water pressure. This system was used to demonstrate the efficient degradation of gluten by a fungal prolyl endopeptidase (AN-PEP) (see Chapter 3, Section 2.1).

Based on the present knowledge of the CD pathomechanism, the following set of structural criteria of CD-active peptides can be defined:

1. a length of at least nine amino acid residues;
2. a high content of proline residues adopting a left-handed polyproline II helical conformation;
3. a high content of glutamine residues capable of deamidation and trans-amidation reactions with TG2.

All gluten protein types contain sequence sections in the form of repetitive sequences (see Chapter 2, Section 2.2) that fulfill these criteria. These proteins are confronted with the digestive power of the gastrointestinal enzymes pepsin, trypsin, and chymotrypsin. The question is how many potentially CD-active digestion products (peptides) reach the intestinal brushborder. The starting point of the following calculations is an average oral intake of 100 g grain or wholemeal flour per meal, corresponding to 8.8–10.6 g of total proteins from the four CD-toxic cereals [278] (Table 1.4). The proportions of storage proteins based on total proteins are around 75% for wheat, rye, and barley and 14% (only prolamins) for oats [279], so that the gluten intake ranges from 1.39 g (oats) to 7.95 g (wheat). As shown in Table 1.4, the proportions of single protein types are strongly different resulting in low amounts of ω5-gliadins (239 mg/100 g) and high amounts of γ-75k-secalins (3168 mg/100 g), for example. As mentioned before, potentially CD-active peptides are almost exclusively located in the repetitive sequence sections of the proteins. These sections are strongly variable in length and proportions ranging from 30% based on total sequences in B-hordeins to 96% in ω-secalins. In consequence, C-hordeins (2471 mg) and γ-75k-secalins (2123 mg) provide the highest amounts of glutamine- and proline-rich structures, whereas those of ω5-gliadins (213 mg), ω1,2-gliadins (293 mg), and D-hordeins (304 mg) are on a very low level. Conditions for the subsequent in silico digestions were the following specificities: cleavage by pepsin before and after hydrophobic amino acids (e.g., X–L–X, X–F–X, but not X = P), cleavage by trypsin after basic amino acids (e.g., K–X, R–X, but not X = P), and cleavage by chymotrypsin after aromatic amino acids (e.g., F–X, Y–X, but not X = P). Proline-rich structures are fairly resistant to the enzymatic attack, so that rather high proportions of the repetitive sequences (69–100%, except avenins = 11%) survive as peptides >8 amino acid residues. Numbers and lengths of these peptides are strongly different. For example, the virtual digestion of B-hordeins yielded only two peptides and that of x-type HMW-GS 33 peptides. The maximum length of peptides was in a range from 10 residues (avenins) to 167 residues (γ-75k-secalins). These results are in agreement with studies performed by Shan et al. [273] and Osorio et al. [274]. With regard to single types, C-hordeins release 2249 mg and γ-75k-secalins 2123 mg peptides per 100 g whole grain. Surprisingly, α-gliadins,

Table 1.4 Estimated (in silico) Quantities of Gluten Proteins and Peptides Arriving at the Intestinal Brushborder after Oral Consumption and Subsequent Digestion with Gastric and Pancreatic Peptidases

	Wheat						Rye				Barley				Oats
Whole grain[a,z]	10,600						8800				10,400				9900
Gluten[b,z] (75%)	7950						6600				7800				1386[c]
Protein types[d]	ω5	ω1,2	α	γ	HMW	LMW	ω	γ-40k	HMW	γ-75k	C	γ	D	B	AVE
% of gluten[d]	3	4	33	27	11	22	18	25	9	48	36	32	5	27	100
Quantity[z]	239	318	2623	2146	875	1749	1188	1650	594	3168	2808	2496	390	2106	1386
Protein section[e]	B	B	I	I	B	I	B	I	B	I	B	I	B	I	I + IV
% of protein type	89	92	35	49	81	35	96	48[f]	81	67	88	47	78	30	43
Quantity[z]	213	293	918	1052	709	612	1140	792	481	2123	2471	1173	304	632	596
No. of peptides >8[g]	8	6	4	3	33/22[h]	5	9	-	32/24[h]	4	9	5	20	2	1
Maximum length	86	94	27	64	50/78	22	73	-	60/44	167	97	32	120	64	10
% of protein section	100	92	79	87	88/85	69	91	87[f]	95/94	100	91	87	90	93	11
Quantity[z]	213	270	725	915	617	422	1037	689	455	2123	2249	1021	274	588	66
Σ[z]	3162						4304				4132				66

[a]*Ref. [278].*
[b]*Prolamins + glutelins.*
[c]*14%, Ref. [279].*
[d]*See Table 2.4.*
[e]*See Figures 2.6–2.8.*
[f]*Taken from γ-gliadin and γ-hordein.*
[g]*Database Uni Prot KB.*
[h]*x/y-type.*
[z]*Quantity in mg/100 g grain.*

frequently characterized as the most immunodominant proteins, are in a medium position (725 mg) similar to γ-40k-secalins (689 mg), B-hordeins (588 mg), and γ-hordeins (1021 mg). Oat avenins provide only one peptide >8 residues (QPYPEQQEPF) corresponding to 66 mg. Summing up, rye is leading as a producer of potentially CD-active peptides (4304 mg), followed by barley (4132 mg) and wheat (3162 mg). The questionable role of oats in CD toxicity is well reflected by the low level of 66 mg.

The following steps of peptide metabolism are structurally and quantitatively uncertain. Are they further digested by brushborder enzymes? Do they pass the tight junctions? How are they endocytosed during the transcellular pathway and deamidated and crosslinked by TG2 in the lamina propria? Last but not least, how do they fit to the mechanisms of innate and adaptive immune responses?

6.2 Epithelial Passage

The intestinal tract is not only responsible for digestion and absorption of nutrients but also has an important barrier function. The single layer of epithelial cells normally permits the absorption of nutrients but restricts the passage of harmful agents such as bacteria, viruses, and other pathogens. Increased intestinal permeability is associated with several different human diseases, including inflammatory bowel disease, irritable bowel syndrome, and CD. Changes in the mucosal permeability are supposed to be an early pathogenic event in the development of CD by exposing the immune system of the lamina propria to the stimulatory gluten peptides. The understanding of intestinal permeability and the control mechanisms that regulate barrier function has increased significantly over the last years. However, it is still not fully understood how gluten peptides reach the lamina propria of the intestine. There is evidence that this occurs both by the paracellular and transcellular routes (step 2 in Figure 1.10). Gluten peptides crossing through the paracellular pathway reach the submucosa unmodified, whereas peptides may be degraded through the transcellular pathway.

Among the most important structures of the paracellular route are the epithelial pore-forming "tight junctions" (TJs) [170,280]. They are in a dynamic balance regulated by intracellular events. TJs are composed of a number of protein components that provide continuous belt-like cell-to-cell junctions and regulate paracellular permeability. The function of these proteins can be subdivided into "tightening" that strengthens barrier properties and "leaking" that selectively mediates permeability. The major protein types of the TJs are occludin, claudins, junctional adhesion molecule A, and tricellulin and the associated protein at the intracellular plaque, the zonula occludens (zonulin-1) (Figure 1.11). The claudin family forms the actual paracellular

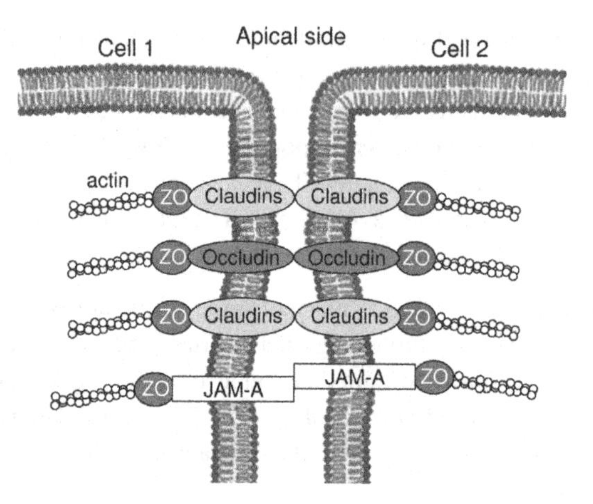

■ **FIGURE 1.11** Schematic representation of the basic structural components of tight junctions consisting of zonulins 1, 2, and 3 (ZO) and the integral membrane proteins occludin, claudins, and junctional adhesion molecule (JAM-) A.

pore and is associated with other transmembrane proteins, such as occludin. Claudin-1, 3, 4, 5, and 8 strengthen the barrier, whereas claudin-2, 7, 10, and 12 weaken it. Zonulin (ZO)-1 and other cytoplasmic proteins, such as ZO-2 and ZO-3, attach to the junctional adhesion molecule (JAM). Occludin and ZO-1 interact directly with the actin cytoskeleton.

ZO-1 (identified as prehaptoglobulin-2 [281]) is an intestinal epithelial protein analog of zonula occludens toxin of *Vibrio cholerae* and is normally expressed and secreted to the surface of intestinal and other epithelia (heart, brain). ZO-1 interacts with the proteins of TJs in a rapid, reversible, and reproducible fashion and links them to the cytoskeletal actin. Zonulin has been characterized as "the only physiological modulator of intercellular TJs described so far that is involved in trafficking of macromolecules and, therefore, in tolerance/immune response balance" [282].

A disturbed intestinal barrier function is considered a key factor in the development of intestinal inflammation and plays an important role in both the pathogenesis and the perpetuation of various intestinal diseases such as CD and inflammatory bowel disease [283]. The most important factor determining the permeability of a probe is its molecular size. The pore size of a healthy intestinal mucosa ranges from around 50 nm (villous tip) to more than 200 nm (crypt base). For example, monosaccharides (molecular mass ≈180) permeate the barrier, whereas nonmetabolized disaccharides (molecular mass ≈340) are not able to pass the barrier. Thus, increased permeability can be measured by a differential sugar absorption test [284]. This test is based on the oral administration of an oligosaccharide (lactulose or cellobiose) and a monosaccharide (mannitol or rhamnose) that differentially cross the intestinal barrier. The quantitative ratio of both sugars in urine samples collected over 5–6 h after oral intake is considered to reflect the loss of barrier function most accurately.

In healthy individuals, gluten peptides are endocytosed by enterocytes and are almost totally degraded by the lysosomal system during epithelial transport. Thus, an excessive activation of the local immune system is likely avoided [285]. In active CD, TJs are opened, showing a reduction of horizontal strands and an increase of strand discontinuities [286]. Consequently, more gluten peptides cross the intestinal mucosa and a significant fraction reaches the lamina propria. Even on a gluten-free diet, the initially enhanced intestinal permeability does not necessarily return to normal. The pathogenic role of intestinal TJs disruption is supported by studies demonstrating that increased intestinal permeability exists prior to CD onset. Increased intestinal permeability persists in asymptomatic patients, who are on a gluten-free diet, and is also present in a significant proportion of healthy first-degree relatives of patients [280].

ZO-1 has been proposed to be one of the initial factors for the pathogenesis of CD [282]. Quantitative immunoblotting of intestinal tissue lysates from patients with active CD revealed an increase in ZO-1 compared with control tissues [287]. ZO-1 upregulation during the acute phase of CD was further confirmed by measuring ZO-1 concentration in the sera of 189 patients with untreated CD [288]. Compared with healthy controls, they had significantly higher concentrations during the active phase of the disease, which decreased following a gluten-free diet. Pharmacological modulation of intestinal permeability by ZO-1 antagonists will possibly enable the treatment of CD (see Chapter 3, Section 2.4).

The chemokine receptor CXCR3 on the luminal side of enterocytes has been identified as the target intestinal receptor for gluten peptides. CXCR3 is overexpressed in active CD patients and induces an increased release of ZO-1 combined with a subsequent increase of permeability [289]. Using an α-gliadin synthetic peptide library, two α-gliadin 20-mer peptides (QVLQQSTYQLLQELCCQHLW and QQQQQQQQQQQQILQQILQQ) were identified that bind to CXCR3 and release ZO-1. In addition, the enhanced intestinal permeability may be caused by the cytokines, especially IFN-γ, produced by activated CD4^{+} T cells [290].

To analyze the relative contribution of the paracellular and transcellular transport pathways, the permeability for labeled gliadin peptides in duodenal biopsy specimens taken from active CD patients was compared by means of Ussing chambers and specific permeability markers (horseradish peroxidase, mannitol) [291]. The transcellular permeability for intact peptides was much higher for peptide α31–49 and the 33-mer peptide (α2/56–88) than for peptides α57–68 and α202–220. The percentage of intact α31–49 and 33-mer peptides crossing the epithelium was 25% and 42%, respectively. The proportion of intact peptides crossing the intestine via the paracellular pathway was negligible. This abnormal passage of intact peptides resulted from an abnormal retrotransport of complexes between anti-gliadin secretory IgA1 and gliadin peptides by CD71, a high avidity receptor for transferrin and polymeric IgA1 [285]. In active CD, CD71 is massively upregulated and expressed at the apex of enterocytes, where it can bind the IgA1-peptide complex present in the lumen. This binding allows gliadin peptides to escape lysosomal degradation and to translocate intact into the lamina propria. Thus, CD71 transforms IgA1 into a "Trojan horse" able to promote the entrance of immunogenic peptides [285]; TG2 participates in this process [292]. The fact that CD can occur in patients with selective IgA deficiency may argue against the mechanism. However, Heyman and colleagues suggested that IgG might play a similar role and transfer peptides via the neonatal Fc receptor [293].

The occurrence of gliadin peptides in enterocytes of patients with active CD was already demonstrated by Zimmer and coworkers in 1998 [294]. Morphological studies using immunofluorescence microscopy showed that increased amounts of gliadin peptides were present in intracellular compartments of enterocytes of CD patients in remission compared with control enterocytes. The intraepithelial transport processes of different gliadin peptides in human duodenal biopsy specimens from CD patients were studied by means of epitope-specific monoclonal AGAs [295]. The toxic peptide α31–49 (LGQQQPFPPQQPYPQPQPF) and the immunogenic peptide α56–68 (LQLQPFPQPQLPY) were compared with the nonactive control peptide α229–246 (LPQFEEIRNLALQTLPAM). The results demonstrated that peptide α31–49 was segregated from the peptides α56–68 and α229–246 along the endosomal pathway. Thus, peptide α31–49 bypassed HLA-DR-positive late endosomes in specimens of CD patients with untreated CD. It was localized in early endosomes and consequently escaped antigen presentation at the basolateral membrane, unlike peptides α56–68 and α229–246 that reached HLA-DR-positive late endosomes. Thus, the endocytic segregation of peptide α31–49 explains why this peptide cannot stimulate gluten-sensitive T cells (see Section 6.3.2). Consistent with these findings, Barone and colleagues found that both peptides α31–43 and α57–68 enter Caco-2 cells and human intestinal biopsies and interact with the endocytic compartment [296]. However, only peptide α31–43 was localized on the enterocyte membrane and interfered with the hepatocyte growth factor-regulated tyrosine kinase substrate (Hrs), which is a key protein of endocytic maturation. Thus, peptide α31–43 delayed vesicle trafficking by interfering with Hrs-mediated maturation of early endosomes in enterocytes of CD patients. In biopsies of healthy controls, the peptide was readily processed by the vesicular compartment. Peptide α31–43 increased IL-15 levels on the cell surface by altering intracellular trafficking [297]. The increased IL-15 protein was bound to IL-15 receptor α with consequent proliferation of crypt enterocytes, an early alteration of CD mucosa causing crypt hyperplasia. In addition, the engulfment of lysosomes containing peptide α31–43 induces cellular stress and the generation of oxidative responses, which are associated with increased TG2 levels [298].

In conclusion, recent data point to a key role for the transcellular pathway. Increased paracellular permeability might rather be the consequence of villous atrophy and local secretion of inflammatory cytokines [293]. However, the question of whether the increased permeability in CD is a cause or consequence of the disease remains to be answered.

6.3 **Immune Response**

The human immune system, built up progressively during evolution to fight against pathogens, involves both innate and adaptive mechanisms. The fast innate system developed very early in primitive multicellular organisms and has gradually gained in complexity to assume a dual function in mammals: a role of immediate barrier albeit with low specificity and no memory and a second role of antigen presentation to the adaptive immune system via MHC molecules [299]. The slow adaptive system emerged much later in vertebrates and relies on B and T lymphocytes to permit a delayed but highly specific response endowed with long-term memory.

The gut-associated lymphoid tissue (GALT) is the largest and probably most complex part of the immune system [300]. It is in continuous contact with a complex mixture of foreign antigens over a surface measuring 400 m^2. The GALT has to discriminate between pathogenic microorganisms and harmless antigens, such as dietary compounds. The default setup of the intestinal immunity is therefore the generation of tolerance, unless specific signals evoke inflammatory reactions. The immunological mechanisms of CD, which cause damage to the intestinal mucosa, are complex, constituting a reaction in which a large number of immune competent cells and immunological mediators participate. The role of gluten peptides in the adaptive immune response in CD is well established. With respect to the innate immune response, a number of open questions exist; in particular, the collaboration between innate and adaptive immunity still remains unclear.

However, the fact that both the adaptive and the innate responses abate on a gluten-free diet suggests ways to probe their possible interdependence.

6.3.1 Adaptive Response

Since the discovery that HLA-DQ2/8 alleles are the main genetic risk factor for CD [301], it has been convincingly established that the adaptive immune response plays a central role in the pathogenesis of CD. Adaptive immunity provides an undisputable link between the main genetic factor (HLA-DQ2/8) and the main environmental factor (gluten). Numerous studies of the last decades contributed to a significant progress in understanding the adaptive immune response to gluten peptides. Major players of the immune cascade in the lamina propria are APCs, T cells, and B cells on the cellular level and TG2, HLA-DQ2/8 heterodimers, T-cell receptors (TCRs), cytokines, and chemokines on the molecular level (Figure 1.10).

6.3.1.1 Transglutaminases

TGs present in the intestinal tissue decisively contribute to the adaptive immune response in CD. TGs (protein glutamine-γ-glutamyltransferases, EC 2.3.2.13) are enzymes that catalyze the acyl transfer of a glutamine side chain (acyl donor) to a primary amine (acyl acceptor). The most important physiological function of TGs is the covalent and irreversible transamidation of a protein with a glutamine residue to another protein with a lysine residue, resulting in the formation of an ε-(γ-glutamyl)-lysine isopeptide bond (Figure 1.12(A)) [302]. The crosslinked products, often highly resistant to mechanical challenge and proteolytic degradation, accumulate in a number of tissues where such properties are crucial, such as skin, hair, cornification of the epidermis, and wound healing. In addition, TGs catalyze transamidation reactions with the incorporation of low-molecular-weight primary amines into proteins. Under certain conditions, particularly when an ε-amino group of lysine or other primary amino groups are not available or at relatively low pH-value, glutamine is deamidated to glutamic acid by reaction with water (Figure 1.12(B)).

TG was first reported in 1959 by Mycek and colleagues as an enzyme in guinea pig liver catalyzing amine incorporation into insulin [303]. Numerous subsequent investigations demonstrated that TGs ubiquitously occur in all eukaryotic organisms, and eight different TGs (TG1-7, factor VIII) have been detected in mammalians. All these different TGs share a common amino acid sequence in the catalytic site and have similar gene structures, although they are encoded by separate genes and show different substrate specifities and functions. Their enzymatic activity is Ca^{2+} dependent, and other factors including guanosine di- and triphosphates (GDP/GTP) can

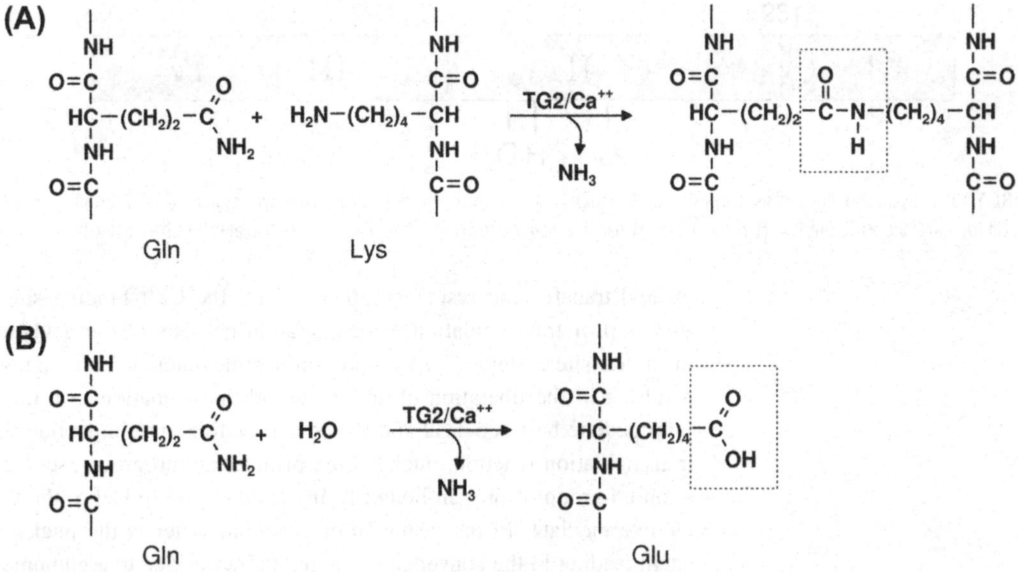

■ **FIGURE 1.12** Possible protein/peptide modifications by tissue transglutaminase (TG2). (A) TG2 catalyzes crosslinking between the side chains of glutamine (Gln) and lysine (Lys). (B) TG2 catalyzes deamidation of the side chain of Gln in the absence of primary amines. *Adapted from Ref. [302].*

also affect the activity of some of the mammalian TGs. Upon activation, the enzyme undergoes a dramatic conformational change, in which the C-terminal residues are displaced by as much as 1.2 pm [304].

TG2, commonly referred to as "tissue transglutaminase," is probably the most ubiquitous and multifunctional member of the TG family [305]. A highly sensitive ELISA developed by Wolf and coworkers enables the detection and quantitation of TG2 [306]. Besides acting as acyl transferase, TG2 can act as G protein, adaptor protein, cell surface adhesion mediator, disulfide isomerase, and serine/threonine kinase [307]. Dysregulation of TG2 activity is associated with several pathologic conditions, such as chronic degenerative disorders, autoimmune diseases, chronic inflammatory disorders, or infectious diseases [308]. Since its identification as the major autoantigen targeted by CD patients' antibodies [113], TG2 has played an important role in the investigation of CD pathogenesis and diagnosis.

TG2 is a monomeric protein of 687 amino acid residues and a molecular weight of around 76,000. It is composed of four different domains: the N-terminal β-sandwich domain (residues 1–139), the α/β catalytic core domain (residues 140–460), and two C-terminal β-barrel domains (residues 461–538 and 539–687, respectively) (Figure 1.13) [305]. Cysteine (C) 277, histidine (H) 335, and aspartic acid (D) 358 form the active site

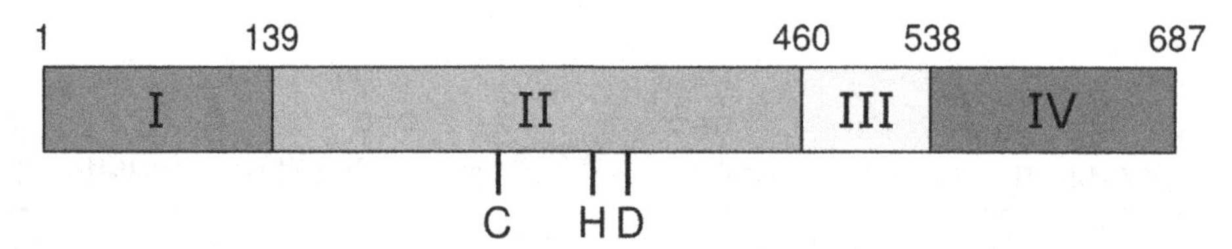

■ **FIGURE 1.13** Different domains of tissue transglutaminase (TG2): I = β-sandwich; II = α/β catalytic core with cysteine (C) 277, histidine (H) 335 and aspartic acid (D) 358 of the active site; III = β-barrel-1; IV = β-barrel-2. *Adapted from Ref. [305].* (Please see color plate at the back of the book.)

of acyl transfer and residues 430–453 form the Ca^{2+} binding site. The first step of transamidation or deamidation consists of the acylation of the active site cysteine 277 by a protein/peptide bound glutamine residue, resulting in the liberation of ammonia and the formation of a thioester intermediate between TG2 and the corresponding protein/peptide. In the transamidation reaction, nucleophilic primary amino groups such as the ε-amino group of protein-bound lysine residues are linked to the thioester intermediate. In the deamidation reaction, water is the nucleophilic agent leading to the conversion of a glutamine residue to a glutamic acid residue. Possibly, gluten peptides involved in CD may become deamidated via a primary transamidation to histamine, the secretion of which is increased in CD patients [309]. A further property of TG2 is its ability to bind and hydrolyze GTP. This activity is independent of the acyl transfer activity, but binding of GTP inhibits substrate binding to the acyl transfer catalytic site.

Originally, TG2 was regarded as an intracellular protein only found in the cytosol that could not be secreted by healthy cells under normal physiological conditions. Only stress or damage of cells may cause the leakage of the enzyme into the extracellular matrix. More recent studies have shown that TG2 can be secreted into the extracellular space under normal conditions, where it contributes to the stabilization and remodeling of the extracellular matrix [310]. However, the mechanism by which TG2 is secreted still remains a mystery and the question, "What comes first, TG2 activity or inflammation?", is still open. Once secreted into the extracellular environment, high Ca^{2+} and low GTP levels will promote activation of the enzyme by conversion of the closed inactive conformation into the open active conformation necessary for catalytic activity. A number of proteins and peptides are potential substrates for crosslinking, including fibronectin, collagen, and gluten peptides (see below).

The first study that described a possible role for TG2 in CD was published by the group of Bruce [311]. It showed that TG2 activity was increased in the jejunal tissue of untreated and treated CD patients in comparison to controls, and that glutamine-rich gliadin peptides represented preferential substrates for TG2. Numerous following investigations have revealed that both crosslinking and deamidation take place, and the physiological significance of deamidation has been established only in association with CD. Gluten proteins and peptides are preferred substrates (acyl donors) of TG2, as glutamine is generally the predominant amino acid residue (see Chapter 2, Section 2.2).

Both deamidation and transamidation are regarded as important during the pathogenic cascade of CD (step 3 in Figure 1.10). First, TG2 is capable of deamidating specific glutamine residues of gluten peptides, creating modified epitopes which bind to HLA-DQ2/8 molecules with increased affinity (see below). Second, TG2 is able to crosslink gluten peptides to other proteins, including several extracellular matrix proteins as well as to itself. Such crosslinking favors the accumulation of gluten peptides in the lamina propria ("hapten-carrier model"). Moreover, conjugates between gluten peptides and TG2 activate the production of TGAs (see Section 4.3). Due to the central role of TG2 within the adaptive immune response, its selective inhibition has been regarded as an alternative therapeutic approach for CD (see Chapter 3, Section 2.5).

The deamidation of glutamine residues is not an absolute requirement for stimulation of $CD4^+$ T cells, especially in the case of HLA-DQ8 heterodimers, but it strongly favors peptide binding to HLA-DQ2/8. Deamidation by TG2 is specific only for selected glutamine residues and depends on the amino acids neighboring the target glutamine. It has been demonstrated by means of synthetic peptide libraries that the relative positions of proline and hydrophobic amino acids to glutamine are crucial [312,313]. The sequences QXP and QXXF (X representing any amino acid and F representing hydrophobic amino acids) have been identified as preferred substrates for TG2, whereas the enzyme is not active on QP and QXXP sequences. Thus, deamidation by TG2 results in a highly selective introduction of negative charges into gluten peptides. Based on these findings, TG2 recognition algorithms have been designed and used to screen databases of various cereal proteins for privileged TG2 recognition sequences, and many deamidation-sensitive epitopes have been identified in wheat gliadins and glutenins, rye secalins, barley hordeins, and oat avenins. Examples for gluten peptide epitopes partially deamidated by TG2 are shown in Table 1.5.

A comprehensive new nomenclature for gluten-sensitive T-cell epitopes restricted by HLA-DQ molecules has been suggested by Sollid and

Table 1.5 Anchor Positions of DQ2- and DQ8-Restricted Epitopes from Different Gluten Protein Types[a]

Epitope	Position								
	1	2	3	4	5	6	7	8	9
DQ2-Restricted Epitopes									
α-Gliadin (DQ2.5-glia-α2)	P	Q	P	**E**	L	P	Y	P	Q
α-Gliadin (DQ2.5-glia-α1a)	P	F	P	Q	P	**E**	L	P	Y
γ-Gliadin (DQ2.5-glia-γ2)	I	Q	P	**E**	Q	P	A	Q	L
γ-Gliadin (DQ2.5-glia-γ4c)	Q	Q	P	**E**	Q	P	F	P	Q
ω1,2-Gliadin (DQ2.5-glia-ω1)	P	F	P	Q	P	**E**	Q	P	F
ω1,2-Gliadin (DQ2.5-glia-ω2)	P	Q	P	**E**	Q	P	F	P	W
LMW-GS (DQ2.5-glut-L1)	P	F	S	**E**	Q	**E**	Q	P	V
LMW-GS (DQ2.5-glut-L2)	F	S	Q	Q	Q	**E**	S	P	F
γ-Secalin (DQ2.5-sec-1)	P	F	P	Q	P	**E**	Q	P	F
γ-Secalin (DQ2.5-sec-2)	P	Q	P	**E**	Q	P	F	P	Q
γ-Hordein (DQ2.5-hor-2)	P	Q	P	**E**	Q	P	F	P	Q
γ-Hordein (DQ2.5-hor-3)	P	I	P	**E**	Q	P	Q	P	Y
Avenin (DQ2.5-ave-1a)	P	Y	P	E	Q	**E**	E	P	F
Avenin (DQ2.5-ave-1b)	P	Y	P	E	Q	**E**	Q	P	F
DQ8-Restricted Epitopes									
α-Gliadin (DQ8-glia-α1)	**E**	G	S	F	Q	P	S	Q	**E**
γ-Gliadin (DQ8-glia-γ1b)	**E**	Q	P	Q	Q	P	Y	P	**E**
HMW-GS (DQ8-glut-H1)	Q	G	Y	Y	P	T	S	P	Q

[a]Glutamic acid residues (E) formed by TG2-mediated deamidation that are important for recognition by T cells are shown in bold.
Adapted from Ref.[314].

coworkers [314]; examples are included in Table 1.5. The nomenclature is based on the following three criteria:

1. reactivity against the epitope must have been defined by at least one specific T-cell clone;
2. the HLA-restriction element involved must have been unequivocally defined;
3. the nine amino acid core of the epitope must have been defined either by analysis with truncated peptides and/or HLA-binding with a lysine scan of the epitope or comparable approach.

A dedicated website (http://www.isscd.net/EpitopeNomenclature.htm) will update the list as more epitopes are identified. However, cleavage of such epitopes by gastrointestinal peptidases, such as peptide bonds between F–S (LMW-GS), Y–Y (HMW-GS), and F–Q (α-gliadins), were not considered by these criteria. For example, Juhasz and colleagues showed by means of proteome-based datasets, collections of CD-relevant epitopes, and in silico enzymatic digestion that the number of CD epitopes in gluten proteins from wheat "Butte-86" was reduced from 549 in the native proteins to 99 in the digests [315].

Beside deamidation, TG2 catalyzes crosslinks between gluten peptides and itself and forms HMW conjugates. The analysis by confocal microscopy showed that TG2 colocalized with gliadin at the epithelial and subepithelial levels in active CD and demonstrated that gliadin was directly bound to TG2 in the duodenal mucosa [316].

The first chemical characterization of a conjugate between TG2 and an immunogenic gluten peptide (α57–68) with the sequence QLQPF-PQPQLPY was reported by Fleckenstein and coworkers in 2004 [317]. Two types of covalently linked conjugates were detected: The peptide was linked (1) through a thioester bond to the active site cysteine of TG2 and (2) through an isopeptide bond to particular lysine residues of TG2. Theoretically, TG2 provides 33 lysine residues (K) and the peptide α57–68 four glutamine residues (Q) for isopeptide bond formation. Only Q65 within the peptide sequences was found to participate in an isopeptide bond. The role of lysine residues within TG2 was shown to be dependent on the molar ratio of TG2 to the peptide. Only K590 was involved at a TG2/peptide ratio of 1:1, K562, K590, and K600 at a ratio of 1:10, and K444, K562, K590, K600, K649, and K677 at a ratio of 1:50 and 1:100. Lysine residues participating in isopeptide bond formation were not randomly distributed. Five out of six residues were located in the C-terminal section IV (Figure 1.13) far from the catalytic site. It can be concluded that the formation of isopeptide bonds between TG2 and gluten peptides occurs strongly directed.

The catalytic activity of TG2 for different gliadins was studied by Dieterich et al. [318]. Eleven α-, six γ-, three ω1,2-gliadins, and one ω5-gliadin were incubated with monodansyl cadaverin (fluorescent acyl acceptor) and TG2 followed by measurements of enhanced fluorescence intensity. The results indicated that all the tested gliadins were good substrates for TG2. No incorporation of monodansyl cadaverin was detected with the control substrates bovine serum albumin and lactalbumin. Using a fluorometric TG2 activity assay, the absolute requirement of Q65 as reactive glutamine in the gliadin peptide α2(56–68) was confirmed by the formation of a TG2/peptide conjugate. A CD-specific relevance of these conjugates can be derived from the production of autoantibodies that are directed against these crosslinked neoepitopes (see below). Furthermore, TG2 catalyzes binding of immunogenic gluten peptides to extracellular matrix proteins such as collagen. This haptenization and long-term immobilization of gluten peptides could be instrumental in the perpetuation of intestinal inflammation in CD [318].

The aim of a study by Dorum and coworkers was to identify the preferred peptide substrates of TG2 in an extremely heterogenous protein complex, namely wheat gluten [319]. Gluten was digested with pepsin, trypsin, chymotrypsin, elastase, and carboxypeptidase and then incubated with TG2 and the primary amino marker 5-biotinamidophenylamin. Peptide/amine conjugates were enriched by streptavidin Dynabeads and identified by mass spectrometry. A total of 31 different gluten peptides were found as preferred substrates of TG2. Strikingly, the majority of these peptides were harboring known gluten T-cell epitopes. The 33-mer peptide was not among the identified TG2 substrates. The same study demonstrated that four α-gliadin peptides and one γ-gliadin peptide carried both a transamidated and a deamidated glutamine residue. For example, peptide α3–24 was deamidated at Q16 and transamidated at Q21.

Despite the major advances in understanding the pathogenic role of TG2 in CD, several issues remain to be elucidated [308]. These include the intracellular regulation of TG2, the mechanism of its externalization, the role of enterocytes as primary sites of gluten modification by TG2, the effect of TGAs on its catalytic activities, and the connection between the two different immune-related functions as a deamidating and crosslinking enzyme and as an autoantigen.

6.3.1.2 HLA-DQ Heterodimers

HLA-DQ2 and -DQ8 alleles are the causative genes for CD (see Section 3.1). DQ2 and DQ8 heterodimers are HLA class II molecules that are expressed on the cellular surface of APCs (mature dendritic cells, macrophages, B cells). The complete amino acid sequences (without signaling peptides) of the α-chains corresponding to alleles A1*0501, 0505, 0201, and 03 and of the β-chains corresponding to alleles B1*0201, 0202, 0301, and 0302 are presented in Figure 1.14. As can be seen, the different proteins within each of the α- and β-chains show a high degree of sequence homology. The α-chains of DQ2 A1*0501 and 0505 are identical except for one amino acid residue in the signaling peptide (not shown).

The combined α- and β-chains bind immunogenic gluten peptides in a "peptide groove" and present them to T cells in the lamina propria (see below). Crystallography of HLA-DQ2.5 in a complex with the immunogenic deamidated gliadin peptide α57–68/E65 (QLQPFPQPELPY) gave an insight into the binding features within the peptide groove of the DQ2.5 molecule (A1*0501/B1*0201). The N-terminal domains of the heterodimer combine to form the groove: a five-turn α-helix from the α-chain runs parallel to a longer but kinked α-helix from the β-chain forming the side wall of the groove (Figure 1.15) [320]. Eleven residues of the peptide (L58–Y65) were clearly visible in the experimental electron density map. There are 13 hydrogen bonds between the main-chain atoms of the peptide and DQ2.5 and four hydrogen bonds between peptide side-chain amides and DQ2.5. The latter is remarkable, given that four of the nine core residues in this peptide are proline residues (P60, P62, P64, P67) that cannot engage in amide hydrogen bonding. The relative contribution of each main chain hydrogen bond interaction was studied by preparing a series of N-methylated peptide analogs [321]. The results demonstrated that hydrogen bonds at phenylalanine F61 and glutamine Q63 are most important for binding, whereas the hydrogen bonds at glutamic acid E65 and tyrosine Y68 make smaller contributions to the overall binding affinity.

The peptide binding specificities of HLA-DQ2.5 and -DQ2.2 are similar, but DQ2.2 seems to have an additional binding pocket at p3 with a preference for serine, threonine, and aspartic acid and with proline being disfavored at this position [322]. Moreover, the much higher disease risk of DQ2.5 compared to DQ2.2 (see Section 3.1) has been explained by the fact that DQ2.5 molecules bind immunogenic peptides much longer (for days) than DQ2.2 molecules (for hours) [36]. The substitution of phenylalanine in DQ2.2 by tyrosine in DQ2.5 at position α22 (Figure 1.14) obviously results in the improved ability of the DQ2.5 molecule to retain its peptide cargo for a longer time. Similarly to HLA-DQ2, the peptide-binding groove of HLA-DQ8 favors the binding of peptides with negatively charged residues. Functional binding studies suggested anchor positions p1 and p9 for glutamic acid and p4 for hydrophobic residues (Table 1.5). The crystallographic structure of HLA-DQ8 complexed with the gluten peptide QQYPSGEGSFQPSQENPQ confirmed the preference for negatively charged residues at binding anchor

(A) α-Chains

```
          1                                               50
0501/5    EDIVADHVASYGVNLYQSYGPSGQYTHEFDGDEQFYVDLGRKETVWCLPV
0201                              F        E     E      K  L
03                                 S       E     E      Q  L

          51                                              100
0501/5    LRQFRFDPQFALTNIAVLKHNLNSLIKRSNSTAATNEVPEVTVFSKSPVT
0201      FHRL                   I
03        F R *                  IV                            *RR

          101                                             150
0501/5    LGQPNILICLVDNIFPPVVNITWLSNGHSVTEGVSETSFLSKSDHSFFKI
0201           T
03             T
          151                                             200
0501/5    SYLTLLPSAEESYDCKVEHWGLDKPLLKHWEPEIPAPMSELTETVVCALG
0201          F    D I           E
03            F   SD I           E           T

          201                            231
0501/5    LSVGLVGIVVGTVFIIRGLRSVGASRHQGPL
0201                   L
03                     L
```

(B) β-Chains

```
          1                                               50
0201      RDSPEDFVYQFKGMCYFTNGTERVRLVSRSIYNREEIVRFDSDVGEFRAV
0202
0301                  A            Y T Y      YA      EVY
0302                                 T Y      YA       VY

          51                                              100
0201      TLLGLPAAEYWNSQKDILERKRAAVDRVCRHNYQLELRTTLQRRVEPTVT
0202
0301       P    D        EV   T  EL T
0302       P  P          EV   T  EL T

          101                                             150
0201      ISPSRTEALNHHNLLVCSVTDFYPAQIKVRWFRNDQEETAGVVSTPLIRN
0202                                        G
0301                                             T
0302                                             T

          151                                             200
0201      GDWTFQILVMLEMTPQRGDVYTCHVEHPSLQSPITVEWRAQSESAQSKML
0202
0301                      H              N
0302                                     N  I

          201                          229
0201      SGIGGFVLGLIFLGLGLIIHHRSQKGLLH
0202
0301
0302
```

■ **FIGURE 1.14** Amino acid sequences of (A) α- and (B) β-chains of human leukocyte antigen (HLA)-DQ2/DQ8 proteins (for designations, see Figure 1.4).

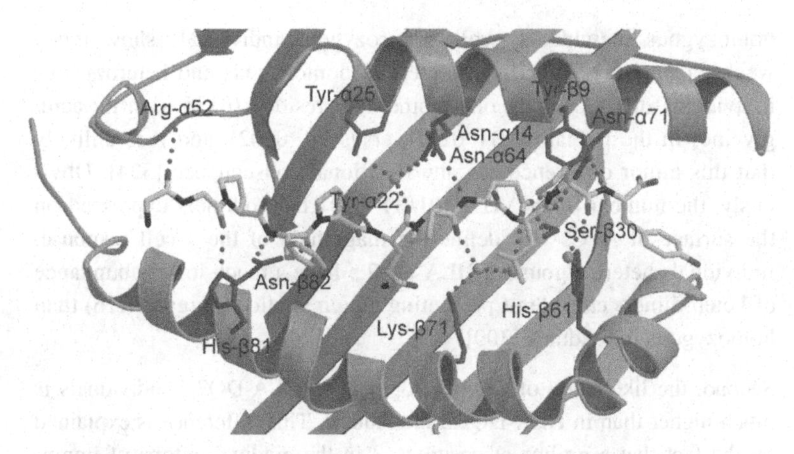

■ **FIGURE 1.15** Putative hydrogen-bonding network in the DQ2.5/peptide complex (shown as red dashes). Peptide α57–68/E65 is shown in yellow, α-chain in green, and β-chain in blue. *According to Ref. [320], copyright 2004 National Academy of Sciences, USA).* (Please see color plate at the back of the book.)

sites p1 and p9, whilst proline residues can be present in p3, p6, and p8 [323]. In contrast to DQ2 requiring only one glutamic acid residue, binding to DQ8 demands two glutamic acid residues. This restraint may explain the lower number of gluten peptides active in DQ8-positive patients as compared to DQ2-positive patients.

The DQ8 heterodimer (A1*03/B1*0302) has a strong structural similarity to the DQ2.5 heterodimer (Figure 1.14). Nevertheless, there are two noticeable differences in the backbone structure. First, the insertion of a second arginine residue (R) in position α56 of DQ8 influences the length of the α-helix stretch in this sequence region. Second, the β-chain of DQ2.5 has a positively charged lysine residue (L) at position β71, which is important for the binding of negatively charged glutamic acid of immunogenic peptides. DQ8 contains threonine (T) at β71 and has an overall neutral electrostatic potential in this region. Consistent with this difference, there are no data available indicating that the epitope α57–68/E65 is recognized by the DQ8 molecule [320].

A model for the correlation between the composition of the HLA-DQ heterodimers and the risk of CD development has been presented by Tjon and colleagues [38]. Accordingly, the level of gluten peptides presented by APCs to T cells critically influences CD development. First, HLA-DQ2.5 homozygous individuals have a fivefold higher risk of CD development than HLA-DQ2.5 heterozygous individuals. This correlates with the very strong T-cell response and IFN-γ production of HLA-DQ2.5

homozygous individuals, while heterozygous individuals show much weaker responses [35]. Heterodimers of homozygous and heterozygous individuals differ only by one amino acid residue (β135 aspartic acid/glycine) in the β-chains (B1*0201 versus B1*0202), and it is unlikely that this minor difference has any functional consequence [324]. Obviously, the number of the A1*0501/B1*0201 heterodimers expressed on the surface of APCs will define the magnitude of the T-cell response. Individuals heterozygous for HLA-DQ2.5 have a much lower abundance of heterodimers capable of presenting gluten peptides (Figure 1.16) than homozygous individuals [300].

Second, the likelihood of CD development in HLA-DQ2.5 individuals is much higher than in HLA-DQ2.2 individuals. This difference is explained by the fact that a proline at position p3 in the binding epitope of immunogenic peptides (Figure 1.17 [325]) has an adverse effect on binding to HLA-DQ2.2 (A1*0201/B1*0202). Consequently, HLA-DQ2.5 is able to present a much broader repertoire of gluten peptides than HLA-DQ2.2. In addition, HLA-DQ2.5 is better in retaining peptides in its binding groove. Third, CD is mainly associated with HLA-DQ2.5 and to a lesser extent with HLA-DQ8. In contrast to the HLA-DQ2.5-restricted peptides (Table 1.5), HLA-DQ8-restricted peptides may not be derived from proline-rich regions and are therefore probably susceptible to degradation in the gastrointestinal

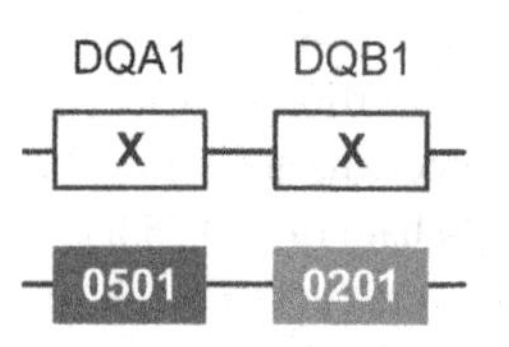

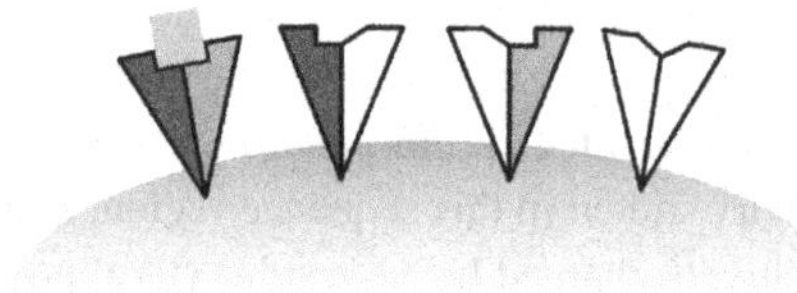

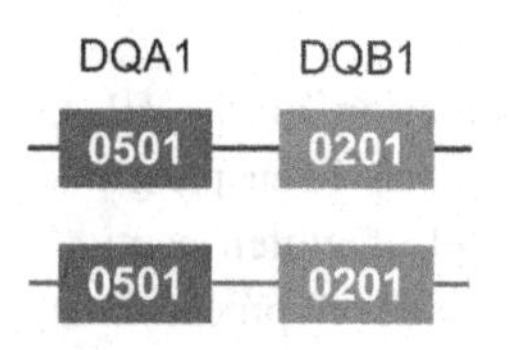

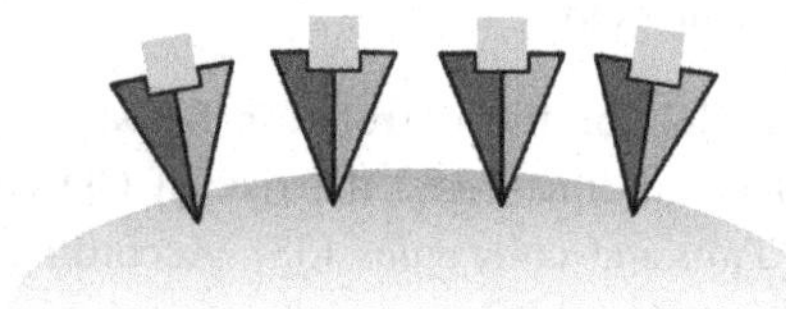

■ **FIGURE 1.16** Gluten peptide binding capacity of antigen-presenting cells heterozygous or homozygous for human leukocyte antigen (HLA)-DQ2. *Reprinted from Ref. [300], with permission from Elsevier.*

tract. Fourth, the fact that most CD patients tolerate oats provides further evidence that the level of gluten presentation is a critical parameter. Avenins contain only two immunogenic epitopes (Table 1.5), while dozens of epitopes are found in the gluten proteins of wheat, rye, and barley. In summary, these data indicate the presence of a threshold for the development of CD. For HLA-DQ2.5 homozygous individuals, the threshold is exceeded most easily, whereas for HLA-DQ2.2 and HLA-DQ8 individuals the threshold is much higher.

6.3.1.3 Cellular Response

Gluten peptides that have passed the enterocyte layer (see Section 6.2) and arrive at the lamina propria are preferred as substrates for extracellular TG2. Where and when deamidation and transamidation take place is still in question. The ratio of deamidation to transamidation has been estimated to be around 1:3 [160]. Released into the extracellular matrix, TG2 usually remains catalytically active only for a short period of time and soon becomes silenced through oxidation. Cys 230, Cys 370, and Cys 371 involved in this inactivation form disulfide bonds linked from Cys 370 either to Cys 230 or to the neighboring Cys 371 [326]. However, a high Ca^{2+} level and an increased reductive environment caused by an ongoing immune response can protect TG2 against inactivation. Another explanation for the presence of extracellular TG2 has been proposed by the group of Tjon [38]. Even if the affinity of native (nondeamidated) gluten peptides to HLA-DQ molecules is weak, their presentation to $CD4^+$ T cells will lead to the production of IFN-γ. The following low-grade inflammation might lead to tissue damage with TG2 release, which enhances the adaptive immune response by deamidation.

Native and deamidated gluten peptides that appear in the lamina propria are selectively bound to the HLA-DQ2/8 molecules expressed on the surface

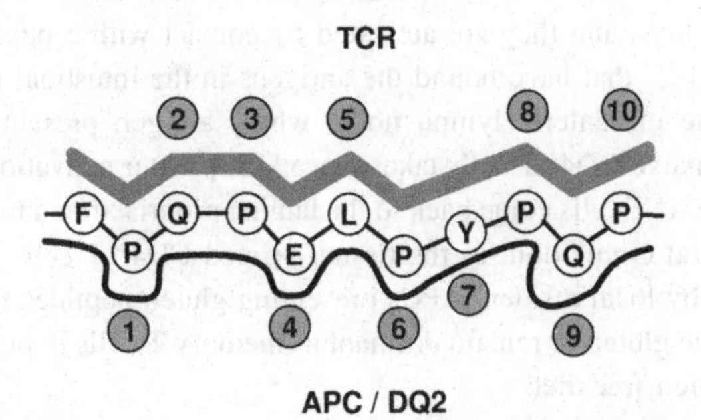

■ **FIGURE 1.17** Binding sites of antigen-presenting cell (APC/DQ2) and T-cell receptor (TCR) for epitope P62–P71 of α2-gliadin (DQ2.5-glia α2; see Table 1.5). *Adapted from Ref.[325].*

of APCs, mainly dendritic cells but also macrophages and B cells (step 4 in Figure 1.10). This provides an explanation for the well-established association between these genetically determined HLA molecules and disease development. DQ2 and DQ8 heterodimers bind the gluten peptides in their peptide grooves and present them to T cells in the lamina propria. Gluten peptides of variable length are bound, usually with nine amino acid residues (p1–p9) and flanked by one or more additional residues, and preferably with a left-handed poly-Pro II helical conformation [327]. Key anchor points in the groove of HLA-DQ2 are at positions p1, p4, p6, p7 and p9 (Figure 1.17). As described before, crystallography of HLA-DQ2.5 complexed with the immunogenic deamidated gliadin peptide α57–68/E65 (QLQPFPQPELPY) demonstrated the presence of an intricate hydrogen-bonding network between the two molecules (Figure 1.15) [320]. The deamidated form of the peptide (E65) had a 25-fold higher affinity compared with the nondeamidated counterpart (Q65). Obviously, the lysine residue at β71 of HLA-DQ2.5 creates a unique positive electrostatic region between the p4 and p6/p7 anchor positions, so that binding of negatively charged glutamic acid residues is favored at these positions.

After binding gluten peptides (native, deamidated, crosslinked with TG2) to the peptide groove of HLA-DQ2/8 molecules on the surface of APCs, the compounds are presented to $CD4^+$ T cells (step 4 in Figure 1.10). T cells assist other white blood cells in immunologic processes, including maturation of B cells into plasma cells and memory cells, and activation of cytotoxic T cells and macrophages. Their response must achieve a certain threshold to be pathogenic, that is, to induce tissue damage (see below). TCRs, heterodimeric proteins membrane-bound to T cells, are responsible for recognizing antigens presented by HLA-DQ2/8. They mostly consist of disulfide-linked α- and β-chains, whereas a minority consists of γ- and δ-chains. TCRs possess unique antigen specificities determined by the structures of the antigen-binding site formed by the α- and β-chains, and they are activated by contact with a peptide/MHC complex. APCs that have bound the antigens in the intestinal tissue can travel to the mesenteric lymph node, where antigen presentation and priming of naïve $CD4^+$ T cells takes place [123]. After activation, gluten-sensitive $CD4^+$ T cells come back to the lamina propria after a brief transit in the general circulation. In the tissue, primed $CD4^+$ T cells are either reactivated by local resident APCs presenting gluten peptides in patients that consume gluten or remain dormant as memory T cells in patients that are on a gluten-free diet.

In 1993, Lundin and colleagues first described the presence of gluten-sensitive T cells in small intestinal biopsies of CD patients [328]. A large number of studies have since established that such T cells can be specific for a large number of peptides derived from gluten, which can differ from patient to patient. Gluten-sensitive $CD4^+$ T cells can be readily isolated from the biopsy specimens of CD patients after in vitro challenge but not from controls [329]. It is, however, difficult to estimate the exact prevalence of gluten-sensitive T cells in the lamina propria due to the lack of specific techniques to visualize and quantify these antigen-specific cells directly. By cloning $CD4^+$ T cells directly from intestinal biopsies of CD patients, Bodd and colleagues found that 0.5–1.8% of $CD4^+$ T cells were gluten-sensitive [330]. About half of these cells were specific for either the immunogenic DQ2.5-glia-α1a or DQ2.5-glia-α2 epitopes. Assessed by flow cytometry, tetramer-positive T cells were present in all 10 untreated CD patients investigated with a frequency of 0.1–1.2% of gluten-sensitive $CD4^+$ T cells. Gluten-sensitive T cells were also detectable in most treated CD patients (7/10). The frequency of gluten-sensitive T cells correlated with the degree of histological damage in the intestinal mucosa and also with IgA TGA levels. The infiltration of T cells in the lamina propria is dominated by $CD4^+$ memory T cells ($CD45R0^+$) bearing the α/β TCR. The minimum length of peptides required for T-cell recognition is nine amino acid residues [324]. Large peptides that contain multiple HLA-DQ2/8 binding epitopes such as the 33-mer peptide have greater T-cell stimulatory activity than small peptides containing only a single binding sequence [273]. Deamidation of glutamine by TG2 is not an absolute requirement for T-cell activation, in particular, early in the CD of children [331]. However, deamidation by TG2 not only increases the level of the DQ2/8-gluten peptide complex, but also directly participates in the selection of the gluten-reactive TCR repertoire in vivo [123].

A common feature among immunogenic epitopes of gluten peptides that activate gluten-sensitive T cells is the presence of multiple glutamine and proline residues (Table 1.5). However, numerous studies with modified peptides have revealed that other amino acid residues also have a strong influence on the stimulatory effect. A well-documented example is the sequence region 56–75 of α-gliadins, one of the most frequently studied epitopes presented by HLA-DQ2 after deamidation of glutamine in position 65 (Q65→E65). The sequence PQPELPYPQPQLPY (α62–75/E65) was modified by alanine at each position except E65 and tested by T-cell stimulation [332]. The results demonstrated that substitution of Q72, L73, P74 or Y75 had no effect on the stimulation index, whereas all the other substitutions abolished activity (Figure 1.18). This showed that each of the residues of the sequence PQPELPYPQP contributed to T-cell stimulation. The authors postulated that Q63, P64, L66, P69, and P71 (anchor positions p2, p3, p5, p8, and p10) may all interact with the TCR and the others are key residues for DQ2 binding (Figure 1.17).

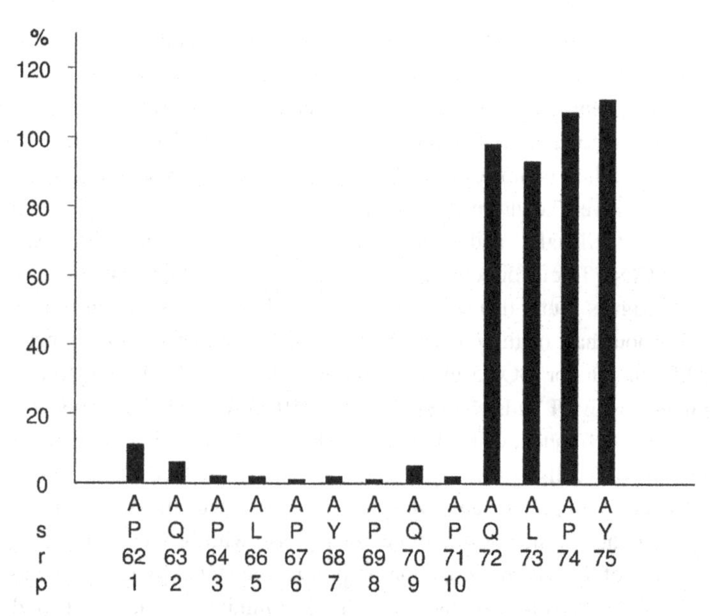

■ **FIGURE 1.18** Response of T-cell clones to alanine-substitutes of DQ2-restricted gliadin peptide α62–75/E65 (nonsubstituted peptide = 100%); s = amino acid sequence; r = position of amino acid residue in the protein sequence; p = anchor positions of the residue (Table 1.5). *Reprinted from Ref. [302].*

The HLA-DQ8-restricted epitope identified in HMW-GS 1Dx2 was shown to have a minimum core region of residues 723–735 (QQGYYPTSPQQSG) (Figure 1.19) and it did not require deamidation for T-cell stimulation [333]. Residues Q724 and Q732 were expected to occupy the anchor positions p1 and p9, respectively, within the DQ8/TCR complex. To identify the residues that contribute to T-cell stimulation, a series of substitution analogs was tested [334]. Any substitution of G725 at p2, Y727 at p4, P728 at p5, and P731 at p8 abrogated T-cell recognition. The critical role of P728 and P731 probably reflects the maintenance of the correct conformation of the peptide in the binding groove. In contrast, substitutions are accepted at p3 (Y726), p6 (T729), and p7 (S730). Substitutions of Q724 at p1, Q733, or S734 had little effect; substitution of Q732 at p9 by alanine (A) or asparagine (N) reduced T-cell stimulation significantly, whereas substitution of Q732 by charged residues such as lysine (K) or glutamic acid (E) abolished stimulation.

Within the adaptive immune system, T cells activated by gluten peptides elicit two different responses, the proinflammatory Th1 response damaging the epithelium and the anti-inflammatory Th2 response promoting B cells to produce antibodies (steps 5 and 6, respectively, in Figure 1.10). The detailed

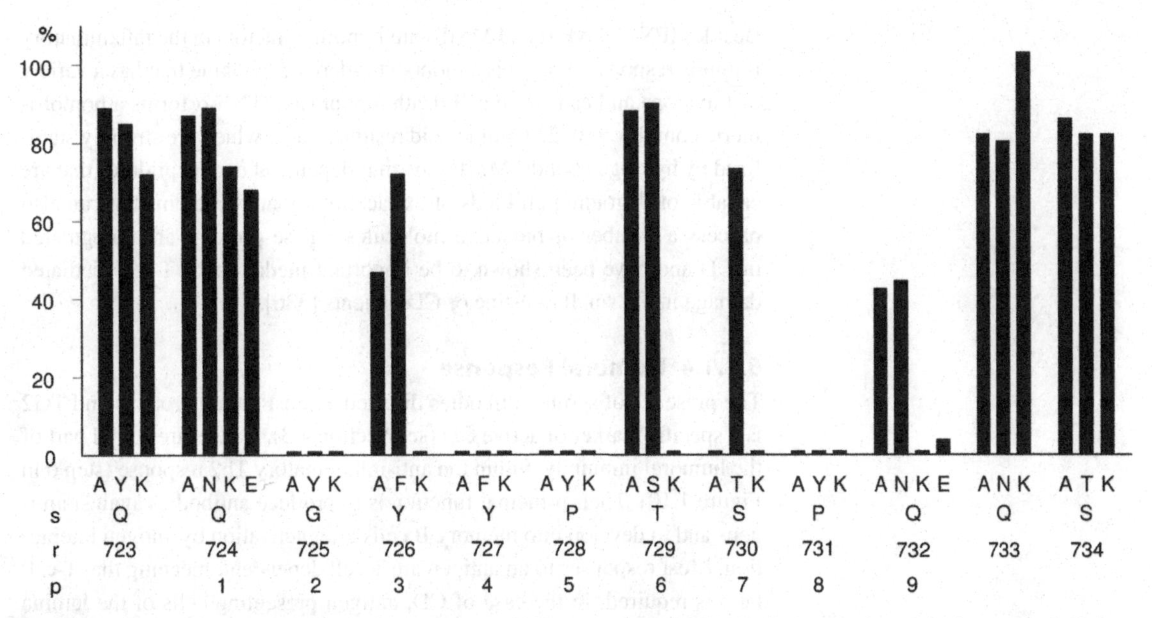

■ FIGURE 1.19 Response of T-cell clones to different substitutes of DQ8-restricted peptide 723-734 of high-molecular-weight glutenin subunit 1Dx2 (nonsubstituted peptide = 100%; s, r, p; see Figure 1.18). *Reprinted from Ref. [302].*

mechanism by which gluten-sensitive T cells exert their cytotoxic effect on the intestinal epithelium is still unclear. $CD4^+$ T cells in the lamina propria become activated upon recognition of gluten peptides and produce many different cytokines and chemokines, such as IFN-γ, IL-4, IL-21, TNF-α, and matrix metalloproteinases (MMPs) (step 5 in Figure 1.10).

The production of IFN-γ is considered to play a key role in the downstream initiation of mucosal damage. IFN-γ is a dimerized soluble cytokine and the only member of the type II class of interferons. The monomer consists of a core of six α-helices and an extended unfolded sequence in the C-terminal region. IFN-γ participates in innate and adaptive immunity against viral and bacterial infections and is an important activator of macrophages. A number of autoinflammatory and autoimmune diseases are associated with aberrant IFN-γ expression. IFN-γ and IL-18, which mediates the synthesis of IFN-γ, are produced in high amounts by gluten-sensitive T cells upon stimulation with gluten peptides and are associated with increased epithelial permeability [335]. Additionally, IFN-γ initiates a higher expression of the HLA-DQ molecules and thereby an increased peptide presentation, which leads to self-amplifying loops of the adaptive immune response [38]. Neutralization of IFN-γ has been shown to prevent gluten-induced mucosal damage, at least in biopsies of CD mucosa maintained in organ culture [336].

Besides IFN-γ, TNF-α and MMPs are important factors in the inflammatory immune response. TNF-α is a monocytic-derived cytokine that has a variety of functions and can cause cell death (apoptosis). TNF-α forms a homotrimeric complex with 233 amino acid residues each, which are strongly stabilized by hydrogen bonds. MMPs are zinc-dependent endopeptidases that are capable of degrading all kinds of extracellular matrix proteins but can also process a number of bioactive molecules. These proteins are upregulated in CD and have been shown to be important mediators of T-cell mediated damage in the small intestine of CD patients [336].

6.3.1.4 Humoral Response

The presence of serum antibodies directed against gluten proteins and TG2 is a specific marker of active CD (see Section 4.3). B cells are a vital part of the humoral immunity within the anti-inflammatory Th2 response (step 6 in Figure 1.10). Their principal function is to produce antibodies against antigens and to develop into memory B cells after activation by antigen interaction. Most responses to an antigen are T-cell dependent, meaning that T-cell help is required. In the case of CD, antigen-presenting cells of the lamina propria present gluten peptides (native or deamidated) to gluten-sensitive T cells, priming them. When B cells present the same antigen to primed helper T cells, T cells release cytokines that help B cells multiply and mature into plasma cells that produce IgA and IgG serum antibodies to gluten proteins and peptides.

Because no TG2-specific T cells providing help to B cells have been found so far, the mechanism of the gluten-dependent production of antibodies against TG2 has not been fully understood. A hypothetical model explaining TG2-antibody formation has been proposed based on the fact that TG2 can crosslink itself to gluten peptides, which then can act as "hapten-carrier-like" complexes (Figure 1.20) [123,300]. Such conjugates could be taken up by TG2-specific B-cell receptors. After intracellular degradation, gluten peptides can be released in endosomes and presented to gluten-sensitive T cells in the context of HLA-DQ2/8 heterodimers. These T cells, in turn, would provide the necessary help for B cells, which differentiate into plasma cells and start secreting TG2-specific autoantibodies. Plasma cells producing TG2-specific antibodies can be visualized in CD lesions and isolated using labeled TG2 antigens [337]. On average, 10% of plasma cells are TG2-specific cells and most produce IgA. This model fits with the observation that the level of TGAs decreases, when patients are treated with a gluten-free diet. In the absence of gluten, gluten-sensitive T cells are not stimulated, so that they cannot provide help to B cells and the antibody production stops [338]. Moreover, the clinical observation of the strict HLA-dependent appearance of TG2-specific antibodies supports

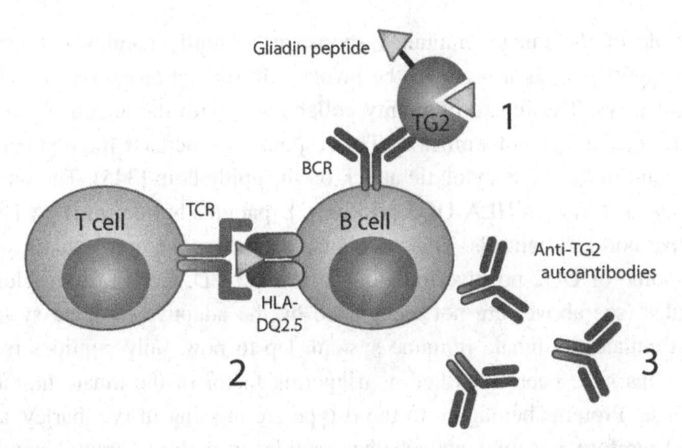

■ **FIGURE 1.20** Model explaining anti-TG2 antibody (TGA) formation. (1) Tissue transglutaminase (TG2)/peptide complex is bound to TG2-specific B-cell receptors (BCR); (2) help from T cells via presentation of peptides to the T-cell receptor (TCR); (3) secretion of TG2-specific autoantibodies after B-cell differentiation into plasma cells. *From Qiao et al. [123], with kind permission from Springer Science and Business Media.* (Please see color plate at the back of the book.)

this model [339]. Although this model has not been formally demonstrated in vivo, di Niro et al. provided in vitro evidence that TG2-specific B-cells can indeed present gluten peptides to gluten-sensitive T cells when offered TG2-gluten peptide conjugates [337]. An alternative hypothesis is that mucosal dendritic cells may also present TG2 to autoreactive TG2-specific T cells that escaped negative selection in the thymus [308]. These TG2-specific T cells could provide direct help to TG2-specific B cells for the production of TGAs. The preliminary demonstration of the existence of TG2-specific HLA-DQ2-restricted T-cell clones from peripheral blood of CD patients seems to confirm this second model, thus suggesting the role of TG2 as T-cell autoantigen.

6.3.2 Innate Response

In the 1980s, CD-toxic peptides were isolated from enzymatic digests of total gliadin [270,340] and A-gliadin [271] for the first time. They were derived from the N-terminal sequences of α-gliadins (α3–55, α3–24, α25–55, α1–30, α31–55) and showed significant toxic effects in organ culture assays (see Chapter 2, Section 3.5). Later on, the toxicity of peptides α31–43, α31–49 and α44–55 was confirmed in vivo by instillation tests [341,342]. However, five overlapping peptides from the N-terminal sequences of α-gliadins (1–19, 11–28, 21–40, 31–49) showed only weak or moderate binding to HLA-DQ2 heterodimers, and no gliadin-sensitive DQ2-restricted T cells recognize these peptides [343]. Maiuri et al. were the first to suggest that these peptides might induce an innate response in CD [344].

The role of the innate immune response is currently gaining extraordinary importance, as it seems to be involved in the pathogenesis of CD in several ways. The innate immunity collaborates with the adaptive immunity to induce a proinflammatory Th1 response, to increase the number of IELs, and to favor the cytolytic attack on the epithelium [345]. The innate response is found in HLA-DQ2 positive CD patients but not in HLA-DQ2 positive non-CD controls. This peculiar innate response may explain why only some of DQ2-positive individuals develop CD. Certain toxic gluten peptides (see above) are not recognized by the adaptive immune system but stimulate the innate immune system. Up to now, only peptides from α-gliadins have been identified as triggering factor of the innate immune response. Proteins belonging to the α-type are missing in rye, barley, and oats. Therefore, it is unknown whether peptides from these cereals can initiate an innate response.

The fact that peptides such as α31–49 activate the innate response implies that a receptor for these peptides should exist. A transcellular transport pathway was proposed where AGAs were able to bind peptide α31–49 [285] (see Section 6.2). This complex would then bind the transferrin receptor CD71, which would provide protected trafficking across the intestinal epithelium. Tjon et al. [38] also assessed the hypothesis that a receptor for peptide α31–49 should be present on intestinal epithelial cells. However, this receptor could not be detected, neither directly nor by either UV-crosslinking or TG2-induced transamidation. In conclusion, robust data demonstrating a direct signaling effect of gliadin peptides on enterocytes are still missing and more work is needed to delineate the mechanism of action of the so-called toxic peptides [293].

An increase in IELs is one of the main features of CD. IELs are phenotypically and functionally different from the lamina propria $CD4^+$ gluten-sensitive T cells. They represent an abundant and heterogenous population of T cells that reside between the intestinal epithelial cells at the basolateral side of the epithelium [299,346]. Their main role is to promote immune protection by preventing the entry and spread of pathogens while avoiding unwanted and excessive inflammatory reactions capable of damaging the intestinal epithelium. They exert both cytolytic functions to eliminate infected and damaged cells and regulatory functions that contribute to epithelium healing and repair. However, they also contribute to inflammatory and tissue destructive reactions such as those seen in CD. IELs are composed of the antigen-experienced memory-effector T-cell subtype $CD8^+$ bearing the αβ or the γδ TCR ($TCR\alpha\beta^+$ or $TCR\gamma\delta^+$) and natural killer (NK) cells [346]. The IEL population of the normal intestine consists of $TCR\alpha\beta^+$ T cells and $TCR\gamma\delta^+$ T cells in a ratio of around 5:1.

The contribution of IELs to villous atrophy in CD has been suggested by several studies and is based on the following facts [299]:

1. $CD8^+$ IELs are the main producers of IFN-γ in active CD;
2. $CD8^+$ IELs are enriched in cytolytic proteins (perforin, granzymes, FasL);
3. expression of the latter proteins is associated with increased epithelial apoptosis.

The epithelial infiltration is highly correlated with gluten ingestion and therefore is considered to be the most sensitive histopathological marker of CD [346]. A count of 20–25 IELs per 100 enterocytes is estimated to be the borderline between normal and CD-damaged biopsies, with values above 30 representing "pathologic intraepithelial lymphocytosis". The distribution of IELs along the villi, particularly at the villous tip, also represents a sensitive morphological feature for the diagnosis of CD. The numbers of $TCR\alpha\beta^+$ IELs return to normal after a gluten-free diet is initiated. In contrast, the numbers of $TCR\gamma\delta^+$ IELs remain high for many years afterwards, indicating that $TCR\alpha\beta^+$ but not $TCR\gamma\delta^+$ IELs can be linked to villous atrophy. The exact role played by $TCR\gamma\delta^+$ IELs in the epithelium of CD patients is still under debate. Baghat and colleagues proposed that $TCR\alpha\beta^+$ IELs have a damaging effect on enterocytes that can be antagonized by $TCR\gamma\delta^+$ IELs [347]. This regulatory function may be overwhelmed in active CD. Whether $TCR\gamma\delta^+$ IEL subsets of CD patients are antigen-driven and what the exact nature of the antigen recognized is have yet to be elucidated. Most IELs express a variety of NK cell receptors. In the healthy small intestine, IELs predominantly express the inhibitory CD94/NKG2A receptor. In contrast, IELs in CD express high levels of activating receptors like CD94/NKG2C and NKG2D [346].

The cytokine IL-15 has been considered to be a central player in this part of the gluten-induced immune response. IL-15, a proinflammatory and anti-apoptotic cytokine, is produced in excess in the intestines of CD patients. The use of organ culture of small intestinal biopsies revealed that neutralization of this cytokine might indeed hamper the CD pathogenesis cascade [344]. IL-15, a glycoprotein with a molecular weight of ≈14,000, is expressed by a large number of cell types and tissues and plays an important role in both innate and adaptive immunity. In particular, it regulates the stimulation and proliferation of T cells and NK cells. In active CD, IL-15 is produced both by epithelial and lamina propria cells but not by T cells and B cells involved in the adaptive immune response. Gluten peptides such as α31–43 or the elongated form α31–49 induce IL-15 secretion directly by the activation of enterocytes [348], macrophages [349], and dendritic cells [350,351]. These peptides do not stimulate HLA-DQ-restricted T cells and activate IL-15 production only in CD patients but not in healthy controls. IL-15 impairs the beneficial suppressor capacity of Tregs and, in the presence of IL-15, retinoic acid (a metabolite of vitamin A) has unexpected coadjuvant properties that induce inflammatory immunity (IL-12 and IL-23) to gliadin in the intestinal mucosa [352]. For this reason, the use of vitamin A supplementation in CD is disapproved.

IL-15 is known to be a potent inducer of the proliferation and survival of IELs. The majority of IL-15 remains bound to the surface of enterocytes, where it can be presented to IELs. IL-15 stimulates IELs to express NKG2D receptors and epithelial cells to express MHC class I chain-related molecule A (MICA), the epithelial ligand of NKG2D [353,354]. Upon engagement of NKG2D receptors with MICA, IELs kill epithelial cells and contribute to tissue destruction. Thus, expression of IL-15 in intestinal epithelial cells entails cell apoptosis, villous atrophy, and intestinal inflammation [355]. It is easy to envisage that the damaged epithelium will not function properly as a selective barrier, so that immunogenic gluten peptides could gain access to the tissue. These findings raise the question of whether the expression of IL-15 would suffice in itself to induce villous atrophy and crypt hyperplasia [120].

It has been suggested that ATIs, present in cereal grains, are coactivators of the innate immune system [162]. ATIs CM3 and O.19, both pest resistance molecules in wheat, were identified as strong activators of the innate immune response in monocytes, macrophages, and dendritic cells. These cells express Toll-like receptors (TLRs), a class of highly conserved membrane-bound molecules, which have a principal role in the recognition of microorganisms and thus act in the first line of defense. ATIs engage the TLR4-MD2-CD14 complex, lead to upregulation of maturation markers, and elicit the release of proinflammatory cytokines in cells from CD and non-CD patients and in CD patients' biopsies. Mice deficient in TLR4 or TLR4 signaling are protected from intestinal and systemic immune responses upon oral challenge with ATIs. These findings define cereal ATIs as novel contributors to CD. Moreover, ATIs may fuel inflammation and immune reactions in other intestinal and nonintestinal immune disorders.

6.4 Concluding Remarks

The improved understanding of different immunological mechanisms allows the creation of a realistic scheme of CD pathogenesis [356]. The key environmental factors in mediating CD are gluten proteins from wheat, rye, barley, and oats. Incomplete gastrointestinal degradation of these proteins leads to the appearance of CD-active (immunogenic, toxic) gluten peptides in the small intestinal lumen. These peptides, rich in glutamine and proline, induce a two-signal immune response, with the first signal being generated by the innate immunity and the second one by the adaptive immunity [357]. Toxic peptides evoke an innate immune response characterized by increased IL-15 expression, IEL proliferation, inflammation of epithelial cells, and increased intestinal permeability. In the adaptive immune response, immunogenic peptides cross the epithelial barrier due to increased permeability and opened tight junctions. After reaching the lamina propria, they are deamidated or crosslinked by TG2. Binding of these modified peptides to HLA-DQ2/8 on APCs and their presentation to gluten-sensitive T cells activates the proinflammatory Th1 response. This response is characterized by the production of different cytokines such as IFN-γ and TNF-α and other immunological molecules, which contribute to the damage to epithelial cells. Both innate and adaptive immune responses result in epithelial apoptosis and mucosal destruction and contribute to the development of intestinal inflammation in CD. In addition, stimulated T cells activate the anti-inflammatory Th2 response by means of B cells that initiate the production of antibodies against gluten and autoantibodies against TG2. While the interplay between genetics and gluten in the induction of the adaptive response is now well understood, further studies are needed to delineate the respective contributions of genetics and environmental factors, particularly gluten peptides, in the induction of the innate response and IL-15 synthesis [346]. How the crosstalk between adaptive and innate immunities is orchestrated is an outstanding question that will need to be addressed to better understand the different stages of CD and gluten sensitivity, design preventive strategies, and develop new therapeutic approaches [299]. Further studies may be expected to elucidate the exact mechanism between innate and adaptive immunity in CD.

REFERENCES

[1] Feldman M, Sears ER. The wild gene resources of wheat. Sci Am 1981:98–109.

[2] Gasbarrini G, Miele L, Corazza GR, Gasbarrini A. When was celiac disease born? The Italian case from the archeological site of Cosa. J Clin Gastroenterol 2010;44:502–3.

[3] Gasbarrini G, Rickards O, Martínez-Labarga C, Pacciani E, Chilleri F, Laterza L, et al. Origin of celiac disease: how old are predisposing haplotypes? World J Gastroenterol 2012;18:5003–4.

[4] Gee S. On the coeliac affection. St Bart's Hosp Rep 1888;24:17–20.

[5] Losowsky MS. A history of coeliac disease. Dig Dis 2008;26:112–20.

[6] Dicke WK. Investigation of the harmful effects of certain types of cereals on patients with coeliac disease [Ph.D. thesis]. University of Utrecht; 1950.

[7] Anderson CM, French JM, Sammons HG, Frazer AC, Gerrard JW, Smellie JM. Coeliac disease; gastrointestinal studies and the effect of dietary wheat flour. Lancet 1952;1:836–42.

[8] Dicke WK, Weijers HA, van de Kamer JH. Coeliac disease. II. The presence in wheat of a factor having a deleterious effect in cases of coeliac disease. Acta Paediatr 1953;42:34–42.
[9] van de Kamer JH, Weijers HA, Dicke WK. Celiac disease. IV. An investigation into the injurious constituents of wheat in connection with celiac disease. Acta Paediatr 1953;42:223–31.
[10] Paulley JW. Observations of the aetiology of idiopathic steatorrhoea; jejunal and lymph-node biopsies. Br Med J 1954;2:1318–21.
[11] Shiner M. Duodenal biopsy. Lancet 1956;270:17–9.
[12] Crosby WH, Kugler HW. Intraluminal biopsy of the small intestine; the intestinal biopsy capsule. Am J Dig Dis 1957;2:336–41.
[13] Davidson LSP, Fountain JR. Incidence of the sprue syndrome; with some observation on the natural history. Br Med J 1950;1:1157–61.
[14] McCarthy CF. Coeliac disease: its Irish dimensions. Ir J Med Sci 1975;144:1–13.
[15] Greco L, Maeki M, di Donato F, Visakorpi JK. Epidemiology of coeliac disease in Europe and the mediterranean area. In: Auricchio S, Visakorpi JK, editors. Common food intolerances 1: epidemiology of coeliac disease. Basel (Switzerland): Karger; 1992. pp. 25–44.
[16] Logan RAF. Problems and pitfalls in epidemiological studies on coeliac disease. In: Auricchio S, Visakorpi JK, editors. Commmon food intolerances 1: epidemiology of coeliac disease. Basel (Switzerland): Karger; 1992. pp. 14–24.
[17] Feighery C. Fortnightly review: coeliac disease. Br Med J 1999;319:236–9.
[18] Biagi F, Trotta L, Alfano C, Balduzzi D, Staffieri V, Bianchi PI, et al. Prevalence and natural history of potential celiac disease in adult patients. Scand J Gastroenterol 2013;48:537–42.
[19] Tanpowpong P, Broder-Fingert S, Katz AJ, Camargo Jr CA. Characteristics of children with positive coeliac serology and normal villous morphology: potential coeliac disease. Acta Pathol Microbiol Immunol Scand 2013;121:266–71.
[20] Mustalahti K, Catassi C, Reunanen A, Fabiani E, Heier M, McMillan S, et al. The prevalence of celiac disease in Europe: results of a centralized, international mass screening project. Ann Med 2010;42:587–95.
[21] Schuppan D, Junker Y, Barisani D. Celiac disease: from pathogenesis to novel therapies. Gastroenterology 2009;137:1912–33.
[22] Catassi C, Ratsch IM, Gandolfi L, Pratesi R, Fabiani E, El Asmar R, et al. Why is coeliac disease endemic in the people of the Sahara? Lancet 1999;354:647–8.
[23] Ludvigsson JF, Rubio-Tapia A, van Dyke CT, Melton III LJ, Zinsmeister AR, Lahr BD, et al. Increasing incidence of celiac disease in a North American population. Am J Gastroenterol 2013;108:818–24.
[24] Lohi S, Mustalahti K, Kaukinen K, Laurila K, Collin P, Rissanen H, et al. Increasing prevalence of coeliac disease overtime. Aliment Pharmacol Ther 2007;26:1217–25.
[25] van den Broeck HC, de Jong HC, Salentijn EMJ, Dekking L, Bosch D, Hamer RJ, et al. Presence of celiac disease epitopes in modern and old hexaploid wheat varieties: wheat breeding may have contributed to increased prevalence of celiac disease. Theor Appl Genet 2010;121:1527–39.
[26] Kasarda DD. Can an increase in celiac disease be attributed to an increase in the gluten content of wheat as a consequence of wheat breeding? J Agric Food Chem 2013;61:1155–9.

[27] Biagi F, Klersy C, Balduzzi D, Corazza GR. Are we over-estimating the prevalence of coeliac disease in the general population? Ann Med 2010;42:557–61.
[28] Goddard CJR, Gillett HR. Complications of coeliac disease: are all patients at risk? Postgrad Med J 2006;82:705–12.
[29] Megiorni F, Mora B, Bonamico M, Barbato M, Montuori M, Viola F, et al. HLA-DQ and susceptibility to celiac disease: evidence for gender differences and parent-of-origin in effects. Am J Gastroenterol 2008;103:997–1003.
[30] Abadie V, Sollid LM, Barreiro LB, Jabri B. Integration of genetic and immunological insights into a model of celiac disease pathogensis. Annu Rev Immunol 2011:29493–525.
[31] Falchuk ZM, Rogentine GN, Strober W. Predominance of histocompatibility antigen HL-A8 in patients with gluten-sensitive enteropathy. J Clin Invest 1972;51:1602–5.
[32] Stokes PL, Asquith P, Holmes GK, Mackintosh P, Cooke WT. Histocompatibility antigens associated with adult coeliac disease. Lancet 1972;2:162–4.
[33] Kooy-Winkelaar Y, van Lummel M, Moustakas AK, Schweizer J, Mearin ML, Mulder CJ, et al. Gluten-specific T cells cross-react between HLA-DQ8 and the HLA-DQ2α/DQ8β transdimer. J Immunol 2011;187:5123–9.
[34] Karell K, Louka AS, Moodie SJ, Ascher H, Clot F, Greco L, et al. HLA types in celiac disease patients not carrying the DQA1*05-DQB1*02 (DQ2) heterodimer: results from the European genetics cluster on celiac disease. Hum Immunol 2003;64:469–77.
[35] Vader W, Stepniak D, Kooy Y, Mearin L, Thompson A, van Rood JJ, et al. The HLA-DQ2 gene dose effect in celiac disease is directly related to the magnitude and breadth of gluten-specific T-cell responses. Proc Natl Acad Sci USA 2003;100:12390–5.
[36] Fallang LE, Bergseng E, Hotta K, Berg-Larsen A, Kim CY, Sollid LM. Differences in the risk of celiac disease associated with HLA-DQ2.5 or HLA-DQ2.2 are related to sustained gluten antigen presentation. Nat Immunol 2009;10:1096–101.
[37] Fabris A, Segat L, Catamo E, Morgutti M, Vendramin A, Crovella S. HLA-G . 14bp deletion/insertion polymorphism in celiac disease. Am J Gastroenterol 2011;106: 139–44.
[38] Tjon JML, Bergen J, Koning F. Celiac disease: how complicated can it get? Immunogenetics 2010;62:641–51.
[39] Hunt KA, Zhernakova A, Turner G, Heap GAR, Franke L, Bruinenberg M, et al. Newly identified genetic risk variants for celiac disease related to the immune response. Nat Genet 2008;40:395–402.
[40] Trynka G, Wijmenga C, van Heel DA. A genetic perspective on coeliac disease. Trends Mol Med 2010;16:537–50.
[41] Gutierrez-Achury J, Coutinho de Almeida R, Wijmenga C. Shared genetics in coeliac disease and other immune-mediated diseases. J Intern Med 2011;269:591–603.
[42] Cotsapas C, Voight BF, Rossin E, Lage K, Neale BM, Wallace C, et al. Pervasive sharing of genetic effects in autoimmune disease. PLoS Genet 2011;7:e1002254.
[43] Kumar V, Wijmenga C, Withoff S. From genome-wide association studies to disease mechanisms: celiac disease as a model for autoimmune diseases. Semin Immunopathol 2012;34:567–80.
[44] Ivarsson A, Myleus A, Wall S. Towards preventing celiac disease – an epidemiological approach. In: Fasano A, Troncone R, Branski D, editors. Frontiers in celiac disease. Basel (Switzerland): Pediatric and Adolescence Medicine; 2008. pp. 198–209.

[45] Stene LC, Honeyman MC, Hoffenberg EJ, Haas JE, Sokol RJ, Emery L, et al. Rotavirus infection frequency and risk of celiac disease autoimmunity in early childhood: a longitudinal study. Am J Gastroenterol 2006;101:2333–40.
[46] Meresse B, Ripoche J, Heyman M, Cerf-Bensussan N. Celiac disease: from oral tolerance to intestinal inflammation, autoimmunty and lymphomagenesis. Mucosal Immunol 2009;2:8–23.
[47] Ivarsson A, Hernell O, Nystrom L, Persson LA. Children born in the summer have increased risk for coeliac disease. J Epidemiol Community Health 2003;57:36–9.
[48] Lebwohl B, Green PHR, Murray JA, Ludvigsson JF. Season of birth in a nationwide cohort of coeliac disease patients. Arch Dis Child 2013;98:48–51.
[49] Tanpowpong P, Obuch JC, Jiang H, McCarty CE, Katz AJ, Leffler DA, et al. Multicenter study on season of birth and celiac disease: evidence for a new theoretical model of pathogenesis. J Pediatr 2013;162:501–4.
[50] Collado MC, Donat E, Ribes-Koninckx C, Calabuig M, Sanz Y. Specific duodenal and faecal bacterial groups associated with paediatric coeliac disease. J Clin Pathol 2009;62:264–9.
[51] Hooper LV, Littman DR, MacPherson AJ. Interactions between the microbiota and the immune system. Science 2012;336:1268–73.
[52] Maynard CL, Elson CO, Hatton RD, Weaver CT. Reciprocal interactions of the intestinal microbiota and immune system. Nature 2012;489:231–41.
[53] de Palma G, Nadal I, Medina M, Donat E, Ribes-Koninckx C, Calabuig M, et al. Intestinal dysbiosis and reduced immunoglobulin-coated bacteria associated with coeliac disease in children. BMC Microbiol 2010;10.
[54] Sanchez E, Ribes-Koninckx C, Calabuig M, Sanz Y. Intestinal Staphylococcus spp. and virulent features associated with coeliac disease. J Clin Pathol 2012;65:830–4.
[55] Medina M, de Palma G, Ribes-Koninckx C, Calabuig M, Sanz Y. Bifidobacterium strains suppress in vitro the pro-inflammatory milieu triggered by the large intestinal microbiota of coeliac patients. J Inflamm 2008;5:19.
[56] Roberts SE, Williams JG, Meddings D, Davidson R, Goldacre MJ. Perinatal risk factors and coeliac disease in children and young adults: a record linkage study. Aliment Pharmacol Ther 2009;29:222–31.
[57] Dominguez-Belloa MG, Costello EK, Contreras M, Magris M, Hidalgo G, Fierer N, et al. Delivery mode shapes the acquisition and structure of the initial microbiota across multiple body habitats in newborns. Proc Natl Acad Sci USA 2010;107:11971–5.
[58] Kondrashova A, Mustalahti K, Kaukinen K, Viskari H, Volodicheva V, Haapala AM, et al. Lower economic status and inferior hygienic environment may protect against celiac disease. Ann Med 2008;40:223–31.
[59] Silano M, Agostini C, Guandalini S. Effect of the timing of gluten introduction on the development of celiac disease. World J Gastroenterol 2010;16:1939–42.
[60] Akobeng AK, Ramanan AV, Buchan I, Heller RF. Effect of breast feeding on risk of coeliac disease: a systematic review and meta-analysis of observational studies. Arch Dis Child 2006;91:39–43.
[61] Henriksson C, Bostrom AM, Wiklund IE. What effect does breastfeeding have on coeliac disease? A systematic review update. Evid Based Med 2013;18:98–103.
[62] Ivarsson A, Persson LA, Nystrom L, Ascher H, Cavell B, Danielsson L, et al. Epidemic of coeliac disease in Swedish children. Acta Paediatr 2000;89:165–71.

[63] Carlsson A, Agardh D, Borulf S, Grodzinsky E, Axelsson I, Ivarsson SA. Prevalence of celiac disease: before and after a national change in feeding recommendations. Scand J Gastroenterol 2006;41:553–8.

[64] Norris JM, Barriga K, Hoffenberg EJ, Taki I, Miao D, Haas JE, et al. Risk of celiac disease autoimmunity and timing of gluten introduction in the diet of infants at increased risk of disease. J Am Med Assoc 2005;293:2343–51.

[65] Agostoni C, Decsi T, Fewtrell M, Goulet O, Kolacek S, Koletzko B, et al. Complementary feeding: a commentary by the ESPGHAN Committee on Nutrition. J Pediatr Gastroenterol Nutr 2008;46:99–110.

[66] Szajewska H, Chmielewska A, Piescik-Lech M, Ivarsson A, Kolacek S, Koletzko S, et al. Systematic review: early infant feeding and the prevention of coeliac disease. Aliment Pharmacol Ther 2012;36:607–18.

[67] Welander A, Tjernberg AR, Montgomery SM, Ludvigsson J, Ludvigsson JF. Infections disease and risk of later celiac disease in childhood. Pediatrics 2010;125:e530–6.

[68] Stoerdal K, White RA, Eggesboe M. Early feeding and risk of celiac disease in a prospective birth cohort. Pediatrics 2013;132:e1201–9.

[69] Nova E, Pozo T, Sanz Y, Marcos A. Dietary strategies of immunomodulation in infants at risk for celiac disease. Proc Nutr Soc 2010;69:347–53.

[70] Mubarak A, Houwen RHJ, Wolters VM. Celiac disease: an overview from pathophysiology to treatment. Minerva Pediatr 2012;64:271–87.

[71] Richey R, Howdle P, Shaw E, Stokes T. Recognition and assessment of coeliac disease in children and adults: summary of NICE guidance. Br Med J 2009;338:b1684.

[72] Mukherjee R, Egbuna I, Brar P, Hernandez L, McMahon DJ, Shane EJ, et al. Celiac disease: similar presentation in the elderly and young adults. Dig Dis Sci 2010;55:3147–53.

[73] Tucker E, Rostami K, Prabhakaran S, Al Dulaimi D. Patients with coeliac disease are increasingly overweight or obese on presentation. J Gastrointestin Liver Dis 2012;21:11–5.

[74] Rewers M. Epidemiology of celiac disease: what are the prevalence, incidence, and progression of celiac disease? Gastroenterology 2005;128:S47–51.

[75] Kaukinen K, Halme L, Collin P, Faerkkilae M, Maeki M, Vehmanen P, et al. Celiac disease in patients with severe liver disease: gluten-free diet may reverse hepatitic failure. Gastroenterology 2002;122:881–8.

[76] Ludvigsson JF, Lindeloef B, Zingone F, Ciacci C. Psoriasis in a nationwide cohort study of patients with celiac disease. J Invest Dermatol 2011;131:2010–6.

[77] Akbulut S, Gur G, Topal F, Senel E, Topal FE, Alli N, et al. Coeliac disease-associated antibodies in psoriasis. Ann Dermatol 2013;25:298–303.

[78] Soni S, Badawy SZA. Celiac disease and its effect on human reproduction: a review. J Reprod Med 2010;55:3–8.

[79] Oezgoer B, Selimoglu MA. Coeliac disease and reproductive disorders. Scand J Gastroenterol 2010;45:395–402.

[80] Tata LJ, Card TR, Logan RFA, Hubbard RB, Smith CJP, West J. Fertility and pregnancy-related events in women with celiac disease: a population-based cohort study. Gastroenterology 2005;128:849–55.

[81] Zugna D, Richiardi L, Akre O, Stephansson O, Ludvigsson JF. A nationwide population-based study to determine whether coeliac disease is associated with infertility. Gut 2010;59:1471–5.

[82] Jackson JR, Eaton WW, Cascella NG, Fasano A, Kelly DL. Neurologic and psychiatric manifestations of celiac disease and gluten sensitivity. Psychiatr Q 2012;83:91–102.

[83] Currie S, Hadjivassiliou M, Clark MJR, Sanders DS, Wilkinson ID, Griffiths PD, et al. Should we be 'nervous' about coeliac disease? Brain abnormalities in patients with coeliac disease referred for neurological opinion. J Neurol Neurosurg Psychiatry 2012;83:1216–21.

[84] Ribaldone DG, Astegiano M, Fagoonee S, Rizzetto M, Pellicano R. Epilepsy and celiac disease: review of literature. Panminerva Med 2011;53:213–6.

[85] Zingone F, Siniscalchi M, Capone P, Tortora R, Andreozzi P, Capone E, et al. The quality of sleep in patients with coeliac disease. Aliment Pharmacol Ther 2010;32:1031–6.

[86] Buie T. The relationship of autism and gluten. Clin Ther 2013;35:578–83.

[87] Ludvigsson JF, Reichenberg A, Hultman CM, Murray JA. A nationwide study of the association between celiac disease and the risk of autistic spectrum disorders. JAMA Psychiatry 2013;70:1224–30.

[88] Chen SJ, Chao YL, Chen CY, Chang CM, Wu ECH, Wu CS, et al. Prevalence of autoimmune diseases in patients with schizophrenia: nationwide population-based study. Br J Psychiatry 2012;200:374–80.

[89] Tio M, Cox MR, Eslick GD. Meta-analysis: coeliac disease and the risk of all-cause mortality, any malignancy and lymphoid malignancy. Aliment Pharmacol Ther 2012;35:540–51.

[90] Biagi F, Corazza GR. Mortality in celiac disease. Nat Rev Gastroenterol Hepatol 2010;7:158–62.

[91] Godfrey JD, Brantner TL, Brinjikji W, Christensen KN, Brogan DL, van Dyke CT, et al. Morbidity and mortality among older individuals with undiagnosed celiac disease. Gastroenterology 2010;139:763–9.

[92] Lohi S, Maeki M, Rissanen H, Knekt P, Reunanen A, Kaukinen K. Prognosis of unrecognized coeliac disease as regards mortality: a population-based cohort study. Ann Med 2009;41:508–15.

[93] Lebwohl B, Granath F, Ekbom A, Montgomery SM, Murray JA, Rubio-Tapia A, et al. Mucosal healing and mortality in coeliac disease. Aliment Pharmacol Ther 2013;37:332–9.

[94] Lohi S, Maeki M, Montonen J, Knekt P, Pukkala E, Reunanen A, et al. Malignancies in cases with screening-identified evidence of coeliac disease: a long-term population-based cohort study. Gut 2009;58:643–7.

[95] Al-Toma A, Verbeek WHM, Hadithi M, von Blomberg BME, Mulder CJJ. Survival in refractory coeliac disease and enteropathy-associated T-cell lymphoma: retrospective evaluation of single-centre experience. Gut 2007;56:1373–8.

[96] Compilato D, Campisi G, Pastore L, Carroccio A. The production of the oral mucosa of anti-endomysial and anti-tissue-tranglutaminase antibodies in patients with celiac disease: a review. Sci World J 2010;10:2385–94.

[97] Bao F, Green PHR, Bhagat G. An update on celiac disease histopathology and the road ahead. Arch Pathol Lab Med 2012;136:735–45.

[98] Marsh MN. Gluten, major histocompatibility complex, and the small intestine. A molecular and immunobiologic approach to the spectrum of gluten sensitivity ('celiac sprue'). Gastroenterology 1992;102:330–54.

[99] Oberhuber G, Granditsch G, Vogelsang H. The histopathology of coeliac disease: time for a standardized report scheme for pathologists. Eur J Gastroenterol Hepatol 1999;11:1185–94.
[100] Corazza GR, Villanacci V. Coeliac disease. J Clin Pathol 2005;58:573–4.
[101] Ensari A. Gluten-sensitive enteropathy (celiac disease): controversies in diagnosis and classification. Arch Pathol Lab Med 2010;134:826–36.
[102] Jos J, Labbe F, Geny B, Griscelli C. Immunoelectron-microscopic localization of immunoglobulin A and secretory component in jejunal mucosa from children with coeliac disease. Scand J Immunol 1979;9:441–50.
[103] Salmi TT, Collin P, Korponay-Szabo IR, Laurila K, Partanen J, Huhtala H, et al. Endomysial antibody-negative coeliac disease: clinical characterisitics and intestinal autoantibody deposits. Gut 2006;55:1746–53.
[104] Koskinen O, Collin P, Lindfors K, Laurila K, Maeki M, Kaukinen K. Usefulness of small-bowel mucosal transglutaminase-2 specific autoantibody deposits in the diagnosis and follow-up of celiac disease. J Clin Gastroenterol 2010;44: 483–8.
[105] Kaukinen K, Peraeahoe M, Collin P, Partanen J, Woolley N, Kaartinen T, et al. Small-bowel mucosal transglutaminase 2-specific IgA deposits in coeliac disease without villous atrophy: a prospective and randomized clinical study. Scand J Gastroenterol 2005;40:564–72.
[106] Koskinen O, Collin P, Korponay-Szabo I, Salmi T, Iltanen S, Haimila K, et al. Gluten-dependent small bowel mucosal transglutaminase 2-specific IgA deposits in overt and mild enteropathy coeliac disease. J Pediatr Gastroenterol Nutr 2008;47:436–42.
[107] Borrelli M, Maglio M, Agnese M, Paparo F, Gentile S, Colicchio B, et al. High density of intraepithelial γδ lymphocytes and deposits of immunoglobulin (Ig) M anti-tissue transglutaminase antibodies in the jejunum of coeliac patients with IgA deficiency. Clin Exp Immunol 2010;160:199–206.
[108] Collin P, Kaukinen K, Vogelsang H, Korponay-Szabo I, Sommer R, Schreier E, et al. Antiendomysial and antihuman recombinant tissue transglutaminase antibodies in the diagnosis of coeliac disease: a biopsy-proven European multicenter study. Eur J Gastroenterol Hepatol 2005;17:85–91.
[109] ten Dam M, van de Wal Y, Mearin ML, Kooy Y, Pena S, Drijfhout JW, et al. Anti-alpha-gliadin antibodies (AGA) in the serum of coeliac children and controls recognize an identical collection of linear epitopes of alpha-gliadin. Clin Exp Immunol 1998;114:189–95.
[110] Schwertz E, Kahlenberg F, Sack U, Richter T, Stern M, Conrad K, et al. Serologic assay based on gliadin-related nonapeptides as a highly sensitive and specific diagnostic aid in celiac disease. Clin Chem 2004;50:2370–5.
[111] Seah PP, Fry L, Rossiter MA, Hoffbrand AV, Holborow EJ. Anti-reticulin antibodies in childhood coeliac disease. Lancet 1971;2:681–2.
[112] Chorzelski TP, Sulej J, Tchorzewska H, Jablonska S, Beutner EH, Kumar V. IgA class endomysium antibodies in dermatitis herpetiformis and coeliac disease. Ann NY Acad Sci 1983;420:325–34.
[113] Dieterich W, Ehnis T, Bauer M, Donner P, Volta U, Riecken EO, et al. Identification of tissue transglutaminase as the autoantigen of celiac disease. Nat Med 1997;3:797–801.

[114] Iversen R, di Niro R, Stamnaes J, Lundin KEA, Wilson PC, Sollid LM. Transglutaminase 2-specific autoantibodies in celiac disease target clustered, N-terminal epitopes not displayed on the surface of cells. J Immunol 2013;190:5981–91.
[115] Byrne G, Ryan F, Jackson J, Feighery C, Kelly J. Mutagenesis of the catalytic triad of tissue transglutaminase abrogates coeliac disease serum IgA autoantibody binding. Gut 2007;56:336–41.
[116] Karponay-Szabo IR, Halttunen T, Szalai Z, Laurila K, Kiraly R, Kovacs JB, et al. In vivo targeting of intestinal and extraintestinal transglutaminase 2 by coeliac autoantibodies. Gut 2004;53:641–8.
[117] Hadjivassiliou M, Maeki M, Sanders DS, Williamson CA, Gruenewald RA, Woodroofe NM, et al. Autoantibody targeting of brain and intestinal transglutaminase in gluten ataxia. Neurology 2006;66:373–7.
[118] Koning F, Schuppan D, Cerf-Bensussan N, Sollid LM. Pathomechanism in celiac disease. Best Pract Res Clin Gastroenterol 2005;19:373–87.
[119] Caja S, Maeki M, Kaukinen K, Lindfors K. Antibodies in celiac disease: implications beyond diagnostics. Cell Mol Immunol 2011;8:103–9.
[120] Lindfors K, Maeki M, Kaukinen K. Transglutaminase 2-targeted autoantibodies in celiac disease: pathogenetic players in addition to diagnostic tools? Autoimmun Rev 2010;9:744–9.
[121] Kaukinen K, Lindfors K, Collin P, Koskinen O, Maeki M. Coeliac disease – a diagnostic and therapeutic challenge. Clin Chem Lab Med 2010;48:1205–16.
[122] Dieterich W, Trapp D, Esslinger B, Leidenberger M, Piper J, Hahn E, et al. Autoantibodies of patients with coeliac disease are insufficient to block tissue transglutaminase activity. Gut 2003;52:1562–6.
[123] Qiao SW, Iversen R, Raki M, Sollid LM. The adaptive immune response in celiac disease. Semin Immunopathol 2012;34:523–40.
[124] Manavalan JS, Hernandez L, Shah JG, Konikkara J, Naiyer AJ, Lee AR, et al. Serum cytokine elevations in celiac disease: association with disease presentation. Hum Immunol 2010;71:50–7.
[125] Rubio-Tapia A, Murray JA. Classification and management of refractory coeliac disease. Gut 2010;59:547–57.
[126] Cellier C, Delabesse E, Helmer C, Patey N, Matuchansky C, Jabri B, et al. Refractory sprue, coeliac disease, and enteropathy-associated T-cell lymphoma. Lancet 2000;356:203–8.
[127] Daum S, Cellier C, Mulder CJJ. Refractory coeliac disease. Best Pract Res Clin Gastroenterol 2005;19:413–24.
[128] Schumann M, Kamel S, Pahlitzsch ML, Lebenheim L, May C, Krauss M, et al. Defective tight junctions in refractory celiac disease. Ann NY Acad Sci 2012;1258:43–51.
[129] Nijeboer P, van Wanrooij RLJ, Tack GJ, Mulder CJJ, Bouma G. Update on the diagnosis and management of refractory coeliac disease. Gastroenterol Res Pract 2013;2013:518483.
[130] Hollon JR, Cureton PA, Martin ML, Puppa ELL, Fasano A. Trace gluten contamination may play a role in mucosal and clinical recovery in a subgroup of diet-adherent non-responsive celiac disease patients. BMC Gastroenterol 2013;13:40.
[131] Mooney PD, Evans KE, Singh S, Sanders DS. Treatment failure in coeliac disease: a practical guide to investigation and treatment of non-responsive and refractory coeliac disease. J Gastrointestin Liver Dis 2012;21:197–203.

[132] Woodward J. The management of refractory coeliac disease. Ther Adv Chronic Dis 2013;4:77–90.

[133] Barret M, Malamut G, Rahmi G, Samaha E, Edery J, Verkarre V, et al. Diagnostic yield of capsule endoscopy in refractory celiac disease. Am J Gastroenterol 2012;107:1546–53.

[134] Malamut G, Afchain P, Verkarre V, Lecomte T, Amiot A, Damotte D, et al. Presentation and long-term follow-up of refractory celiac disease: comparison of type I with type II. Gastroenterology 2009;136:81–90.

[135] Verbeek WHM, Goerres MS, von Blomberg BME, Oudejans JJ, Scholten PET, Hadithi M, et al. Flow cytometric determination of aberrant intra-epithelial lymphocytes predicts T-cell lymphoma development more accurately than T-cell clonality analysis in refractory celiac disease. Clin Immunol 2008;126:48–56.

[136] Daum S, Ipczynski R, Heine B, Schulzke JD, Zeitz M, Ullrich R. Therapy with budesonide in patients with refractory sprue. Digestion 2006;73:60–8.

[137] Jamma S, Leffler DA, Dennis M, Najarian RM, Schuppan DB, Sheth S, et al. Small intestinal release mesalamine for the treatment of refractory celiac disease type I. J Clin Gastroenterol 2011;45:30–3.

[138] Tack GJ, van Asseldonk DP, van Wanrooij RLJ, van Bodegraven AA, Mulder CJ. Tioguanine in the treatment of refractory coeliac disease - a single centre experience. Aliment Pharmacol Ther 2012;36:274–81.

[139] Tack GJ, Verbeek WHM, Al-Toma A, Kuik DJ, Schreurs MWJ, Visser O, et al. Evaluation of cladribine treatment in refractory celiac disease type II. World J Gastroenterol 2011;17:506–13.

[140] Ludvigsson JF, Leffler DA, Bai JC, Biagi F, Fasano A, Green PHR, et al. The Oslo definitions for coeliac disease and related terms. Gut 2013;62:43–52.

[141] Pietzak M. Celiac disease, wheat allergy, and gluten sensitivity: when gluten free is not a fad. J Parenter Enteral Nutr 2012;36:68S–75S.

[142] Sapone A, Bai JC, Ciacci C, Dolinsek J, Green PHR, Hadjivassiliou M, et al. Spectrum of gluten-related disorders: consensus on new nomenclature and classification. BMC Med 2012;10:13.

[143] Reunala T, Maeki M. Dermatitis herpetiformis: a genetic disease. Eur J Dermatol 1993;3:519–26.

[144] Caproni M, Bonciolini V, D'Errico A, Antiga E, Fabbri P. Celiac disease and dermatologic manifestations: many skin clue to unfold gluten-sensitive enteropathy. Gastroenterol Res Pract 2012;2012:952753.

[145] Borroni G, Biagi F, Ciocca O, Vassallo C, Carugno A, Cananzi R, et al. IgA anti-epidermal transglutaminase autoantibodies: a sensible and sensitive marker for diagnosis of dermatitis herpetiformis in adult patients. J Eur Acad Dermatol Venereol 2013;27:836–41.

[146] Plotnikova N, Miller JL. Dermatitis herpetiformis. Skin Therapy Lett 2013;18:1–3.

[147] Bolotin D, Petronic-Rosic V. Dermatitis herpetiforms. Part I. Epidemiology, pathogenesis, and clinical presentation. J Am Acad Dermatol 2011;64:1017–24.

[148] Hadjivassiliou M, Sanders DS, Gruenewald RA, Woodroofe N, Boscolo S, Aeschlimann D. Gluten sensitivity: from gut to brain. Lancet Neurol 2010;9:318–30.

[149] Hadjivassiliou M, Aeschlimann P, Strigun A, Sanders DS, Woodroofe N, Aeschlimann D. Autoantibodies in gluten ataxia recognize a novel neuronal transglutaminase. Ann Neurol 2008;64:332–43.

[150] Hadjivassiliou M, Aeschlimann P, Sanders DS, Maeki M, Kaukinen K, Gruenewald RA, et al. Transglutaminase 6 antibodies in the diagnosis of gluten ataxia. Neurology 2013;80:1740–5.
[151] Hadjivassiliou M, Rao DG, Wharton SB, Sanders DS, Gruenewald RA, Davies-Jones AGB. Sensory ganglionopathy due to gluten sensitivity. Neurology 2010;75:1003–8.
[152] Tatham AS, Shewry PR. Allergens in wheat and related cereals. Clin Exp Allergy 2008;38:1712–26.
[153] Matsuo H, Morita E, Tatham AS, Morimoto K, Horikawa T, Osuna H, et al. Identification of the IgE-binding epitope in omega-5 gliadin, a major allergen in wheat-dependent exercise-induced anaphylaxis. J Biol Chem 2004;279:12135–40.
[154] Morita E, Kunie K, Matsuo H. Food-dependent exercise-induced anaphylaxis. J Dermatol Sci 2007;47:109–17.
[155] Matsuo H, Morimoto K, Akaki T, Kaneko S, Kusatake K, Kuroda T, et al. Exercise and aspirin increase levels of circulatory gliadin peptides in patients with wheat-dependent exercise-induced anaphylaxis. Clin Exp Allergy 2005;35:461–6.
[156] Biesiekierski JR, Newnham ED, Irving PM, Barrett JS, Haines M, Doecke JD, et al. Gluten causes gastrointestinal symptoms in subjects without celiac disease: a double-blind, randomized, placebo-controlled trial. Am J Gastroenterol 2011;106:508–14.
[157] Newnham ED. Does gluten cause gastrointestinal symptoms in subjects without coeliac disease? J Gastroenterol Hepatol 2011;26:132–4.
[158] Brottveit M, Vandvik PO, Wojniusz S, Loevik A, Lundin KEA, Boye B. Absence of somatization in non-coeliac gluten sensitivity. Scand J Gastroenterol 2012;47:770–7.
[159] Volta U, Tovoli F, Cicola R, Parisi C, Fabbri A, Piscaglia M, et al. Serological tests in gluten sensitivity (nonceliac gluten intolerance). J Clin Gastroenterol 2012;46:680–5.
[160] Bizzaro N, Tozzoli R, Villalta D, Fabris M, Tonutti E. Cutting-edge issues in coeliac disease and in gluten intolerance. Clin Rev Allergy Immunol 2012;42:279–87.
[161] Brottveit M, Beitnes ACR, Tollefsen S, Bratlie JE, Jahnsen FL, Johansen FE, et al. Mucosal cytokine response after short-term gluten challenge in celiac disease and non-celiac gluten sensitivity. Am J Gastroenterol 2013;108:842–50.
[162] Junker Y, Zeissig S, Kim SJ, Barisani D, Wieser H, Leffler DA, et al. Wheat amylase trypsin inhibitors drive intestinal inflammation via activation of toll-like receptor 4. J Exp Med 2012;209:2395–408.
[163] Biesiekierski JR, Peters SL, Newnham ED, Rosella O, Muir JG, Gibson PR. No effects of gluten in patients with self-reported non-celiac gluten sensitivity after dietary reduction of fermentable, poorly absorbed, short-chain carbohydrates. Gastroenterology 2013;145:320–8.
[164] Sapone A, Lammers KM, Casolaro V, Cammarota M, Giuliano MT, de Rosa M, et al. Divergence of gut permeability and mucosal immune gene expression in two gluten-associated conditions: celiac disease and gluten sensitivity. BMC Med 2011;9:23.
[165] Volta U, Caio G, Tovoli F, de Giorgio R. Non-celiac gluten sensitivity: questions still to be answered despite increasing awareness. Cell Mol Immunol 2013;10:383–92.
[166] Aziz I, Sanders DS. The irritable bowel syndrome-celiac disease connection. Gastrointest Endosc Clin N Am 2012;22:623–37.

[167] Thompson WG, Heaton KW, Smyth GT, Smyth C. Irritable bowel syndrome in general practice: prevalence, characteristics, and referral. Gut 2000;46:78–82.

[168] Hillila MT, Faerkkilae MA. Prevalence of irritable bowel syndrome according to different diagnostic criteria in a non-selected adult population. Aliment Pharmacol Ther 2004;20:339–45.

[169] Longstreth GF, Thompson WG, Chey WD, Houghton LA, Mearin F, Spiller RC. Functional bowel disorders. Gastroenterology 2006;130:1480–91.

[170] Camilleri M, Madsen K, Spiller R, van Meerveld BG, Verne GN. Intestinal barrier function in health and gastrointestinal disease. Neurogastroenterol Motil 2012;24:503–12.

[171] Piche T, Barbara G, Aubert P, Bruley des Varannes S, Dainese R, Nano JL, et al. Impaired intestinal barrier integrity in the colon of patients with irritable bowel syndrome: involvement of soluble mediators. Gut 2009;58:196–201.

[172] Mereiles L, Li M, Loo D, Lin E. Celiac disease and intestinal endocrine autoimmunity. In: Eisenbarth GS, editor. Immunoendocrinology: scientific and clinical aspects, contemporary. Springer Science+Business Media; 2011. pp. 535–45.

[173] Ventura A, Magazzu G, Greco L. Duration of exposure to gluten and risk for autoimmune disorders in patients with celiac disease. Gastroenterology 1999;117:297–303.

[174] Armstrong MJ, Hegade VS, Robins G. Advances in coeliac disease. Curr Opin Gastroenterol 2012;28:104–12.

[175] Smyth DJ, Plagnol V, Walker NM, Cooper JD, Downes K, Yang JHM, et al. Shared and distinct genetic variants in type 1 diabetes and celiac disease. N Engl J Med 2008;359:2767–77.

[176] Concannon P, Rich SS, Nepom GT. Genetics of type 1A diabetes. N Engl J Med 2009;360:1646–54.

[177] Aggarwal S, Lebwohl B, Green PHR. Screening for celiac disease in average-risk and high-risk populations. Therap Adv Gastroenterol 2012;5:37–47.

[178] Sollid LM, Jabri B. Triggers and drivers of autoimmunity: lessons from coeliac disease. Nat Rev Immunol 2013;13:294–302.

[179] Rubio-Tapia A, Murray JA. Celiac disease. Curr Opin Gastroenterol 2010;26: 116–22.

[180] Evans KE, Hadjivassiliou M, Sanders DS. Is it time to screen for adult coeliac disease? Eur J Gastroenterol Hepatol 2011;23:833–8.

[181] Virta LJ, Kaukinen K, Collin P. Incidence and prevalence of diagnosed coeliac disease in Finland: results of effective case finding in adults. Scand J Gastroenterol 2009;44:933–8.

[182] Working Group of European Society of Paediatric Gastroenterology and Nutrition. Revised criteria for diagnosis of coeliac disease. Arch Dis Child 1990;65: 909–11.

[183] Klapp G, Masip E, Bolonio M, Donat E, Polo B, Ramos D, et al. Celiac disease: the new proposed ESPGHAN diagnostic criteria do work well in a selected population. J Pediatr Gastroenterol Nutr 2013;56:351–6.

[184] Makovicky P, Rimarova K, Boor A, Makovicky P, Vodicka P, Samasca G, et al. Correlation between antibodies and histology in celiac disease: incidence of celiac disease is higher than expected in the pediatric population. Mol Med Rep 2013;8:1079–83.

[185] Fernandez-Banares F, Alsina M, Modolell I, Andujar X, Piqueras M, García-Puig R, et al. Are positive serum-IgA-tissue-transglutaminase antibodies enough to diagnose coeliac disease without a small bowel biopsy? Post-test probability of coeliac disease. J Crohns Colitis 2012;6:861–6.

[186] Husby S, Koletzko S, Korponay-Szabo IR, Mearin ML, Phillips A, Shamir R, et al. European Society for Pediatric Gastroenterology, Hepatology, and Nutrition guidelines for the diagnosis of coeliac disease. J Pediatr Gastroenterol Nutr 2012;54:136–60.

[187] Cotton D, Taichman D, Williams S, Crowe SE. Celiac disease. Ann Intern Med 2011. ITC5-2-16.

[188] Leffler D, Schuppan D, Pallav K, Najarian R, Goldsmith JD, Hansen J, et al. Kinetics of the histological, serological and symptomatic responses to gluten challenge in adults with coeliac disease. Gut 2013;62:996–1004.

[189] Ukkola A, Maeki M, Kurppa K, Collin P, Huhtala H, Kekkonen L, et al. Patients' experiences and perceptions of living with coeliac disease – implications for optimizing care. J Gastrointestin Liver Dis 2012;21:17–22.

[190] Lebwohl B, Rubio-Tapia A, Assiri A, Newland C, Guandalini S. Diagnosis of celiac disease. Gastrointest Endosc Clin N Am 2012;22:661–77.

[191] Lalkhen AG, McCluskey A. Clinical tests: sensitivity and specificity. Contin Educ Anaesth Crit Care Pain 2008;8:221–3.

[192] Buergin-Wolff A, Hernandez R, Just M, Signer E. Immunofluorescent antibodies against gliadin: a screening test for coeliac disease. Helv Paediatr Acta 1976;31:375–80.

[193] O'Farrelly C, Kelly J, Hekkens W, Bradley B, Thompson A, Feighery C, et al. Alpha gliadin antibody levels: a serological test for coeliac disease. Br Med J 1983;286:2007–10.

[194] Leffler DA, Schuppan D. Update on serologic testing in celiac disease. Am J Gastroenterol 2010;105:2520–4.

[195] Hill ID, Dirks MH, Liptak GS, Colletti RB, Fasano A, Guandalini S, et al. Guideline for the diagnosis and treatment of celiac disease in children: recommendations of the North American Society for Pediatric Gastroenterology, Hepatology and Nutrition. J Pediatr Gastroenterol Nutr 2005;40:1–19.

[196] Giersiepen K, Lelgemann M, Stuhldreher N, Ronfani L, Husby S, Koletzko S, et al. Accuracy of diagnostic antibody tests for coeliac disease in children: summary of an evidence report. J Pediatr Gastroenterol Nutr 2012;54:229–41.

[197] Foucher B, Johanet C, Jego-Desplat S, Sanmarco M, Dubucquoi S, Fily-Nalewajk S, et al. Are immunoglobulin A anti-gliadin antibodies helpful in diagnosing coeliac disease in children younger than 2 years? J Pediatr Gastroenterol Nutr 2012;54:110–2.

[198] Richter T, Bossuyt X, Vermeersch P, Uhlig HH, Stern M, Hauer A, et al. Determination of IgG and IgA antibodies against native gliadin is not helpful for the diagnosis of coeliac disease in children up to 2 years old. J Pediatr Gastroenterol Nutr 2012;55:21–5.

[199] Parizade M, Bujanover Y, Weiss B, Nachmias V, Shainberg B. Performance of serology assays for diagnosing celiac disease in a clinical setting. Clin Vaccine Immunol 2009;16:1576–82.

[200] Dahlbom I, Korponay-Szabo I, Kovacs JB, Szalai Z, Maeki M, Hansson T. Prediction of clinical and mucosal severity of coeliac disease and dermatitis herpetiformis

by quantification of IgA/IgG serum antibodies to tissue transglutaminase. J Pediatr Gastroenterol Nutr 2010;50:140–6.

[201] Abrams JA, Diamond B, Rotterdam H, Green PHR. Seronegative celiac disease: increased prevalence with lesser degrees of villous atrophy. Dig Dis Sci 2004;49:546–50.

[202] Raivio T, Korponay-Szabo I, Collin P, Laurila K, Huhtala H, Kaartinen T, et al. Performance of a new rapid whole blood coeliac test in adult patients with low prevalence of endomysial antibodies. Dig Liver Dis 2007;39:1057–63.

[203] Popp A, Jinga M, Jurcut C, Balaban V, Bardas C, Laurila K, et al. Fingertip rapid point-of-care test in adult case-finding in coeliac disease. BMC Gastroenterol 2013;13:115.

[204] Mooney PD, Kurien M, Sanders DS. Simtomax, a novel point of care test for coeliac disease. Expert Opin Med Diagn 2013;7:645–51.

[205] Rostom A, Dube C, Cranney A, Saloojee N, Sy R, Garritty C, et al. The diagnostic accuracy of serological tests for celiac disease: a systemic review. Gastroenterology 2005;128:S38–46.

[206] Lewis NR, Scott BB. Meta-analysis: deamidated gliadin peptide antibody and tissue transglutaminase antibody compared as screening tests for coeliac disease. Aliment Pharmacol Ther 2010;31:73–81.

[207] Amarri S, Alvisi P, Giorgio R, Gelli MC, Cicola R, Tovoli F, et al. Antibodies to deamidated gliadin peptides: an accurate predictor of coeliac disease in infancy. J Clin Immunol 2013;33:1027–30.

[208] Vivas S, Ruiz de Morales JG, Riestra S, Arias L, Fuentes D, Alvarez N, et al. Duodenal biopsy may be avoided when high transglutaminase antibody titers are present. World J Gastroenterol 2009;15:4775–80.

[209] Rozenberg O, Lerner A, Pacht A, Grinberg M, Reginashvili D, Henig C, et al. A novel algorithm for the diagnosis of celiac disease and a comprehensive review of celiac disease diagnostics. Clin Rev Allergy Immunol 2012;42:331–41.

[210] Buergin-Wolff A, Buser M, Hadziselimovic F. Intestinal biopsy is not always required to diagnose celiac disease: a retrospective analysis of combined antibody tests. BMC Gastroenterol 2013;13:19.

[211] Pallav K, Leffler DA, Bennett M, Tariq S, Xu H, Kabbani T, et al. Open conformation tissue transglutaminase testing for celiac dietary assessment. Dig Liver Dis 2012;44:375–8.

[212] Tozzoli R, Kodermaz G, Tampoia M, Visentini D, Tonutti E, Bizzaro N. Detection of autoantibodies specific for transglutaminase-gliadin peptides complex: a new way to explore the celiac iceberg? Riv Ital Med Lab 2010;6:28–35.

[213] Carroccio A, Iacono G, di Prima L, Pirrone G, Cavataio F, Ambrosiano G, et al. Antiendomysium antibodies assay in the culture medium of intestinal mucosa: an accurate method for celiac disease diagnosis. Eur J Gastroenterol Hepatol 2011;23:1018–23.

[214] Collin P, Kaukinen K, Maeki M. Duodenal intraepithelial lymphocytosis: celiac disease or not? Am J Gastroenterol 2009;104:1847.

[215] Korponay-Szabo IR, Szabados K, Pusztai J, Uhrin K, Ludmany E, Nemes E, et al. Population screening for coeliac disease in primary care by distric nurses using a rapid antibody test: diagnostic accuracy and feasibility study. Br Med J 2007;335:1244–7.

[216] Baviera LCB, Aliaga ED, Ortigosa L, Litwin N, Pena-Quintana L, Mendez V, et al. Celiac disease screening by immunochromatographic visual assays: results of a multicenter study. J Pediatr Gastroenterol Nutr 2007;45:546–50.
[217] Balkenhohl T, Lisdat F. An impedimetric immunosensor for the detection of autoantibodies directed against gliadins. Analyst 2007;132:314–22.
[218] Balkenhohl T, Lisdat F. Screen-printed electrodes as impedimetric immunosensors for the detection of anti-transglutaminase antibodies in human sera. Anal Chim Acta 2007;597:50–7.
[219] West N, Baker P, Priscilla GL, Arotiba OA, Hendricks NR, Baleg AA, et al. Overoxidized polypyrrole incorporated with gold nanoparticles as platform for impedimetric anti-transglutaminase immunosensors. Anal Lett 2011;44:1956–66.
[220] Pividori MI, Lermo A, Bonanni A, Alegret S, del Valle M. Electrochemical immunosensor for the diagnosis of celiac disease. Anal Biochem 2009;388:229–34.
[221] Kergaravat SV, Beltramino L, Garnero N, Trotta L, Wagener M, Pividori MI, et al. Electrochemical magneto immunosensor for the detection of anti-TG2 antibody in celiac disease. Biosens Bioelectron 2013;48:203–9.
[222] Adornetto G, Volpe G, de Stefano A, Martini S, Gallucci G, Manzoni A, et al. An ELIME assay for the rapid diagnosis of coeliac disease. Anal Bioanal Chem 2012;403:1191–4.
[223] Dulay S, Lozano-Sanchez P, Iwuoha E, Katakis I, O'Sullivan CK. Electrochemical detection of celiac disease-related anti-tissue transglutaminase antibodies using thiol based surface chemistry. Biosens Bioelectron 2011;26:3852–6.
[224] Cennamo N, Varriale A, Pennacchio A, Staiano M, Massarotti D, Zeni L, et al. An innovative plastic optical fiber-based biosensor for new bio/applications. The case of celiac disease. Sens Actuators B Chem 2013;176:1008–14.
[225] Neves MMPS, Gonzales-Garcia MB, Delerue-Matos C, Costa-Garcia A. Multiplexed electrochemical immunosensors for detection of celiac disease serological markers. Sens Actuators B Chem 2013;187:33–9.
[226] Neves MMPS, Gonzalez-García MB, Nouws HPA, Costa-García A. An electrochemical deamidated gliadin antibody immunosensor for celiac disease clinical diagnosis. Analyst 2013;138:1956–8.
[227] Fleur du Pre M, van Berkel LA, Raki M, van Leeuwen MA, de Ruiter LF, Broere F, et al. CD62LnegCD38^{+} expression on circulating CD4^{+} T cells identifies mucosally differentiated cells in protein fed mice and in human celiac disease patients and controls. Am J Gastroenterol 2011;106:1147–59.
[228] Collin P, Rondonotti E, Lundin KEA, Spada C, Keuchel M, Kaukinen K, et al. Video capsule endoscopy in celiac disease: current clinical practice. J Dig Dis 2012;13:94–9.
[229] Kurien M, Evans KE, Aziz I, Sidhu R, Drew K, Rogers TL, et al. Capsule endoscopy in adult celiac disease: a potential role in equivocal cases of celiac disease? Gastrointest Endosc 2013;77:227–32.
[230] Tennyson CA, Ciaccio EJ, Lewis SK. Video capsule endoscopy in celiac disease. Gastrointest Endosc Clin N Am 2012;22:747–58.
[231] Pallav K, Leffler DA, Tariq S, Kabbani T, Hansen J, Peer A, et al. Noncoeliac enteropathy: the differential diagnosis of villous atrophy in contemporary clinical practice. Aliment Pharmacol Ther 2012;35:380–90.
[232] Bao F, Bhagat G. Histopathology of celiac disease. Gastrointest Endosc Clin N Am 2012;22:679–94.

[233] Gonzalez S, Gupta A, Cheng J, Tennyson C, Lewis SK, Bhagat G, et al. Prospective study of the role of duodenal bulb biopsies in the diagnosis of celiac disease. Gastrointest Endosc 2010;72:758–65.

[234] Tanpowpong P, Broder-Fingert S, Katz AJ, Camargo Jr CA. Predictors of duodenal bulb biopsy performance in the evaluation of coeliac disease in children. J Clin Pathol 2012;65:791–4.

[235] Arguelles-Grande C, Tennyson CA, Lewis SK, Green PHR, Bhagat G. Variability in small bowel histopathology reporting between different pathology practice settings: impact on the diagnosis of coeliac disease. J Clin Pathol 2012;65: 242–7.

[236] Mohamed BM, Feighery C, Coates C, O'Shea U, Delaney D, O'Briain S, et al. The absence of a mucosal lesion on standard histological examination does not exclude diagnosis of celiac disease. Dig Dis Sci 2008;53:52–61.

[237] Not T, Ziberna F, Vatta S, Quaglia S, Martelossi S, Villanacci V, et al. Cryptic genetic gluten intolerance revealed by intestinal antitransglutaminase antibodies and response to gluten-free diet. Gut 2011;60:1487–93.

[238] Rathsman S, Tysk C, Eriksson S, Hultgren O, Aaberg AK, Olcen P. Elution of antitransglutaminase antibodies from duodenal biopsies: a novel approach in the diagnosis of celiac disease. APMIS 2012;120:666–74.

[239] Tosco A, Aitoro R, Auricchio R, Ponticelli D, Miele E, Paparo F, et al. Intestinal anti-tissue transglutaminase antibodies in potential coeliac disease. Clin Exp Immunol 2013;171:69–75.

[240] Picarelli A, di Tola M, Marino M, Libanori V, Borghini R, Salvi E, et al. Usefulness of the organ culture system when villous height/crypt depth ratio, intraepithelial lymphocyte count, or serum antibody tests are not diagnostic for celiac disease. Transl Res: J Lab Clin Med 2013;161:172–80.

[241] Ravelli A, Villanacci V. Tricks of the trade: how to avoid histological pitfalls in celiac disease. Pathol Res Pract 2012;208:197–202.

[242] Leon F. Flow cytometry of intestinal intraepithelial lymphocytes in celiac disease. J Immunol Methods 2011;363:177–86.

[243] Hadithi M, von Blomberg BME, Crusius JBA, Bloemena E, Kostense PJ, Meijer JWR, et al. Accuracy of serologic tests and HLA-DQ typing for diagnosing celiac disease. Ann Intern Med 2007;147:294–302.

[244] Romanos J, Rosen A, Kumar V, Trynka G, Franke L, Szperl A, et al. Improving coeliac disease risk prediction by testing non-HLA variants additional to HLA variants. Gut 2014;63:415–22.

[245] Ludvigsson JF, Green PH. Clinical management of coeliac disease. J Intern Med 2011;269:560–71.

[246] Hadithi M, Pena AS. Current methods to diagnose the unresponsive and complicated forms of coeliac disease. Eur J Intern Med 2010;21:247–53.

[247] Mubarak A, Spierings E, Wolters V, van Hoogstraten I, Kneepkens CMF, Houwen R. Human leukocyte antigen DQ2.2 and celiac disease. J Pediatr Gastroenterol Nutr 2013;56:428–30.

[248] Lavant EH, Carlson J. HLA DR-DQ genotyping by capillary electrophoresis for risk assessment for celiac disease. Methods Mol Biol 2013;919:297–307.

[249] Brottveit M, Raki M, Bergseng E, Fallang LE, Simonsen B, Loevik A, et al. Assessing possible coeliac disease by an HLA-DQ2-gliadin tetramer test. Am J Gastroenterol 2011;106:1318–24.

[250] Tsuji NM, Kosaka A. Oral tolerance: intestinal homeostasis and antigen-specific regulatory T cells. Trends Immunol 2008;29:532–40.

[251] Brazowski E, Cohen S, Yaron A, Filip I, Eisenthal A. FOXP3 expression in duodenal mucosa in pediatric patients with celiac disease. Pathobiology 2010;77:328–34.

[252] Zanzi D, Stefanile R, Santagata S, Iaffaldano L, Iaquinto G, Giardullo N, et al. IL-15 interferes with suppressive activity of intestinal regulatory T cells expanded in celiac disease. Am J Gastroenterol 2011;106:1308–17.

[253] Marietta EV, Murray JA. Animal models to study gluten sensitivity. Semin Immunopathol 2012;34:497–511.

[254] Kagnoff MF, Austin RK, Hubert JJ, Bernardin JE, Kasarda DD. Possible role for a human adenovirus in the pathogenesis of celiac disease. J Exp Med 1984;160:1544–57.

[255] Nieuwenhuizen WF, Pieters RJH, Knippels LMJ, Jansen MCJF, Koppelman SJ. Is *Candida albicans* a trigger in the onset of coeliac disease? Lancet 2003;361:2152–4.

[256] Food and Agricultural Organization of the United Nations. http://faostat.fao.org [accessed December 2013].

[257] Hischenhuber C, Crevel R, Jarry B, Maeki M, Moneret-Vautrin DA, Romano A, et al. Review article: safe amounts of gluten for patients with wheat allergy and coeliac disease. Aliment Pharmacol Ther 2006;23:559–75.

[258] Akobeng AK, Thomas AG. Systematic review: tolerable amount of gluten for people with coeliac disease. Aliment Pharmacol Ther 2008;27:1044–52.

[259] Jansson UH, Gudjonsdottir AH, Ryd W, Kristansson B. Two different doses of gluten show a dose-dependent response of enteropathy but not of serological markers during gluten challenge in children with celiac disease. Acta Paediatr 2001;90:255–9.

[260] Ciclitira PJ, Evans DJ, Fagg NL, Lennox ES, Dowling RH. Clinical testing of gliadin fractions in coeliac patients. Clin Sci 1984;66:357–64.

[261] Ciclitira PJ, Cerio R, Ellis HJ, Maxton D, Nelufer JM, Macartney JM. Evaluation of a gliadin-containing gluten-free product in coeliac patients. Hum nutr Clin Nutr 1985;39:303–8.

[262] Ejderhamn J, Veress B, Strandvik B. The long-term effect of continual ingestion of wheat starch-containing gluten-free products in celiac patiens. In: Kumar PJ, Walker-Smith JA, editors. Coeliac disease: one hundred years. Leeds (UK): Leeds University Press; 1990. pp. 294–7.

[263] Kaukinen K, Collin P, Holm K, Rantala I, Vuolteenaho N, Reunala T, et al. Wheat starch-containing gluten-free flour products in the treatment of coeliac disease and dermatitis herpetiformis. A long-term follow-up study. Scand J Gastroenterol 1999;34:163–9.

[264] Peraeaho M, Kaukinen K, Paasikivi K, Sievanen H, Lohiniemi S, Maeki M, et al. Wheat-starch-based gluten-free products in the treatment of newly detected coeliac disease: prospective and randomized study. Aliment Pharmacol Ther 2003;17:587–94.

[265] Catassi C, Rossini M, Ratsch IM, Bearzi I, Santinelli A, Castagnani R, et al. Dose dependent effects of protracted ingestion of small amounts of gliadin in coeliac disease children: a clinical and jejunal morphometric study. Gut 1993;34:1515–9.

[266] Catassi C, Fabiani E, Iacono G, D'Agate C, Francavilla R, Biagi F, et al. A prospective, double-blind, placebo-controlled trial to establish a safe gluten threshold for patients with celiac disease. Am J Clin Nutr 2007;85:160–6.

[267] Frazer AC. The malabsorption syndrome, with special reference to the effects of wheat gluten. Adv Clin Chem 1962;5:69–106.

[268] Marsh MN, Loft DE. Coeliac sprue: a centennial overview 1888–1988. Dig Dis 1988;6:216–28.

[269] Douglas AP, Booth CC. Digestion of gluten peptides by normal human jejunal mucosa and by mucosa from patients with adult coeliac disease. Clin Sci 1970;38:11–25.

[270] Wieser H, Belitz HD, Idar D, Ashkenazi A. Coeliac activity of the gliadin peptides CT-1 and CT-2. Z Lebensm Unters Forsch 1986;182:115–7.

[271] de Ritis G, Auricchio S, Jones HW, Lew EJL, Bernardin JE, Kasarda DD. In vitro (organ culture) studies of the toxicity of specific A-gliadin peptides in celiac disease. Gastroenterology 1988;94:41–9.

[272] Shan L, Molberg O, Parrot I, Hausch F, Filiz F, Gray GM, et al. Structural basis for gluten intolerance in celiac sprue. Science 2002;297:2275–9.

[273] Shan L, Qiao SW, Arentz-Hansen H, Molberg O, Gray GM, Sollid LM, et al. Identification and analysis of multivalent proteolytically resistant peptides from gluten: implications for celiac sprue. J Proteome Res 2005;4:1732–41.

[274] Osorio C, Wen N, Gemini R, Zemetra R, Wettstein D, Rustgi S. Targeted modification of wheat grain protein to reduce the content of celiac causing epitopes. Funct Integr Genomics 2012;12:417–38.

[275] Wieser H. Studies on the acid deamidation of glutamine by means of a tripeptide from α-gliadins. In: Stern M, editor. Proceedings of the 19th meeting of the working group on prolamin analysis and toxicity. Zwickau (Germany): Verlag Wissenschaftliche Scripten; 2005. pp. 23–6.

[276] Bethune MT, Khosla C. Oral therapy for celiac sprue. Methods Enzymol 2012;502:241–71.

[277] Mitea C, Havenaar R, Drijfhout JW, Edens L, Dekking L, Koning F. Efficient degradation of gluten by a prolyl endoproteinase in a gastrointestinal model: implications for coeliac disease. Gut 2008;57:25–32.

[278] Der kleine Souci-Fachmann-Kraut: Lebensmitteltabelle für die Praxis. Stuttgart (Germany): Wissenschaftliche Verlagsgesellschaft mbH; 2011. p. 223, 225, 233, 241.

[279] Wieser H, Seilmeier W, Belitz HD. Vergleichende Untersuchungen über partielle Aminosäuresequenzen von Prolaminen und Glutelinen verschiedener Getreidearten. I. Proteinfraktionierung nach Osborne. Z Lebensm Unters Forsch 1980;170:17–26.

[280] Assimakopoulos SF, Papageorgiou I, Charonis A. Enterocytes´ tight junctions: from molecule to disease. World J Gastrointest Pathol 2011;2:123–37.

[281] Tripathi A, Lammers KM, Goldblum S, Shea-Donohue T, Netzel-Arnett S, Buzza MS, et al. Identification of human zonulin, a physiological modulator of tight junctions, as prehaptoglobulin-2. Proc Natl Acad Sci USA 2009;106:16799–804.

[282] Fasano A. Zonulin and its regulation of intestinal barrier function: the biological door to inflammation, autoimmunity, and cancer. Physiol Rev 2011;91:151–75.

[283] Arrieta MC, Bistritz L, Meddings JB. Alterations in intestinal permeability. Gut 2006;55:1512–20.

[284] Grootjans J, Thuijls G, Verdam F, Derikx JPM, Lenaerts K, Buurman WA. Non-invasive assessment of barrier integrity and function of the human gut. World J Gastrointest Surg 2010;2:61–9.

[285] Matysiak-Budnik T, Candalh C, Dugave C, Namane A, Cellier C, Cerf-Bensussan N, et al. Alterations of the intestinal transport and processing of gliadin peptides in celiac disease. Gastroenterology 2003:696–707.

[286] John LJ, Fromm M, Schulzke JD. Epithelial barriers in intestinal inflammation. Antioxid Redox Signal 2011;15:1255–70.

[287] Drago S, El Asmar R, di Pierro M, Grazia-Clemente M, Sapone ATA, Thakar M, et al. Gliadin, zonulin and gut permeability: effects on celiac disease and non-celiac intestinal mucosa and intestinal cell lines. Scand J Gastroenterol 2006;41:408–19.

[288] Fasano A, Not T, Wang W, Uzzau S, Berti I, Tommasini A, et al. Zonulin, a newly discovered modulator of intestinal permeability, and its expression in coeliac disease. Lancet 2000;355:1518–9.

[289] Lammers KM, Lu R, Brownley J, Lu B, Gerard C, Thomas K, et al. Gliadin induces an increase in intestinal permeability and zonulin release by binding to the chemokine receptor CXCR3. Gastroenterology 2008;135:194–204.

[290] Nilsen EM, Lundin KEA, Krajci P, Scott H, Sollid LM, Brandtzaeg P. Gluten specific, HLA-DQ restricted T cells from celiac mucosa produce cytokines with Th1 or Th0 profile dominated by interferon γ. Gut 1995;37:766–76.

[291] Menard S, Lebreton C, Schumann M, Matysiak-Budnik T, Dugave C, Bouhnik Y, et al. Paracellular versus transcellular intestinal permeability to gliadin peptides in active celiac disease. Am J Pathol 2012;180:608–15.

[292] Lebreton C, Menard S, Abed J, Moura IC, Coppo R, Dugave C, et al. Interactions among secretory immunoglobulin A, CD 71, and transglutaminase-2 affect permeability of intestinal epithelial cells to gliadin peptides. Gastroenterology 2012;143:698–707.

[293] Heyman M, Abed J, Lebreton C, Cerf-Bensussan N. Intestinal permeability in coeliac disease: insight into mechanisms and relevance to pathogenesis. Gut 2012;61:1355–64.

[294] Zimmer KP, Naim H, Weber P, Ellis HJ, Ciclitira PJ. Targeting of gliadin peptides, CD8, α/β-TCR, and γ/δ-TCR to Golgi complexes and vacuoles within celiac disease enterocytes. FASEB J 1998;12:1349–57.

[295] Zimmer KP, Fischer I, Mothes T, Weissen-Plenz G, Schmitz M, Wieser H, et al. Endocytotic segregation of gliadin peptide 31–49 in enterocytes. Gut 2010;59:300–10.

[296] Barone MV, Nanayakkara M, Paolella G, Maglio M, Vitale V, Troiano R, et al. Gliadin peptide P31–43 localises to endocytic vesicles and interferes with their maturation. PLoS One 2010;5:e12246.

[297] Barone MV, Zanzi D, Maglio M, Nanayakkara M, Santagata S, Lania G, et al. Gliadin-mediated proliferation and innate immune activation in celiac disease are due to alterations in vesicular trafficking. PLoS One 2011;6:e17039.

[298] Maiuri L, Luciani A, Villella VR, Vasaturo A, Giardino I, Pettoello-Mantovani M, et al. Lysosomal accumulation of gliadin p31-43 peptide induces oxidative stress and tissue transglutaminase-mediated PPARγ downregulation in intestinal epithelial cells and coeliac mucosa. Gut 2010;59:311–9.

[299] Meresse B, Malamut G, Amar S, Cerf-Bensussan N. Innate immunity and celiac disease. In: Fasano A, Troncone R, Branski D, editors. Frontiers in celiac disease. Basel (Switzerland): Karger; 2008. pp. 66–81.

[300] Stepniak D, Koning F. Celiac disease – sandwiched between innate and adaptive immunity. Hum Immunol 2006;67:460–8.

[301] Sollid LM, Markussen G, Ek J, Gjerde H, Vartdal F, Thorsby E. Evidence for a primary association of celiac disease to particular HLA-DQ α/β heterodimer. J Exp Med 1989;169:345–50.

[302] Wieser H, Koehler P. The biochemical basis of celiac disease. Cereal Chem 2008;85:1–13.

[303] Mycek MJ, Clarke DD, Neidle A, Waelsch H. Amine incorporation into insulin as catalyzed by transglutaminase. Arch Biochem Biophys 1959;84:528–40.

[304] Pinkas DM, Strop P, Brunger AT, Khosla C. Transglutaminase 2 undergoes a large conformational change upon activation. PLoS Biol 2007;5:2788–96.

[305] Wang Z, Griffin M. TG2, a novel extracellular protein with multiple functions. Amino Acids 2012;42:939–49.

[306] Wolf J, Lachmann I, Wagner U, Osman A, Mothes T. Immunoassay of in vitro activated human tissue transglutaminase. Anal Biochem 2011;411:10–5.

[307] Park D, Choi SS, Ha KS. Transglutaminase 2: a multi-functional protein in multiple subcellular compartments. Amino Acids 2010;39:19–31.

[308] di Sabatino A, Vanoli A, Giuffrida P, Luinetti O, Solcia E, Corazza GR. The function of tissue transglutaminase in celiac disease. Autoimmun Rev 2012;11: 746–53.

[309] Qiao SW, Piper J, Haraldsen G, Oynebraten I, Fleckenstein B, Molberg O, et al. Tissue transglutaminase-mediated formation and cleavage of histamine-gliadin complexes: biological effects and implications for celiac disease. J Immunol 2005;174:1657–63.

[310] Verderio EAM, Johnson T, Griffin M. Tissue transglutaminase in normal and abnormal wound healing: review article. Amino Acids 2004;26:387–404.

[311] Bruce SE, Bjarnason I, Peters TJ. Human jejunal transglutaminase: demonstration of activity, enzyme kinetics and substrate specificity with special relation to gliadin and coeliac disease. Clin Sci 1985;68:573–9.

[312] Fleckenstein B, Molberg O, Qiao SW, Schmid DG, von der Mulbe F, Elgstoen K, et al. Gliadin T cell epitope selection by tissue transglutaminase in celiac disease. Role of enzyme specificity and pH influence on the transamidation versus deamidation reactions. J Biol Chem 2002;277:34109–16.

[313] Vader LW, de Ru A, van der Wal Y, Kooy YMC, Benckhuijsen W, Mearin ML, et al. Specificity of tissue transglutaminase explains cereal toxicity in celiac disease. J Exp Med 2002;195:643–9.

[314] Sollid LM, Qiao SW, Anderson RP, Gianfrani C, Koning F. Nomenclature and listing of celiac disease relevant gluten T-cell epitopes restricted by HLA-DQ molecules. Immunogenetics 2012;64:455–60.

[315] Juhasz A, Gell G, Bekes F, Balazs E. The epitopes in wheat proteins for defining toxic units relevant to human health. Funct Integr Genomics 2012;12:585–98.

[316] Ciccocioppo R, di Sabatino A, Ara C, Biagi F, Perilli M, Amicosante G, et al. Gliadin and tissue transglutaminase complexes in normal and coeliac duodenal mucosa. Clin Exp Immunol 2003;134:516–24.

[317] Fleckenstein B, Qiao SW, Larsen MR, Jung G, Roepstorff P, Sollid LM. Molecular characterization of covalent complexes between tissue transglutaminase and gliadin peptides. J Biol Chem 2004;279:17607–16.

[318] Dieterich W, Esslinger B, Trapp D, Hahn E, Huff T, Seilmeier W, et al. Cross linking to tissue transglutaminase and collagen favours gliadin toxicity in coeliac disease. Gut 2006;55:478–84.

[319] Dorum S, Arntzen M, Qiao SW, Holm A, Koehler CJ, Thiede B, et al. The preferred substrates for transglutaminase 2 in a complex wheat gluten digest are peptide fragments harboring celiac disease T-cell epitopes. PLoS One 2010;5: e14056.
[320] Kim CY, Quarsten H, Bergseng E, Khosla C, Sollid LM. Structural basis for HLA-DQ2-mediated presentation of gluten epitopes in celiac disease. Proc Natl Acad Sci USA 2004;101:4175–9.
[321] Bergseng E, Xia J, Kim CY, Khosla C, Sollid LM. Main chain hydrogen bond interactions in the binding of proline-rich gluten peptides to the celiac disease-associated HLA-DQ2 molecule. J Biol Chem 2005;280:21791–6.
[322] van de Wal Y, Kooy YMC, Drijfhout JW, Amons R, Papadopoulos GK, Koning F. Unique peptide binding characteristics of the disease-associated DQ(α1*0501, β1*0201) vs. the non-disease-associated DQ(α1*0201, β1*0202) molecule. Immunogenetics 1997;46:484–92.
[323] Henderson KN, Tye-Din JA, Reid HH, Chen Z, Borg NA, Beissbarth T, et al. A structural and immunological basis for the role of human leukocyte antigen DQ8 in celiac disease. Immunity 2007;27:23–34.
[324] Sollid LM. Coeliac disease: dissecting a complex inflammatory disorder. Nat Rev Immunol 2002;2:647–55.
[325] Wieser H, Konitzer K, Koehler P. Celiac disease – multidisciplinary approaches. Cereal Foods World 2012;57:215–24.
[326] Stamnaes J, Pinkas DM, Fleckenstein B, Khosla C, Sollid LM. Redox regulation of transglutaminase 2 activity. J Biol Chem 2010;285:25402–9.
[327] Kagnoff MF. Celiac disease: pathogenesis of a model immunogenetic disease. J Clin Invest 2007;117:41–9.
[328] Lundin KEA, Scott H, Hansen T, Paulsen G, Halstensen TS, Fausa O, et al. Gliadin-specific HLA-DQ(α1*0501, β1*0201) restricted T cells isolated from the small intestinal mucosa of celiac disease patients. J Exp Med 1993;178: 187–96.
[329] Molberg O, Kett K, Scott H, Thorsby E, Sollid LM, Lundin KEA. Gliadin specific, HLA DQ2-restricted T cells are commonly found in small intestinal biopsies from celiac disease patients, but not from controls. Scand J Immunol 1997;46:103–8.
[330] Bodd M, Raki M, Bergseng E, Jahnsen J, Lundin KEA, Sollid LM. Direct cloning and tetramer staining to measure the frequency of intestinal gluten-reactive T cells in celiac disease. Eur J Immunol 2013;43:2605–12.
[331] Vader W, Kooy Y, van Veelen P, de Ru A, Harris D, Benckhuijsen W, et al. The gluten response in children with celiac disease is directed toward multiple gliadin and glutenin peptides. Gastroenterology 2002;122:1729–37.
[332] Ellis HJ, Pollock EL, Engel W, Fraser JS, Rosen-Bronson S, Wieser H, et al. Investigation of the putative immunodominant T cell epitopes in coeliac disease. Gut 2003;52:212–7.
[333] van de Wal Y, Kooy YMC, van Veelen P, Vader W, August SA, Drijfhout JW, et al. Glutenin is involved in the gluten-driven mucosal T cell response. Eur J Immunol 1999;29:3133–9.
[334] Moustakas AK, van de Wal Y, Routsias J, Kooy YMC, van Veelen P, Drijfhout JW, et al. Structure of celiac disease-associated HLA-DQ8 and non-associated HLA-DQ9 alleles in complex with two disease-specific epitopes. Int Immunol 2000;12:1157–66.

[335] Beaurepaire C, Smyth S, McKay DM. Interferon-γ regulation of intestinal epithelial permeability. J Interferon Cytokine Res 2009;29:133–44.

[336] Przemioslo RT, Lundin KEA, Sollid LM, Nelufer J, Ciclitira PJ. Histological changes in small bowel mucosa induced by gliadin sensitive T lymphocytes can be blocked by anti-interferon gamma antibody. Gut 1995;36:874–9.

[337] di Niro R, Mesin L, Zheng NY, Stamnaes J, Morrissey M, Lee JH, et al. High abundance of plasma cells secreting transglutaminase 2-specific IgA autoantibodies with limited somatic hypermutation in celiac disease intestinal lesions. Nat Med 2012;18:441–5.

[338] Sollid LM, Molberg O, McAdam S, Lundin KEA. Autoantibodies in coeliac disease: tissue transglutaminase – guilt by association? Gut 1997;41:851–2.

[339] Bjorck S, Brundin C, Lorinc E, Lynch KF, Agardh D. Screening detects a high proportion of celiac disease in young HLA-genotyped children. J Pediatr Gastroenterol Nutr 2010;50:49–53.

[340] Wieser H, Belitz HD, Ashkenazi A. Amino-acid sequence of the coeliac active peptide B3142. Z Lebensm Unters Forsch 1984;179:371–6.

[341] Sturgess R, Day P, Ellis HJ, Lundin KEA, Gjertsen HA, Kontakou M, et al. Wheat peptide challenge in coeliac disease. Lancet 1994;343:758–61.

[342] Marsh MN, Morgan S, Ensari A, Wardle T, Lobley R, Mills C, et al. In-vivo activity of peptides 31–43, 44–55, 56–68 of α-gliadin in gluten sensitive enteropathy (GSE). Gastroenterology 1995;108:A871.

[343] Johansen BH, Gjertsen HA, Vartdal F, Buus S, Thorsby E, Lundin KEA, et al. Binding of peptides from the N-terminal region of α-gliadin to the celiac disease-associated HLA-DQ2 molecule assessed in biochemical and T cell assays. Clin Immunol Immunopathol 1996;79:288–93.

[344] Maiuri L, Ciacci C, Ricciardelli I, Vacca L, Raia V, Auricchio S, et al. Association between innate response to gliadin and activation of pathogenic T cells in coeliac disease. Lancet 2003;362:30–7.

[345] Gianfrani C, Auricchio S, Troncone R. Adaptive and innate immune responses in celiac disease. Immunol Lett 2005;99:141–5.

[346] Abadie V, Discepolo V, Jabri B. Intraepithelial lymphocytes in celiac disease immunopathology. Semin Immunopathol 2012;34:551–66.

[347] Baghat G, Naiyer AJ, Sha JG, Harper J, Jabri B, Wang TC, et al. Small intestinal $CD8^{+}TCR\gamma\delta^{+}NKG2A^{+}$ intraepithelial lymphocytes have attributes of regulatory cells in patients with coeliac disease. J Clin Invest 2008;118:281–93.

[348] Maiuri L, Troncone R, Mayer M, Coletta S, Picarelli A, de Vincenzi M, et al. In vitro activities of A-gliadin-related synthetic peptides. Scand J Gastroenterol 1996;31:247–53.

[349] Tuckova L, Novotna J, Novak P, Flegelova Z, Kveton T, Jelinkova L, et al. Activation of macrophages by gliadin fragments: isolation and characterization of active peptide. J Leukoc Biol 2002;71:625–31.

[350] Nikulina M, Habich C, Flohe SB, Scott FW, Kolb H. Wheat gluten causes dendritic cell maturation and chemokine secretion. J Immunol 2004;173:1925–33.

[351] Palova-Jelinkova L, Rozkova D, Pecharova B, Bartova J, Sediva A, Tlaskalova-Hogenova H, et al. Gliadin fragments induce phenotypic and functional maturation of human dendritic cells. J Immunol 2005;175:7038–45.

[352] de Paolo RW, Abadie V, Tang F, Fehlner-Peach H, Hall JA, Wang W, et al. Co-adjuvant effects of retinoic acid and IL-15 induce inflammatory immunity to dietary antigens. Nature 2011;471:220–4.

[353] Huee S, Mention JJ, Monteiro RC, Zhang SL, Cellier C, Schmitz J, et al. A direct role for NKG2D/MICA interaction in villous atrophy during celiac disease. Immunity 2004;21:367–77.

[354] Meresse B, Chen Z, Ciszewski C, Tretiakova M, Bhagat G, Krausz TN, et al. Coordinated induction by IL15 of a TCR-independent NKG2D signaling pathway converts CTL into lymphokine-activated killer cells in celiac disease. Immunity 2004;21:357–66.

[355] Yokoyama S, Watanabe N, Sato N, Perera PY, Filkoski L, Tanaka T, et al. Antibody-mediated blockade of IL-15 reverses the autoimmune intestinal damage in transgenic mice that overexpress IL-15 in enterocytes. Proc Natl Acad Sci USA 2009;106:15849–54.

[356] Lindfors K, Laehdeaho ML, Kalliokoski S, Kurppa K, Collin P, Maeki M, et al. Future treatment strategies for celiac disease. Expert Opin Ther Targets 2012;16:665–75.

[357] Brandtzaeg P. The changing immunological paradigm in coeliac disease. Immunol Lett 2006;105:127–39.

Chapter 2

Gluten—The Precipitating Factor

CHAPTER OUTLINE

1. OVERVIEW ON CEREALS

Cereals are the most important staple foods worldwide. The major cereals are wheat, corn, rice, barley, sorghum, millet, oats, and rye. They are grown on nearly 60% of the cultivated area in the world. Corn, rice, and wheat take up the largest part of areas under cultivation for cereals and yield the largest quantities of grains (875, 718, and 675 million metric tons (t), respectively, in 2012 [1]), which are predominantly used for food and animal feed production.

Cereals produce dry one-seeded fruits, called kernels or grains, in the form of a caryopsis, in which the fruit coat (pericarp) is strongly bound to the seed coat (testa). Grain size and weight can vary widely from rather large corn grains to small millet grains. The anatomy of cereal grains is fairly uniform: Fruit and seed coats (bran) enclose the germ and the

Celiac Disease and Gluten. http://dx.doi.org/10.1016/B978-0-12-420220-7.00002-X

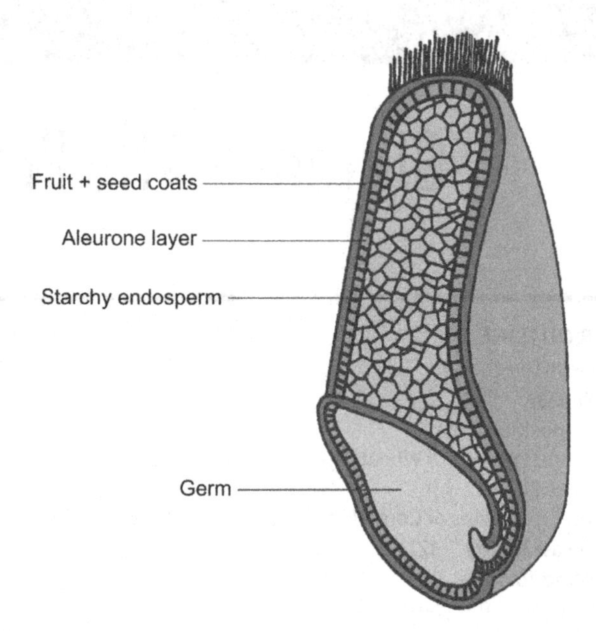

■ **FIGURE 2.1** Cross-section of a wheat grain consisting of its main compartments: starchy endosperm, aleurone layer, bran (fruit and seed coats), and germ.

endosperm, the latter consisting of the starchy endosperm and the aleurone layer (Figure 2.1). In oats, barley, rice, and some wheat species (e.g., spelt, emmer, einkorn), the husk is fused with the fruit coat and cannot be removed simply by threshing, as with "naked" cereals such as common wheat and rye.

Botanically, cereals are grasses belonging to the monocot family *Poaceae* (grass family). Wheat (*Triticum*), rye (*Secale*), and barley (*Hordeum*) are closely related members of the subfamily *Pooideae* and the tribe *Triticeae* (Figure 2.2) [2]. Oats (*Avena*) is a distant relative to the *Triticeae* within the subfamily *Pooideae*, whereas rice (*Oryza*), corn (*Zea*), sorghum (*Sorghum*), and millet (*Pennisetum*) show separate evolutionary lines. Cultivated wheat consists of five species: the hexaploid (genome AABBDD) common wheat (*Triticum aestivum* L.) and spelt wheat (*Triticum spelta* L.); the tetraploid (genome AABB) durum wheat (*Triticum durum* Desf.) and emmer (*Triticum dicoccon* (Schrank) Schübler), and the diploid (genome AA) einkorn (*Triticum monococcum* L.). Common wheat, also called bread wheat, was developed by spontaneous hybridization of *Triticum turgidum* (genome AABB) and *Aegilops tauschii* (genome DD) about 10,000 years ago. Triticale is a man-made hybrid of durum wheat and rye (genome AABBRR). Rarely used cereals are Kamut®, teff, ragi,

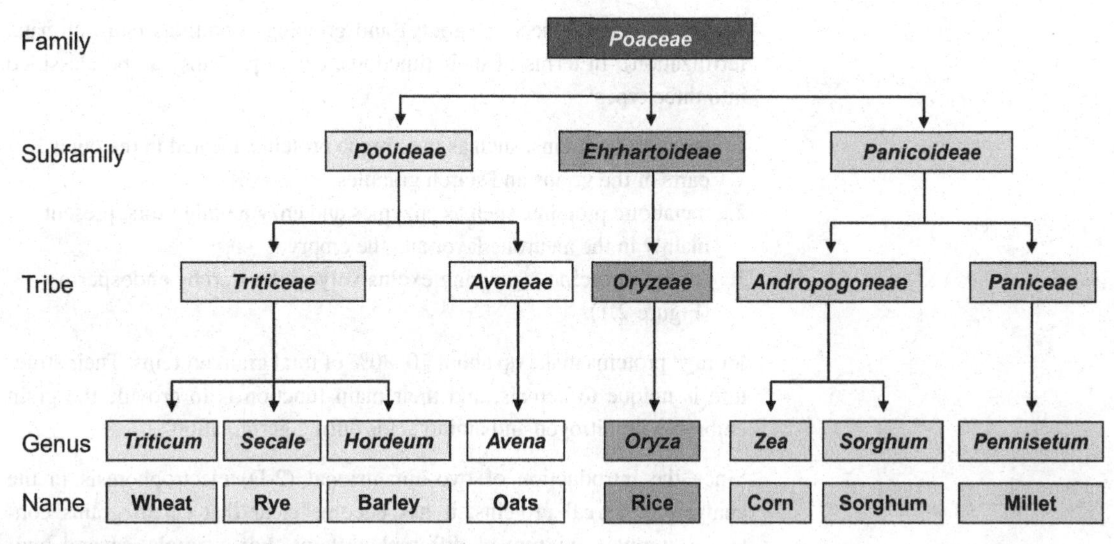

■ **FIGURE 2.2** Phylogeny of cereals belonging to the monocot family *Poaceae*.

and Job's tears. Within each cereal species, numerous varieties exist, produced by breeding to optimize agronomical, technological, and nutritional properties.

The chemical composition of cereal grains is characterized by the high content of carbohydrates in the form of polysaccharides [3]. Among the nutritionally available carbohydrates, starch deposited in the endosperm is predominant (56–74%). Nonavailable fiber (e.g., arabinoxylans, β-glucans, cellulose), located mainly in the bran, ranges from 2% to 13%. The second important group of constituents is protein, which falls within an average range of 8–12%. In particular, the storage proteins of some cereals have been identified as precipitating factors in celiac disease (CD). Therefore, cereal proteins will be considered in detail in the following sections. Cereal lipids belong to minor constituents (2–4%), with the exception of oat lipids (≈7%). The mineral content ranges from 1.0% to 2.5%. Cereals are good sources of B-vitamins and tocopherols. Both minerals and vitamins are concentrated in the aleurone layer and the germ.

2. CEREAL PROTEINS

2.1 Composition

Since the 1950s, it has been known that cereal proteins are the antigens for CD-specific immune response. The protein content of cereal grains covers a broad variable range, from less than 6% to more than 20%, depending on genotype (cereal, species, variety) and growing conditions (soil, climate, fertilization). In terms of their functions, cereal proteins can be classified into three types:

1. structural proteins, such as membrane proteins, located in the outer parts of the grains and starch granules;
2. metabolic proteins, such as enzymes and enzyme inhibitors, present mainly in the aleurone layer and the embryo;
3. storage proteins, occurring exclusively in the starchy endosperm (Figure 2.1).

Storage proteins make up about 70–80% of total grain proteins. Their structure is unique to cereals, and their main function is to provide the grain embryo with nitrogen and amino acids during germination.

Since the introduction of two-dimensional (2-D) electrophoresis in the analysis of cereal proteins, it has become clear that cereal grains contain a complex mixture of different proteins. For example, several hundreds of protein components have been detected in wheat flour [4] (Figure 2.3). Traditionally, cereal proteins have been classified into four fractions (Osborne fractions) according to their differences in solubility: (1) albumins, (2) globulins, (3) prolamins, and (4) glutelins [5]. Albumins are soluble in water and dilute salt solutions. Globulins are insoluble in pure water but soluble in salt solutions. Both fractions mainly consist of metabolic proteins. Prolamins classically are defined as cereal proteins that are insoluble in water and salt solution but soluble in aqueous alcohols (e.g., 60–70% ethanol); they mainly occur as monomers. Glutelins are polymerized by interchain disulfide bonds. Originally, they were described by Osborne as remaining insoluble after the extraction of albumins, globulins, and prolamins but extractable with dilute acids or bases [5]. However, notable portions of glutelins are insoluble in weak acids such as acetic acid, and extraction with strong acids or bases may affect their primary structure. Nowadays, complete extraction of glutelins is achieved at increased temperatures (e.g., 50°C) by solvents containing a mixture of aqueous alcohols (e.g., 60% ethanol or 50% propanol), reducing agents (e.g., 2-mercaptoethanol or dithiothreitol), and disaggregating compounds (e.g., urea or guanidine) [6]. Using this treatment, disulfide bonds are cleaved, and glutelins are obtained as monomeric subunits that are soluble in aqueous alcohols like the prolamins. Both prolamins and glutelins are storage proteins. A small group of flour proteins does not fall into any of the four solubility fractions. With starch, they remain in the insoluble residue after Osborne fractions have been extracted; they mainly belong to the structural protein type.

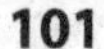

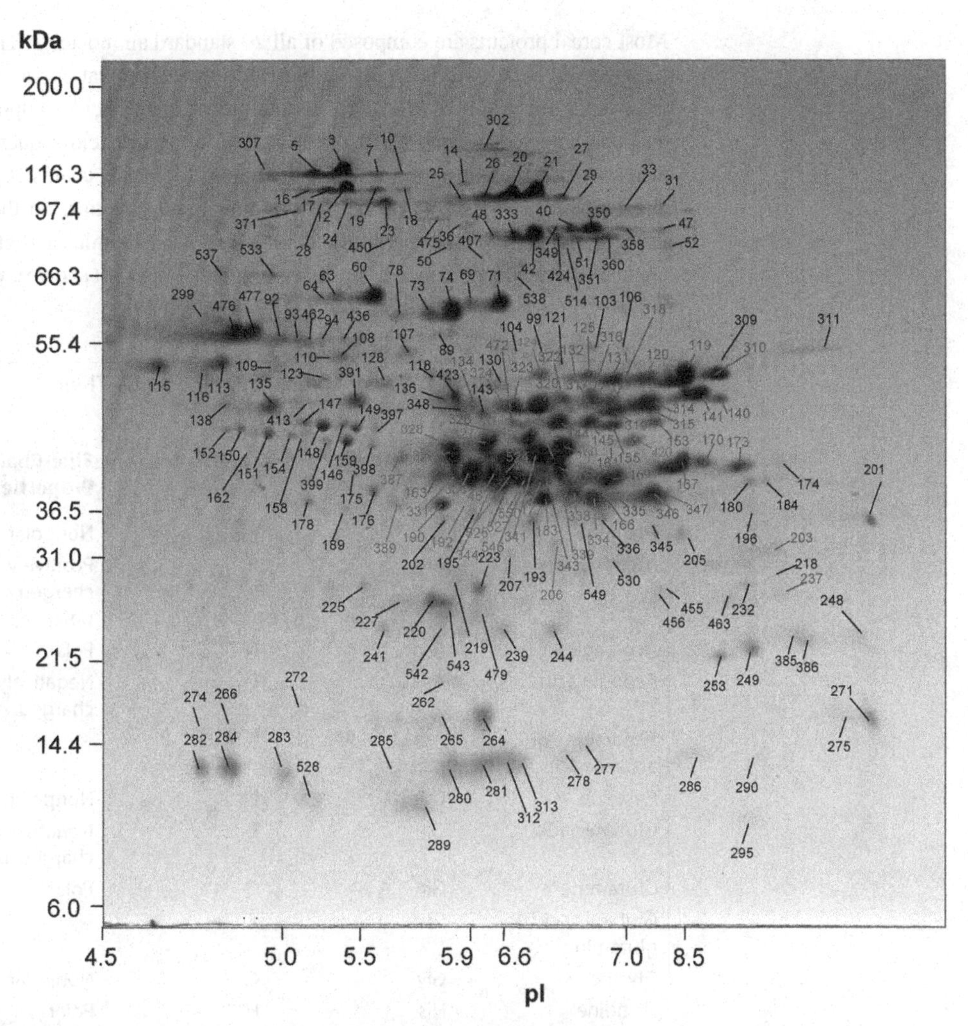

FIGURE 2.3 Two-dimensional electrophoresis of wheat flour proteins. *From Dupont et al. [4], with permission of BioMed Central.*

The storage proteins of the various cereals have been given common names: wheat, gliadins (prolamins) and glutenins (glutelins); rye, secalins; barley, hordeins; oat, avenins; corn, zeins; rice, oryzins; and millet and sorghum, kafirins. The proteinaceous mass that remains after wheat dough is washed with water to remove starch and soluble constituents consists of gliadins and glutenins and is called gluten in the field of cereal chemistry and technology.

Most cereal proteins are composed of all 20 standard amino acids. These are listed in Table 2.1. Additionally, Table 2.1 shows abbreviations as a three-letter code (usually used for the presentation of amino acid compositions) and one-letter code (used for the presentation of amino acid sequences); it also shows the chemical properties of their amino acid side chains. Albumins and globulins, on the one hand, and prolamins and glutelins, on the other, differ significantly in their amino acid compositions. Albumins and globulins are characterized by balanced, "ordinary" compositions (not shown), whereas

Table 2.1 Common Names of Standard Amino Acids, Their Abbreviations, and Side-Chain Properties

Amino Acid	Three-Letter Code	One-Letter Code	Side-Chain Properties
Alanine	Ala	A	Nonpolar
Arginine	Arg	R	Positively charged, polar
Asparagine	Asn	N	Polar
Aspartic acid	Asp	D	Negatively charged, polar
Asparagine or aspartic acid	Asx	B	–
Cysteine	Cys	C	Nonpolar
Glutamic acid	Glu	E	Negatively charged, polar
Glutamine	Gln	Q	Polar
Glutamic acid or glutamine	Glx	Z	–
Glycine	Gly	G	Nonpolar
Histidine	His	H	Polar
Isoleucine	Ile	I	Nonpolar
Leucine	Leu	L	Nonpolar
Lysine	Lys	K	Positively charged, polar
Methionine	Met	M	Nonpolar
Phenylalanine	Phe	F	Nonpolar
Proline	Pro	P	Nonpolar
Serine	Ser	S	Polar
Threonine	Thr	T	Polar
Tryptophan	Trp	W	Nonpolar
Tyrosine	Tyr	Y	Polar
Valine	Val	V	Nonpolar

prolamins and glutelins show unbalanced, "extraordinary" compositions (Tables 2.2 and 2.3) [7]. Typical to all prolamin and glutelin fractions is their high grade of amidation of the acidic amino acids, particularly of glutamic acid. Thus, glutamic acid almost entirely occurs in its amidated form as glutamine, and this amino acid is generally predominating (15.5–37.1 mol%). Additional common features of all storage proteins are low contents of the essential amino acids lysine (0.0–4.0%), methionine (0.5–2.4%), and tryptophan (0.0–0.8%). For this reason, the biological value of cereal storage proteins is rather low. Considering this aspect from a nutritional point of view, a gluten-free diet (GFD) is not disadvantageous for consumers.

The name "prolamins" reflects the characteristics of amino acid compositions with high contents of *pro*line and glut*amine*, which is particularly true for prolamins of wheat, rye, and barley (35–37% glutamine and 17–23% proline). Both amino acids glutamine and proline (Figure 2.4) play significant but different roles in the functions of storage proteins. In contrast to

Table 2.2 Amino Acid Composition (mol%) of Prolamins of Different Cereals [7][a]

AA	WH	RY	BA	OA	RI	MI	CO
Ala	2.8	3.0	2.3	5.5	9.1	13.5	13.6
Arg	1.7	1.9	2.0	2.7	4.7	0.8	1.2
Asx	2.7	2.4	1.7	2.3	7.3	6.8	4.9
Cys	2.2	2.2	1.9	3.3	0.8	1.1	1.0
Glx	37.1	35.4	35.3	34.1	19.6	21.8	19.4
Gly	2.9	4.5	2.2	2.7	5.8	1.5	2.6
His	1.7	1.2	1.2	1.1	1.5	1.3	1.1
Ile	4.1	3.0	3.6	3.3	4.6	5.2	3.9
Leu	6.9	5.8	6.1	10.6	11.8	13.4	18.5
Lys	0.8	1.0	0.5	1.0	0.5	0.0	0.0
Met	1.1	1.0	0.9	2.1	0.5	1.7	1.1
Phe	4.6	4.5	5.8	5.3	4.8	4.9	4.9
Pro	16.6	18.4	23.0	10.2	5.1	7.8	10.2
Ser	5.9	6.6	4.6	3.8	7.5	6.4	6.9
Thr	2.3	2.6	2.1	2.3	2.9	3.8	3.1
Trp	0.4	0.4	0.6	0.3	0.5	1.5	0.0
Tyr	2.0	1.7	2.3	1.7	6.1	2.1	3.6
Val	4.2	4.4	3.9	7.7	6.9	6.4	4.0
Amide[b]	37.5	34.7	34.9	31.6	23.3	23.0	23.0

[a]*AA, amino acid; WH, wheat; RY, rye; BA, barley; OA, oats; RI, rice; MI, millet; CO, corn.*
[b]*Sum of asparagine (Asn) and glutamine (Gln).*

Table 2.3 Amino Acid Composition (mol%) of Glutelins (+Residual Proteins) of Different Cereals [7][a]

AA	WH	RY	BA	OA	RI	MI	CO
Ala	4.4	7.3	5.6	6.5	7.9	10.1	9.4
Arg	2.7	3.8	2.5	6.0	6.1	3.5	3.2
Asx	3.7	7.1	4.9	9.3	9.5	7.6	5.5
Cys	1.4	0.8	0.5	1.2	1.2	1.7	1.8
Glx	30.1	19.7	24.2	19.0	15.5	16.8	16.0
Gly	7.9	9.2	6.4	7.9	7.4	6.9	6.9
His	1.8	2.0	2.0	2.4	2.1	2.3	3.3
Ile	3.5	3.7	4.0	4.6	4.5	4.1	3.4
Leu	6.9	7.4	7.5	7.8	8.4	9.1	10.9
Lys	2.1	4.0	2.8	3.2	3.3	3.1	2.4
Met	1.3	1.6	1.3	1.3	2.4	1.6	2.8
Phe	3.6	3.8	4.0	4.8	4.3	3.7	3.3
Pro	11.9	9.4	14.2	5.5	5.1	8.4	11.5
Ser	7.3	6.9	6.7	6.6	6.7	5.9	6.1
Thr	3.6	4.7	4.2	4.2	4.2	5.1	4.2
Trp	0.6	0.4	0.3	0.7	0.8	0.6	0.3
Tyr	2.4	2.3	1.7	2.8	3.6	2.9	2.9
Val	4.8	5.9	7.2	6.2	7.0	6.6	6.1
Amide[b]	31.0	21.3	23.6	20.2	16.6	16.4	16.4

[a]*AA, amino acid; WH, wheat; RY, rye; BA, barley; OA, oats; RI, rice; MI, millet; CO, corn.*
[b]*Sum of asparagine (Asn) and glutamine (Gln).*

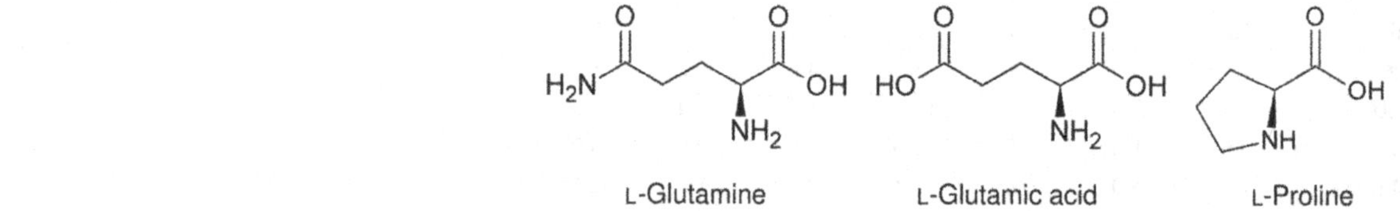

L-Glutamine L-Glutamic acid L-Proline

■ **FIGURE 2.4** Structures of the amino acids L-glutamine, L-glutamic acid, and L-proline.

most amino acids, glutamine contains two nitrogen (N) atoms, which are important for the nitrogen supply of the embryo during the first stage of germination. Unique to proline is the secondary amino group, which causes kinks within the protein chains and, therefore, allows a dense packing of the protein strands in the starchy endosperm. Moreover, proline residues prevent the storage proteins from degradation by external enzymatic attack.

In the context of CD, glutamine and proline also are of outstanding importance (see Chapter 1, Section 6). Their proline-rich nature makes gluten proteins resistant to complete proteolytic degradation in the gastrointestinal lumen, and, therefore, long peptide fragments survive in the stomach and small intestine. Moreover, proline residues contribute to the formation of left-handed poly–Pro II helical conformations of peptides, which are preferred for human leukocyte antigen (HLA)-DQ binding. Glutamine-rich peptides are good substrates for the intestinal tissue enzyme transglutaminase 2 (TG2). Proline influences the specificity of the enzyme toward glutamine and, thus, only specific glutamine residues are substrates for deamidation and transamidation, both typical for the CD pathomechanism.

Prolamins of wheat, rye, and barley show the highest values for glutamine (35–37%) and proline (17–23%), followed by leucine (6–7%) and phenylalanine (5–6%). Histidine (1–2%), lysine (≈1%), methionine (≈1%), and tryptophan (<1%) occur only in traces. Prolamins of rice, millet, sorghum, and corn are lower in glutamine (19–22%) and proline (5–10%) but rich in leucine (12–19%) and alanine (9–14%). Prolamins of oats are in a medium position: their glutamine content (34%) is similar to that of the *Triticeae* prolamins, and the values of proline (10%) and leucine (11%) are close to those of rice, millet, and corn. Thus, the amino acid compositions of prolamins show a close relationship to the phylogeny of the cereals (Figure 2.2) as well as to their CD toxicity [8] (see Section 3.2). Compared with prolamins, glutelins and residual proteins show a more balanced amino acid composition, mainly with less glutamine and proline and increased values for most of the other amino acids. Similar to prolamins, distinct differences are obvious between wheat, rye, and barley—on the one hand—and rice, millet, and corn—on the other—with oats in an intermediate position.

The content of Osborne fractions varies considerably and depends on genotype and growing conditions. Moreover, the results of the stepwise Osborne fractionation are strongly influenced by experimental conditions, and the fractions obtained are not clear-cut. Therefore, data from the literature on the qualitative and quantitative compositions of Osborne fractions differ and are partly contradictory. On average, the smallest proportion of total proteins is present in the globulin fraction, followed by the albumin fraction. An exception is oat globulins, which amount to more than 50% of total proteins. In most cereals, prolamins are the dominating fraction. Oat prolamins, however, are minor proteins, and rice is almost free of prolamins. Each Osborne fraction consists of numerous, partly related proteins. Nowadays, efficient methods for their separation are available, for example, methods based on electrophoresis such as acid polyacrylamide gel electrophoresis (PAGE), sodium dodecylsulfate (SDS-) PAGE, isoelectrofocusing (IEF) alone or in combination with SDS-PAGE (2-D electrophoresis; Figure 2.3), and high-performance liquid chromatography (HPLC) such as reversed-phase (RP-) and gel permeation (GP-) HPLC. All of these methods confirm the complex protein composition of each fraction. Preparation of single components using these methods has allowed further structural characterization and classification and, in addition, tests on functionality, allergenicity, and CD toxicity.

2.2 **Storage Proteins of Wheat, Rye, Barley, and Oats**

The prolamin and glutelin fractions of wheat, rye, barley, and oats consist of numerous, partly closely related proteins. The reason for this heterogeneity is gene mutations (substitution, deletion, and insertion of DNA nucleobases) during the evolution of the cereals, resulting in many modifications in the amino acid sequences. To illustrate, the N-terminal amino acid sequences (positions 1–40) of nine selected α-gliadins are shown in Figure 2.5. Because of sequence homologies, the high number of protein components can be reduced to a small number of different protein types.

Along with the progress of protein separation techniques, the nomenclature of prolamin monomers and glutelin subunits has been developed step by step and is, therefore, rather confusing and inconsistent. On the one hand, the proteins were named based on differences in electrophoretic mobility (e.g., ω-, α-, β-, and γ-gliadins or ω- and γ-secalins). And on the other hand, the terms were based on differences in molecular weights (e.g., high-molecular-weight glutenin subunits (HMW-GS) and low-molecular-weight glutenin subunits (LMW-GS); or D-, C-, and B-hordeins). The nomenclature based on electrophoretic or chromatographic mobility does not always agree with the classification according to the primary structures (amino acid sequences) determined

	1 — 40
a	VRVPVPQLQPQNPSQQQPQEQVPLVQQQQFPGQQQQFPPQ
b	VRVPVPQLQPQ**S**PSQQQPQEQVPLVQQQQFPGQQQQFPPQ
c	VRVPVPQLQP**K**NPSQQQPQEQVPLVQQQQFPGQQQQFPPQ
d	VRVPVPQLQPQNPSQQQPQ**K**QVPLVQQQQFPGQQQ**P**FPPQ
e	VRVPVPQ**P**QPQNPSQ**P**QPQ**R**QVPLVQQQQFPGQQQQFPPQ
f	VRVPVPQ**P**QPQNPSQ**P**QPQ**G**QVPLVQQQQFPGQQQQFPPQ
g	VRVPVPQLQ**L**QNPSQQQPQEQVPLVQ**E**QQF**Q**GQQQ**P**FPPQ
h	VR**F**PVPQLQPQNPSQQQPQEQVPLVQQQQF**L**GQQQ**P**FPPQ
i	VRVPVPQLQPQNPSQQQPQEQVPLVQQQQF**L**GQQQ**P**FPPQ

■ **FIGURE 2.5** Examples of N-terminal amino acid sequences of α-gliadins. Modifications labeled in bold indicate point mutations within the DNA.

later. For example, studies on amino acid sequences revealed that α- and β-gliadins fall into one type, mostly termed α-type and sometimes α/β-type.

The most important criterion for protein classification is the primary structure (amino acid sequence). In the past decades, numerous sequences of cereal storage proteins, almost entirely determined by DNA sequencing, have been published either in original publications or in databases. The data indicate that, in accordance with phylogeny (Figure 2.2) and amino acid compositions (Tables 2.2 and 2.3), the storage proteins of wheat, rye, barley, and, partly, oats (only prolamins) are closely related and differ decisively from those of other cereals.

Based on homologous amino acid sequences and similar molecular weights, the storage proteins of the *Triticeae* and oats (only prolamins) can be divided into three groups (Table 2.4) [12]:

1. HMW group;
2. Medium-molecular-weight (MMW) group;
3. LMW group.

Each group contains numerous related proteins that can be assigned to different types. The proteins partly occur as monomers and partly as polymers linked by interchain disulfide bonds.

The HMW group consists of three types: (1) HMW-GS of wheat, (2) HMW-secalins of rye, and (3) D-hordeins of barley. Oats is missing from this group. HMW-GS and HMW-secalins can be subdivided into the x- and y-types, which

Table 2.4 Classification and Proportions of *Pooideae* Storage Proteins[a]

Group	Wheat	Rye	Barley	Oats
HMW	HMW-GS (p) 11%	HMW-Secalins (p) 9%	D-Hordeins (p) 5%	–
MMW	ω1,2-Gliadins (m) 4%	ω-Secalins (m) 18%	C-Hordeins (m) 36%	–
	ω5-Gliadins (m) 3%	–	–	–
LMW	LMW-GS (p) 22%	γ-75k-Secalins (p) 48%	B-Hordeins (p) 27%	–
	γ-Gliadins (m) 27%	γ-40k-Secalins (m) 25%	γ-Hordeins (m) 32%	Avenins 100%
	α-Gliadins (m) 33%	–	–	–

HMW, high-molecular-weight; MMW, medium-molecular-weight; LMW, low-molecular-weight; GS, glutenin subunit.
[a]Wheat, Monopol [9]; rye, Halo [10]; barley, Golden Promise [11]; m = monomeric; p = polymeric.

differ in molecular weights and number of repetitive units. Proteins of the HMW group consist of around 600–800 amino acid residues, corresponding to molecular weights of 70,000–90,000. The amino acid compositions are characterized by high contents of glutamine (≈26–36%), glycine (≈16–20%), and proline (≈10–15%), which account for approximately 60% of total amino acid residues (Table 2.5). The amino acid sequences can be separated into three structural domains (Figure 2.6): (1) a nonrepetitive N-terminal domain A of ≈100 residues, (2) a repetitive central domain B of ≈500–700 residues, and (3) a nonrepetitive domain C of ≈40 residues. Domains A and C are characterized by relatively balanced amino acid compositions, including most or all cysteines and charged amino acids (glutamic acid, arginine). Domain B contains numerous repetitive hexapeptides such as QQPGQG as a backbone. These are frequently modified and interspersed by hexapeptides such as YYPTSP and tripeptides such as QQP

Table 2.5 Amino Acid Compositions (mol%) of High-Molecular-Weight Group Proteins of Wheat, Rye, and Barley[a]

AA	HMW-GSx	HMW-GSy	HMW-SECx	HMW-SECy	D-HOR
Ala	2.9	3.8	2.4	3.5	3.2
Arg	1.2	2.7	1.6	2.1	1.6
Asn	0.0	0.0	0.0	0.0	0.9
Asp	0.5	0.6	0.7	0.7	0.6
Cys	0.5	1.1	0.5	1.1	1.4
Gln	35.8	32.3	33.5	33.9	25.7
Glu	2.1	2.7	2.5	3.9	2.2
Gly	20.0	17.9	20.1	17.7	15.8
His	0.5	2.3	0.8	2.5	3.1
Ile	0.5	1.1	0.5	0.8	0.7
Leu	4.4	3.8	3.7	3.2	4.1
Lys	0.7	1.1	0.9	1.0	1.2
Met	0.3	0.6	0.3	0.6	0.4
Phe	0.3	0.3	0.3	0.3	1.3
Pro	13.0	11.0	14.7	12.4	10.5
Ser	6.0	6.6	5.3	5.5	10.8
Thr	2.9	3.6	3.8	3.6	7.1
Trp	1.0	0.9	0.5	0.6	1.2
Tyr	5.7	5.2	6.4	4.8	4.1
Val	1.7	2.4	1.5	1.8	4.1
Residues	815	637	760	716	686
Code[b]	Q6R2V1	Q52JL3	Q94IK6	Q94IL4	Q40054

[a]*AA, amino acid; HMW-GSx, wheat high-molecular-weight glutenin subunit x-type; HMW-GSy, wheat high-molecular-weight glutenin subunit y-type; HMW-SECx, rye high-molecular-weight secalin x-type; HMW-SECy, rye high-molecular-weight secalin y-type; D-HOR, D-hordein.*
[b]*Accession number of proteins in database Uni Prot KB used for calculation.*

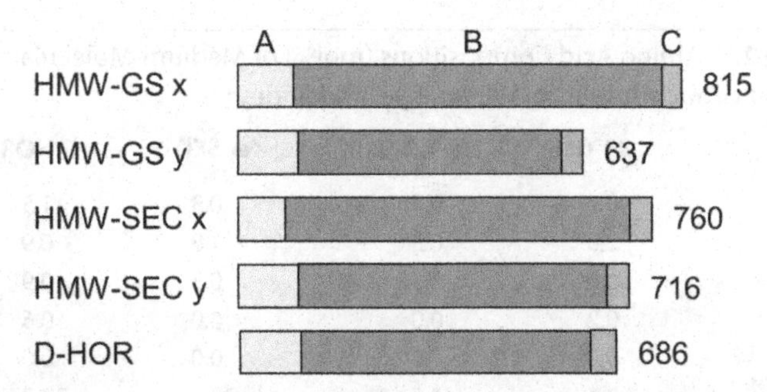

■ **FIGURE 2.6** Schematic architecture of proteins of the high-molecular-weight (HMW) group of wheat, rye, and barley (A, N-terminal domain; B, repetitive domain; C, C-terminal domain; individual proteins correspond to accessions given in Table 2.5; HMW-GSx, wheat high-molecular-weight glutenin subunit x-type; HMW-GSy, wheat high-molecular-weight glutenin subunit y-type; HMW-SECx, rye high-molecular-weight secalin x-type; HMW-SECy, rye high-molecular-weight secalin y-type; D-HOR, D-hordein). (Please see color plate at the back of the book.)

and QPG. Differences among the subunits of the HMW group are mainly due to modifications of single residues and to the number and arrangement of repeats. For example, the x-type differs from the y-type by a shorter domain A and a longer domain B. Because of the importance of HMW-GS for the bread-making quality of wheat, single subunits have been numbered according to the coding genome (1A, 1B, or 1D), the protein type (x or y), and the mobility on SDS-PAGE (originally from no. 1 to no. 12). Examples of nomenclature are HMW-GS 1Ax1, 1Bx7, and 1Dy10 [13]. In general, proteins of the HMW group do not occur as monomers in the prolamin fractions, but are polymerized by interchain disulfide bonds and are present in glutelin fractions. After reduction of disulfide bonds, the resulting subunits are alcohol-soluble like the prolamins.

The MMW group consists of the homologous ω1,2-gliadins of wheat, ω-secalins of rye, and C-hordeins of barley. These proteins contain between 300 and 400 residues, which correspond to molecular weights of around 40,000. Additionally, wheat contains unique ω5-gliadins with more than 400 residues and molecular weights of around 50,000. Proteins corresponding to the MMW group are not present in oats. Proteins of the MMW group have extremely unbalanced amino acid compositions with typically high contents of glutamine, proline, and phenylalanine, which together account for about 80% of total amino acid residues (Table 2.6). They occur mainly as monomers and are readily soluble in aqueous alcohols and, partly, even in water. They consist almost entirely of repetitive sequences with only short nonrepetitive N-terminal and C-terminal domains (up to ≈30 residues) (Figure 2.7). The central domains contain repeats consisting mainly of glutamine, proline, and phenylalanine. Typical repetitive units of ω1,2-gliadins, ω-secalins, and C-hordeins are heptapeptides such as QPQQPFP. Those of ω5-gliadins are different in number and composition (QQQPF) of repeats.

Table 2.6 Amino Acid Compositions (mol%) of Medium-Molecular-Weight Group Proteins of Wheat, Rye, and Barley[a]

AA	ω5-GLI	ω1,2-GLI	ω-SEC	C-HOR
Ala	0.2	0.5	0.3	1.5
Arg	1.0	0.5	1.8	0.9
Asn	0.0	0.5	0.3	0.9
Asp	0.2	0.0	0.0	0.6
Cys	0.0	0.0	0.0	0.0
Gln	53.1	41.6	39.6	37.3
Glu	1.9	1.4	2.7	1.5
Gly	0.7	0.8	0.6	0.6
His	1.4	0.5	0.3	0.6
Ile	4.3	1.6	4.7	3.4
Leu	3.1	4.0	4.4	8.6
Lys	0.7	0.5	0.3	0.9
Met	0.0	0.0	0.0	0.0
Phe	9.3	8.4	7.4	7.7
Pro	19.8	29.0	29.3	29.1
Ser	2.9	5.9	4.4	2.5
Thr	0.5	2.4	0.9	1.2
Trp	0.0	0.3	0.0	0.6
Tyr	0.7	1.6	1.2	1.8
Val	0.2	0.5	1.8	0.3
Residues	420	373	338	328
Code[b]	Q40215	Q6DLC7	Q04365	Q40055

[a]AA, amino acid; ω5-GLI, ω5-gliadin; ω1,2-GLI, ω1,2-gliadin; ω-SEC, ω-secalin; C-HOR, C-hordein.
[b]Accession number of proteins in database Uni Prot KB used for calculation.

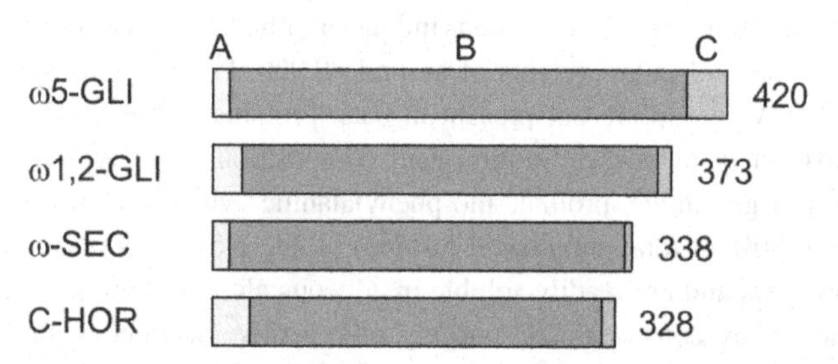

■ **FIGURE 2.7** Schematic architecture of proteins of the medium-molecular-weight group of wheat, rye, and barley (A, N-terminal domain; B, repetitive domain; C, C-terminal domain; individual proteins correspond to accessions given in Table 2.6; ω5-GLI, ω5-gliadin; ω1,2-GLI, ω1,2-gliadin; ω-SEC, ω-secalin; C-HOR, C-hordein). (Please see color plate at the back of the book.)

The LMW group can be divided into monomeric and polymeric proteins. The monomeric proteins include α- and γ-gliadins (wheat), γ-40k-secalins (rye), γ-hordeins (barley), and avenins (oats). The polymeric proteins are LMW-GS (wheat), γ-75k-secalins (rye), and B-hordeins (barley). Their sequences consist of approximately 300 amino acid residues corresponding to molecular weights of around 28,000–35,000, with the exception of γ-75k-secalins (≈430 residues, molecular weights ≈50,000) and avenins (≈200 residues, molecular weights ≈23,000). The amino acid compositions are characterized by relatively high contents of hydrophobic amino acids such as leucine (5–9%) and valine (5–8%), in addition to the predominating glutamine (28–36%) and proline (11–22%) (Table 2.7). According to structural homologies, amino acid sequences can be subdivided into an N-terminal domain containing sections I and II and a C-terminal domain containing sections III, IV, and V (Figure 2.8).

Table 2.7 Amino Acid Compositions (mol%) of Low-Molecular-Weight Group Proteins of Wheat, Rye, Barley, and Oats[a]

AA	α-GLI	γ-GLI	LMW-GS	γ-75k-SEC	γ-HOR	B-HOR	AVE
Ala	2.2	2.9	3.9	2.3	2.1	2.6	5.2
Arg	2.2	1.3	2.5	0.9	1.7	2.6	3.0
Asn	2.6	1.3	0.7	1.4	1.7	0.7	1.5
Asp	0.4	0.7	0.3	0.0	0.7	0.0	0.5
Cys	2.2	2.6	2.8	2.0	3.5	2.9	4.0
Gln	35.9	36.1	32.2	38.3	28.0	30.3	33.0
Glu	1.8	0.7	1.8	1.4	2.5	1.8	2.5
Gly	2.6	2.9	3.2	1.6	3.2	2.9	1.8
His	2.2	1.3	1.1	1.4	1.4	1.5	0.5
Ile	4.7	4.9	4.3	3.0	3.9	4.4	4.0
Leu	8.0	7.2	8.2	4.8	7.0	8.0	8.9
Lys	0.4	0.7	0.3	0.5	1.7	0.7	0.5
Met	0.7	1.6	1.8	0.9	1.7	1.1	2.0
Phe	3.7	4.9	4.3	5.0	5.6	4.7	6.4
Pro	14.3	17.5	12.8	21.8	16.8	19.4	10.8
Ser	5.1	5.5	8.9	6.9	5.6	4.7	2.5
Thr	1.8	2.0	3.5	1.6	2.8	2.2	2.5
Trp	0.4	1.0	0.7	0.0	0.7	0.7	0.0
Tyr	3.7	0.3	1.4	0.9	2.1	2.6	2.0
Val	5.1	4.6	5.3	5.3	7.3	6.2	8.4
Residues	273	308	282	436	286	274	203
Code[b]	Q9M4M5	Q94G91	Q52NZ4	Q9FR41	P17990	P06470	Q09072

[a]*AA, amino acid; α-GLI, α-gliadin; γ-GLI, γ-gliadin; LMW-GS, wheat low-molecular-weight glutenin subunit; γ-75k-SEC, γ-75k-secalin; γ-HOR, γ-hordein; B-HOR, B-hordein; AVE, avenin.*
[b]*Accession number of proteins in database Uni Prot KB used for calculation.*

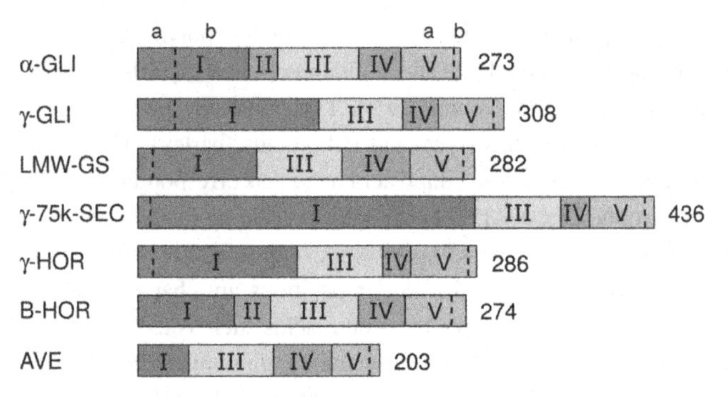

■ **FIGURE 2.8** Schematic architecture of proteins of the low-molecular-weight (LMW) group of wheat, rye, barley, and oats (sections I–II, N-terminal domain; sections III–V, C-terminal domain; individual proteins correspond to accessions given in Table 2.7; α-GLI, α-gliadin; γ-GLI, γ-gliadin; LMW-GS, wheat low-molecular-weight glutenin subunit; γ-75k-SEC, γ-75k-secalin; γ-HOR, γ-hordein; B-HOR, B-hordein; AVE, avenin). (Please see color plate at the back of the book.)

The N-terminal domains are rich in glutamine and proline, whereas the C-terminal domains possess a more balanced composition with less glutamine and a strongly reduced proline content, but more charged residues (glutamic acid, lysine, arginine) and hydrophobic side chains (leucine, isoleucine, valine). The N-terminal domains start with relatively short nonrepetitive sequences (section Ia), which are up to 32 residues long and unique to each type; section Ia is missing in B-hordeins. Section Ib is rich in glutamine, proline, and phenylalanine and consists exclusively of repetitive units such as QPQPFPPQQPY (α-gliadins), QQPQQPFP (γ-gliadins, γ-75k-secalins, γ- and B-hordeins), QQPPFS (LMW-GS), or PFVQQQQ (avenins). Depending on the protein type, the length of section Ib varies widely and ranges from 22 residues (avenins) to 273 residues (γ-75k-secalins). Section II is present only in α-gliadins and B-hordeins and, thus, is unique to these protein types.

Whereas α-gliadins contain a polyglutamine sequence of up to 18 residues long, B-hordeins consist of sequences of 30 amino acid residues rich in glutamine and leucine. Section III shows a high degree of homology in length (68–73 residues) and composition. Regarding section IV, proteins of the LMW group have partly homologous, partly unique sequences of different lengths (25–55 residues). Section V can be divided into a homologous section Va and a short unique section Vb. Their length is similar (42–55 residues), but their degree of homology is lower compared to section III.

The most characteristic features of all HMW, MMW, and LMW groups of proteins are repetitive sequences, and most CD-active peptides identified up to now are derived from these sections (see Section 3.5). Their compositions are predominated by glutamine (Q) and proline (P). Moreover, hydrophobic amino acid residues such as phenylalanine (F), tyrosine (Y), and leucine (L) occur frequently. Exceptions are the repetitive sequences of HMW group proteins that are additionally characterized by high glycine (G) contents. The repetitive units vary in length and frequency and are modified by exchange, insertion, or deletion of single amino acid residues. Each protein type has a unique profile of repetitive units. Figure 2.9 shows examples for repetitive sequences of the storage protein types of wheat and avenins of oats. The peptide motif QQPQQPFP present in ω1,2- and γ-gliadins is obviously one of the ancestral motifs of repetitive sequences. These are modified into QQQFP units of ω5-gliadins and into QPQPFP and PQQPYP units of α-gliadins. LMW-GS differ significantly due to repetitive units such as QQQPPFS. HMW-GS are characterized by a backbone formed by QQPGQG units and insertion of tripeptides (QPG or QQG) and hexapeptides (YYPTSP). The storage proteins of rye (secalins) and barley (hordeins) are homologous to the different gliadin and glutenin types of wheat (Table 2.4) and include corresponding repetitive sequences. Two various repetitive sequence units occur in oat avenins: PFVQQQQ and QPQLQQVF (Figure 2.9). They differ strongly from those of wheat, rye, and barley protein types.

The spatial conformation of proteins containing proline-rich repetitive sequences is characterized by missing α-helices and β-sheet structures. They have a stretched conformation including poly-L-proline I and II structures. An important conformational feature of these structures are reversed turns (β-turns or β-bends). They occur at corners, where the peptide chain abruptly changes direction. In the case of HMW-GS, such corners involve four amino acids, mainly including proline, glutamine, and glycine. Tatham and coworkers proposed that the regularly repeated β-turns of these subunits (QPGQ) are organized to form a loose spiral structure (β-spiral) similar to the connective tissue protein elastin (VPGV) [14]. Both spirals are thought to confer elastic properties to the proteins. Proline-poor, nonrepetitive sequences of gluten proteins are rich in α-helices and form compact globular structures stabilized by intrachain disulfide bonds.

Protein sections consisting of proline-rich repetitive sequences are resistant to enzymatic degradation in the gastrointestinal tract (see Chapter 1, Section 6.1). Trypsin, which cleaves peptide bonds after lysine and arginine residues (K–X, R–X), is ineffective owing to the scarcity of these amino acids. The activities of pepsin and chymotrypsin, which usually cleave after (pepsin, also before) hydrophobic amino acid residues (e.g., L–X, F–X, Y–X), are restricted because these residues are frequently followed

ω5 (Q40215) (191–274)[a]	**ω1,2 (Q6DLC7) (167–285)**[a]	**α(Q9M4M5) (33–95)**[b]
^{191}QQQFP	^{167}QPQQPIP	^{33}QQQPFP--PQQPYP
^{196}QQQFP	^{174}VQPQQSFP	^{45}QPQPFP--SQQPYL
^{201}QQQFP	^{182}QQSQQSQQPFA	^{57}QLQPFP-QPQLPYS
^{206}QQQFP	^{193}QPQQLFP	^{70}QPQPFR--PQQPYP
^{211}QQEFP	^{200}ELQQPIP	^{82}QPQPQYSQPQQPIS
^{216}QQQQFP	^{207}QQPQQPFP	**AVE (Q09072) (21–41/125–161)**[b]
^{222}QQQIA	^{215}LQPQQPFP	
^{227}RQPQQLP	^{223}QQPQQPFP	
^{234}QQQQIP	^{231}QQPQQSFP	^{21}PFVQQQQ
^{240}QQPQQFP	^{239}QQPQQPYP	^{28}PFVQQQQ
^{247}QQQQFP	^{247}QQQQSFP	^{35}PFVQQQQ
^{253}QQQSP	^{254}QQPQQPFP	^{125}QPQLQ--QQVF
^{258}QQQQFP	^{262}PTTTKPFP	^{134}QPQLQLQQQVF
^{264}QQQQLP	^{270}QQPQQPFP	^{145}QPQLQ--QQVF
^{270}QKQFP	^{278}LRPQQPFP	^{154}QPQLQ---QVF
γ (Q94691) (20–147)[b]	**LMW (Q52NZ4) (14–100)**[b]	**HMW (Q6R2V1) (241–390)**[a]
^{20}QLQQPLS	^{14}QQQPLPP	^{241}QQPGQGQQG
^{28}QQPQQTFP	^{21}QQTLFP	^{250}QQLGQGQQG
^{35}QPQQTFP	^{27}QQQPFP	^{259}YYPTSLQQSGQGQPG
^{42}HQPQQQVP	^{33}QQQPPFS	^{274}YYPTSLQQLGQGQSG
^{50}QPQQPQQPFL	^{40}QQQPSFS	^{289}YYPTSPQQPGQG
^{60}QPQQPFP	^{47}QQQPPFS	^{301}QQPGQL
^{67}QQPQQPFP	^{54}QQQPILP	^{307}QQPAQG
^{75}QTQQPQQPFP	^{61}QPPFS	^{313}QQPGQGQQG
^{85}QQPQQPFP	^{66}LQQQPVLP	^{322}QQPGQGQQG
^{93}QTQQPQQPFP	^{74}QQSPFS	^{331}QQPGQG
^{103}QQPQQPFP	^{80}QQQQLILP	^{337}QQPGQGQPG
^{111}QTQQPQQPFP	^{88}PQQQQQLP	^{346}YYPTSPQQSGQGQPG
^{121}QLQQPQQPFP	^{96}QQQIP	^{361}YYPTSSQQPTQS
^{131}QPQQQLP		^{373}QQPGQGQQG
^{138}QPQQPQQSFP		^{382}QQVGQGQQA

■ **FIGURE 2.9** Repetitive units of wheat gluten protein types and oat avenins (proteins corresponding to Tables 2.5–2.7); [a]part of repetitive sequences; [b]complete repetitive sequences.

by proline (e.g., L–P, F–P, Y–P), and these particular peptide bonds are hardly cleaved by pepsin and chymotrypsin. Such bonds are specifically cleaved only by prolyl endopeptidases, which are active in germinating cereal grains or produced by special bacteria and fungi (see Chapter 3, Section 2.1) but are absent in the human gastrointestinal tract. Judging by the differences in the repetitive sequences, proteins of the HMW group and LMW-GS appear to be most sensitive to an enzymatic digest because cleavable peptide bonds such as Y–Y (HMW-GS) and F–S (LMW-GS) are frequently present.

As mentioned earlier, the quantitative composition of storage proteins is strongly dependent on genotype and growing conditions. Nevertheless, some constant data can be observed (Table 2.4). Proteins of the HMW group belong to the minor components and those of the LMW group are most abundant. Within the LMW group, monomeric proteins exceed polymeric proteins, such as in the case of wheat, whereas rye and barley are characterized by more polymeric than monomeric proteins. The proportions of the MMW group proteins are significantly different with ω-gliadins in a low range, ω-secalins in a medium range, and C-hordein in a high range. Avenins belonging to the LMW group represent the only type of oat storage proteins because oat glutelins correspond to globulin-like proteins.

2.3 Wheat Gluten

In 1745, wheat gluten (Figure 1.2) was described by the Italian biochemist Jacopo Beccari [15] in his article "De frumento" (*Concerning grain*) as the first protein of plant origin. Before that time, it was believed that proteins were present only in materials of animal origin. Based on the worldwide yield of wheat, an estimated 50 million metric tons of wheat gluten are produced annually, making it the predominant class among plant proteins. The special physical and chemical properties of wheat gluten account for the exceptional position of wheat among cereals, which is due to the unique baking properties of wheat flour. Gluten is not soluble in water under normal conditions. Despite its insolubility and its hydrophobic nature, gluten absorbs approximately twice its dry weight in water. Because of the formation of a hydrated gluten network, wheat flour forms a cohesive, viscoelastic dough when mixed with water. Thus, the dough retains gas produced during fermentation, and this results in a leavened loaf of bread with an evenly pored, elastic crumb after baking.

Gluten mainly consists of the two major protein fractions of wheat flour: (1) gliadins and (2) glutenins [16] (see Section 2.1). It is commonly accepted that both fractions decisively account for the physical properties (cohesiveness, viscosity, extensibility, elasticity) of wheat dough. They are important contributors to these properties, but their functions are divergent. Hydrated gliadins have little elasticity and are less cohesive than glutenins; they contribute mainly to the viscosity and extensibility of dough. In contrast, hydrated glutenins are cohesive and elastic and are responsible for dough strength and elasticity. Thus, wheat gluten is a "two-component glue", in which gliadins act as plasticizer or solvent for glutenins [6] (Figure 2.10). A proper mixture (≈2:1) of the two is essential to give desirable dough and bread properties.

Gluten is characterized by an extremely complex chemical structure. It consists of several hundred protein components that correspond to wheat storage proteins and are preformed in the starchy endosperm of wheat grains. Correspondingly, they are classified into the different gliadin types (ω5-, ω1,2-, α-, and γ-gliadins) and glutenin types (HMW- and LMW-GS) [16] (see Section 2.2). In addition to the amino acid sequences, covalent and noncovalent linkages of proteins and molecular weight distribution determine the unique chemical and physical properties of gluten. Disulfide bonds are one of the most important determinants of gluten structure. They are formed between sulfhydryl groups of cysteine residues, either within a single protein (intrachain) or between proteins (interchain) [17]. With a few exceptions, ω5- and ω1,2-gliadins are free of cysteine and occur as monomers. Most α- and γ-gliadins contain six and eight cysteines, respectively, and form three or four homologous intrachain disulfide bonds, present within or between sequence sections III and V (Figure 2.8). A 2-D model of the α-gliadin structure is shown in Figure 2.11. The N-terminal domain (sections I and II) is free of cysteine and, consequently, free of disulfide bonds. The C-terminal domain (sections III, IV, and V) contains six cysteine residues that are involved in three intrachain disulfide bonds forming two small rings (AB and C) and a large ring (D) [18]. γ-Gliadins having eight cysteines form four intrachain disulfide bonds with separate rings A and B [19]. LMW-GS include eight cysteine residues, six of which form three intrachain disulfide bonds homologous to those of α- and γ-gliadins. Two cysteine residues located in sections I and IV are unique to LMW-GS, and

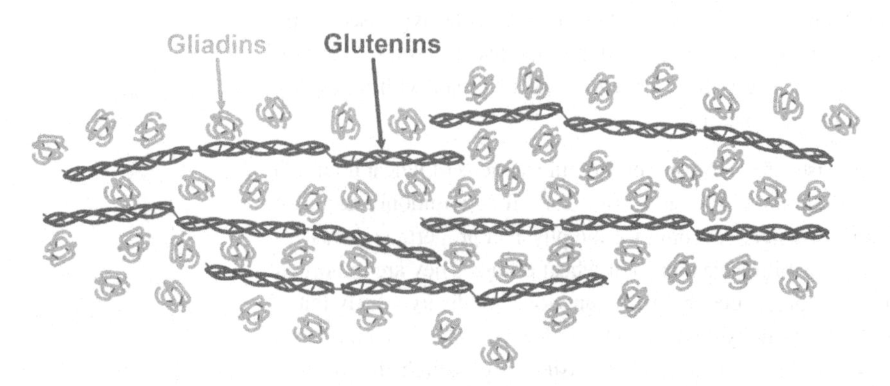

■ **FIGURE 2.10** Schematical representation of gluten as a two-component glue formed by gliadins and glutenins.

they are involved in interchain bonds mainly with cysteines of the same type. Similarly, HMW-GS form both intra- and interchain disulfide bonds, the latter being involved in end-to-end polymerization. Thus, the glutenin aggregate consists of LMW-GS polymers and HMW-GS polymers that are linked by interchain disulfide bonds (Figure 2.12). Polymerization is stopped by so-called terminators, such as glutathione or cysteine.

Besides disulfide bonds, noncovalent bonds, such as hydrogen bonds, and to a lesser degree ionic and hydrophobic bonds, contribute to the complex gluten structure [6]. A further characteristic feature of gluten is the broad molecular weight distribution of the proteins [3]. Monomeric gliadins (ω5-, ω1,2-, α-, γ-gliadins) have molecular weights of approximately 30,000 to 55,000. Besides monomers, the alcohol-soluble gliadin fraction contains oligomers with molecular weights roughly ranging from 60,000 to 600,000. They consist of modified gliadins (with an odd number of cysteines) and LMW-GS linked by interchain disulfide bonds. They have been named differently as HMW-gliadins, aggregated gliadins, or ethanol-soluble glutenins. The alcohol-insoluble glutenin fraction contains polymers of LMW- and HMW-GS linked together and resulting in molecular weights from 600,000 to more than 10 million. The largest polymers, called glutenin macropolymer, may belong to the largest proteins in nature [20]. Although rye flour contains proteins homologous to wheat flour proteins, its ability to form gluten is missing. Structural differences (e.g., disulfide structure, molecular weight distribution, and ratio of monomers to polymers) have been discussed as reasons [21]. Additionally, the high arabinoxylan content of rye flour seems to prevent the agglomeration of storage proteins from forming rye gluten during dough mixing [22].

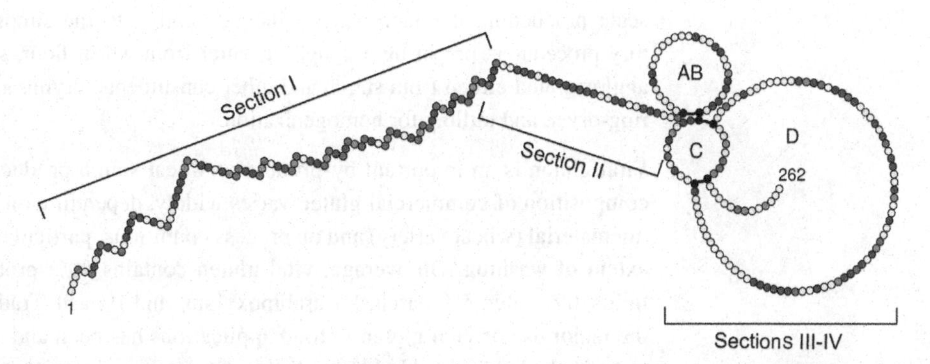

■ **FIGURE 2.11** Two-dimensional structure of an α-gliadin divided into sections I, II, and III–V (see Figure 2.8). (Please see color plate at the back of the book.)

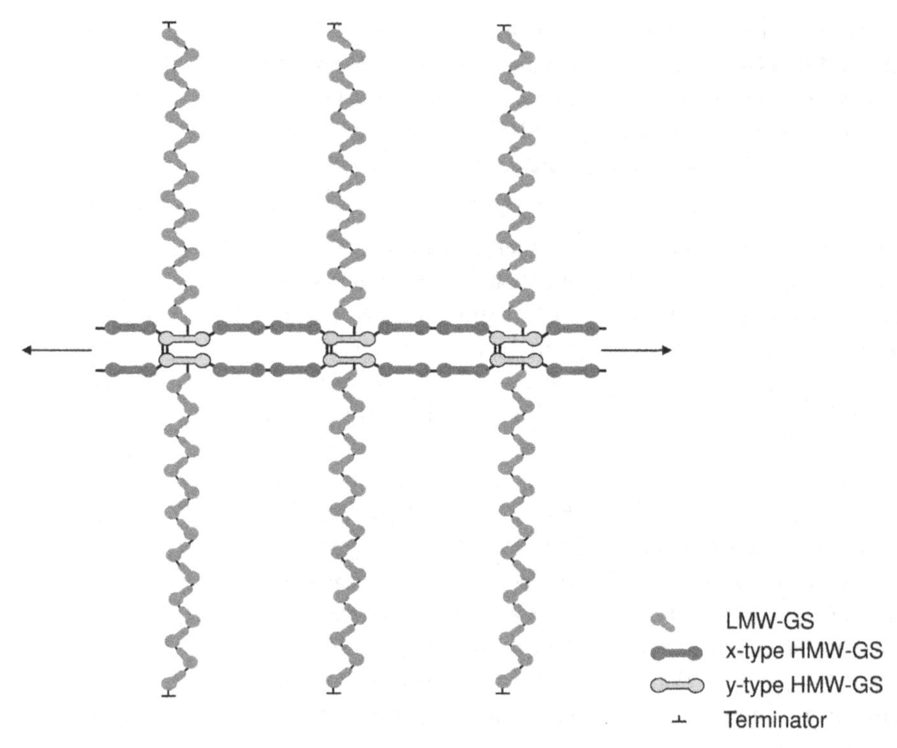

■ **FIGURE 2.12** Model of polymeric glutenin building blocks consisting of x- and y-type HMW-GS and LMW-GS. (Please see color plate at the back of the book.)

Wheat gluten can be prepared easily in the laboratory by mixing wheat flour with water into a dough and washing out the starch and the solubles in a stream of water, either manually or by a specific instrument (Glutomatic®, Perten Instruments). This process yields the so-called wet gluten that can be dried and ground into a product known as vital gluten. Industrial large-scale production of gluten is, in principle, similar to the simple laboratory procedures: preparing a dough or batter from wheat flour, separating agglomerated gluten from starch and other constituents, drying gluten in a ring-dryer, and milling for homogenization.

Vital gluten is an important by-product of wheat starch production. The composition of commercial gluten varies widely, depending on the starting material (wheat variety) and on process conditions, particularly on the extent of washing. On average, vital gluten contains 80% proteins, 7% lipids, 6% water, 5% starch, 1% arabinoxylans, and 1% ash. Traditionally, the major use of vital gluten in food applications has been and continues to be in the bakery and baking industry. Gluten is an important constituent of flour-improving products that guarantee high protein content and water absorption, improved dough handling, and increased bread quality. Moreover, bakers can meet the requirements of many different baked products with varying amounts of added gluten and, thus, can standardize the bread-making process, even if the flours used have different baking qualities. In addition, significant quantities of gluten are used in the pet food industry.

CD patients should be aware that "hidden" gluten is unexpectedly present in numerous composite foods [23,24]. The meat and fish industry uses the unique adhesive and thermosetting properties of wheat gluten in products such as extended ground meat, textured meats, meat analogs, canned hams, sausages, poultry rolls, and seafood analogs. The unique viscoelastic properties of hydrated gluten can be exploited in the manufacture of synthetic cheese, such as imitation mozzarella. The water-binding and thickening properties of gluten are used to improve the quality of ice cream, instant puddings, soups, sauces, ketchup, marinades, and dressings. Gluten is also applied in the production of breakfast cereals, such as cornflakes or puffed rice, where gluten helps to bind the vitamin and mineral supplements and to improve strength and crispness of the product. Gluten proteins partially hydrolyzed by acid have a high emulsifying capacity and a good solubility and are used as an additive, such as in coffee creamers.

Wheat gluten also has many applications in the nonfood industry (e.g., as adhesives, coatings, detergents, and foils) (Figure 2.13). After edible gluten foils (e.g., for coating fruits and cheese) were introduced into the market, Codex Standard 163-1987 prohibited the use of these foils for foods that are gluten-free by nature (see Chapter 4, Section 3.1). Gluten may be present in some medications, postage stamp glue, and cosmetics (e.g., lipsticks). The chemical modification of amino, carboxy, carboxamido, and thiol groups or enzymatic treatment allows numerous variations of the viscoelastic properties of gluten. There also is an interest in gluten as a substitute for petroleum-based polymers because it is readily biodegradable and produced from a renewable and sustainable raw material.

2.4 Storage Proteins of Corn, Rice, Sorghum, and Millet

The storage proteins of corn, rice, sorghum, and millet differ significantly from those of wheat, rye, barley, and oats. The amino acid compositions contain less glutamine and proline and more hydrophobic amino acids, such as leucine (Tables 2.2 and 2.3) [7]. Corn storage proteins (zeins) can

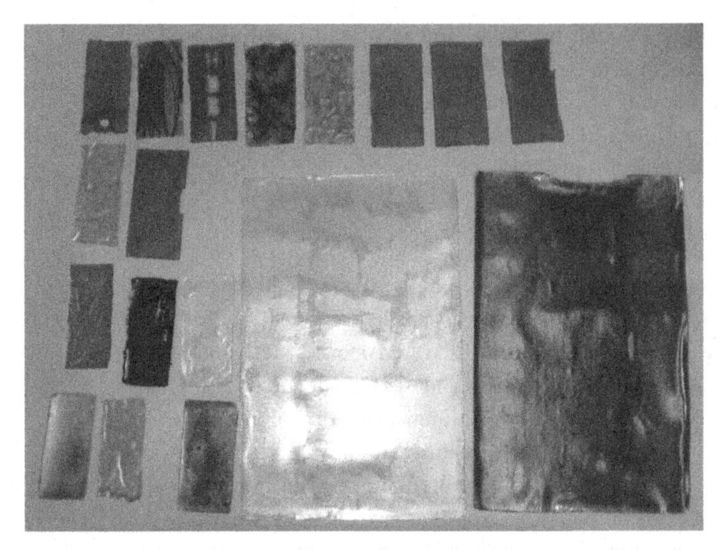

■ **FIGURE 2.13** Gluten foils produced by high-pressure treatment and colored by food dyes. (Please see color plate at the back of the book.)

be grouped into alcohol-soluble monomeric zeins and crosslinked zeins which are alcohol-soluble only upon heating or after reduction of disulfide bonds. According to structural differences, zeins are subdivided into four subclasses [25]: α-Zeins, the major subclass (71–85% of total zeins), followed by γ-zeins (10–20%), and β- and δ-zeins (1–5% each). α-Zeins are monomeric proteins with molecular weights of 19,000 and 22,000. Their amino acid sequences contain up to 10 repetitive units, rich in glutamine and proline, which, however, are different from those of the *Triticeae* and oats. Zeins from the other subclasses are crosslinked by disulfide bonds, and their subunits have molecular weights of 18,000 and 27,000 (γ-zeins), 18,000 (β-zeins), and 10,000 (δ-zeins).

The storage proteins of sorghum and millet (kafirins) are closely related and similar to zeins. Kafirins also are subdivided into α-, β-, γ-, and δ-subclasses based on solubility, molecular weight, and amino acid sequences [26]. α-Kafirins are monomeric proteins and represent the major subclass, accounting for around 65% to 85% of total kafirins. Proteins of the other subclasses are highly crosslinked and alcohol-soluble only after reduction of disulfide bonds. On average, each of these accounts for less than 10% of total kafirins. The storage proteins of rice (oryzins) are characterized by the highly unbalanced ratio of prolamins to glutelins (≈1:30). Both fractions show the lowest proline content (≈5 mol%) among cereal storage proteins [27]. The molecular weights of the prolamin components range from 17,000 to 23,000, and those of glutelin subunits range from 20,000 to 38,000.

1 FIIP**Q**CSLAPSASIPQFLPPVTSMGFEHPAVQAYRL**Q**LAL

41 AASAL**Q**QPIAQLQ**Q**QSLAHLTLQTIATQQ**QQ**QFLPSLSH

81 LAMVNPVTYL**QQ**QLLASNPLALANVAAYQQ**Q**QQL**Q**QFMPV

121 LS**Q**LAMVNPAVYLQLLSSSPLAVGNAPTYL**QQ**QLL**Q**QIVP

161 ALT**Q**LAVANPAAYL**Q**QLLPFN**Q**LAVSNSAAYLQQR**Q**QLLN

201 PLAVANPLVATFLQQ**QQ**QLLPYN**Q**FSLMNPAL**Q**QPIVGGA

241 IF

■ **FIGURE 2.14** Amino acid sequence of corn zein cZ22A1 [28] (accession number Q9SBC4: database Uni Prot KB) (Glutamine residues (Q) potentially deamidated by TG2 are shown in bold).

The amino acid sequences of storage proteins from corn, rice, sorghum, and millet are, as far as is known, entirely different from those of gluten proteins. Figure 2.14 shows the sequence of zein cZ22A1 (α-zein) as an example [28]. According to the algorithms of glutamine deamidation (see Chapter 1, Section 6.3.1), zeins are frequently deamidated by TG2. However, this protein type is digested well by gastrointestinal enzymes. In silico fragmentation with pepsin, trypsin, and chymotrypsin (see Chapter 1, Section 6.1) yields only three peptides with a length of more than 8 amino acid residues (8–18, 63–74, 233–241). Their structures do not fit the requirements for HLA-DQ binding (see Chapter 1, Section 6.3.1). In contrast, Chabrera-Chavez and coworkers identified a few immunoreactive α-zein peptides in a peptic-tryptic digest of zein by in silico analysis [29]. They postulated that corn prolamins could be harmful for a limited subgroup of CD patients and that this subgroup should follow a corn-free diet, in addition to a GFD [30]. However, comprehensive in vivo and in vitro tests on immunogenicity and toxicity have to be performed before zeins and, correspondingly, corn are called into question as food components harmless to CD patients.

3. CELIAC DISEASE TOXICITY

3.1 Testing Toxicity

Numerous in vivo and in vitro methods have been developed to identify CD toxicity and immunogenicity of different cereal and noncereal raw materials, cereal proteins and peptides and to test novel therapies (see Chapter 3, Section 2). The tests can be differentiated into (1) in vivo challenge of CD patients; (2) in vitro tests with tissues and cells of CD patients; and (3) animal models [31,32]. Before testing, the material should be well characterized by chemical analysis.

3.1.1 Material to be Tested

Cereal-derived protein and peptide preparations should be chemically characterized before testing toxicity and immunogenicity to guarantee reliable statements. Crude material, such as wheat gluten, has to be analyzed—using, for example, the Kjeldahl or Dumas method—for the content of nitrogen, which can be converted to crude protein content by the factor 5.7. Further studies on protein composition, such as prolamin and glutelin proportions and content of impurities, are desirable because gluten composition can vary to a considerable degree due to different origins and conditions of preparation or processing. For example, a combined extraction/liquid chromatography procedure can be used for a detailed analysis of different protein fractions [33]. For in vitro tests, proteins should be partially hydrolyzed by enzymes such as pepsin, trypsin, chymotrypsin, or pancreatin to mimic gastrointestinal digestion and to convert the insoluble proteins into soluble peptides. When salts are present (e.g., resulting from a neutralization step during enzymatic digestion), the protein/peptide content of the dried hydrolyzate has to be analyzed by nitrogen determination. Purified proteins and peptides available in small amounts can be quantitated by RP-HPLC [3]. For calibration, a defined reference (e.g., PWG-gliadin [34]) should be used. Isolated or synthesized peptides have to be checked for purity and identity; RP-HPLC and mass spectrometry are recommended for this purpose [35].

3.1.2 In vivo Testing

Most researchers would agree that in vivo testing is the gold standard for assessing CD toxicity. This is performed in celiac volunteers who have been on a GFD for some years and, thus, can be expected to have normal morphology of the small intestine. Initially, CD patients were challenged with cereal products and crude protein fractions by feeding tests followed by measuring xylose and fat malabsorption or by monitoring symptoms such as steatorrhea [36]. These tests, however, have been considered unsatisfactory owing to the uncertainty of the optimal amount of challenge material and duration of challenge. Moreover, the effect on xylose malabsorption and fat balance is secondary and does not provide information about the reaction on the epithelial surface. In most studies, only few CD patients were tested, and controls were not included. In the 1970s, the technique of intestinal biopsy was introduced, and bigger cohorts of patients and controls were challenged, resulting in more precise conclusions on toxicity. The in vivo study of Janatuinen and coworkers on oat toxicity may be an example for test performance [37]. They conducted a randomized study on CD patients challenged with a selected diet containing defined quantities of oats. The primary method of evaluation was endoscopy with duodenal biopsy before the application of the special diet and after the tests, accompanied by serological tests. The patients ($n=92$) were divided into an oat-eating group and a control group. Patients in the oat group consumed about 50 g of oats per day for 6 or 12 months. Once completed, duodenal biopsies with subsequent histological and morphometrical measurements and serological tests were performed.

Such extensive testing can be carried out only with material (e.g., cereal grains or flour, wheat gluten) available in high amounts, but not with purified proteins or peptides difficult to prepare. The introduction of oral challenge by direct instillation into the small intestine of CD patients in remission, followed by biopsy at the beginning of and after several hours of testing, allowed the reduction of the amount of proteins and peptides to about 1 g [38] or even less [35,39]. As an example, the in vivo test with the gliadin peptide α56–75 is described in the following process [35,39]: a cannula is attached to a Quinton® hydraulic, multiple biopsy capsule. The capsule is positioned in the distal duodenum of a sedated CD patient under fluoroscopic control. The solution of a peptic-tryptic protein digest or a gluten peptide is infused into the duodenum for 2 h by a syringe driver. Biopsies are taken before infusion and at 2, 4, and 6 h after the start of infusion. The tissues are then removed from the capsule and fixed in formalin for morphometric analysis. Sections of the tissues are partly stained and partly snap frozen. The stained sections are measured for villous height, crypt depth, and height of enterocytes. The frozen sections are used for measuring the number of intraepithelial lymphocytes (IELs) per 100 enterocytes by means of a special antibody test. Changes in villous height, ratio of villous height to crypt depth, and the number of IELs are considered to be reliable parameters for toxicity assessment (Figure 2.15) [35].

To avoid invasive biopsy testing, the measurement of intestinal permeability or the examination of peripheral blood T cells after oral challenge with potentially CD-toxic agents can be used for testing. The permeability test is based on the oral administration of an oligosaccharide (e.g., lactulose) and a monosaccharide (e.g., mannitol) that differentially cross the intestinal barrier to the blood circulation [40] (see Chapter 1, Section 6.2). The smaller molecule (monosaccharide) is thought to traverse the intestinal barrier freely, independent of barrier function loss, whereas the larger molecule (oligosaccharide) traverses only during barrier function loss. The ratio of both saccharides in urine samples collected over 5 to 6 h after oral intake is considered to reflect the loss of barrier function and, thus, the CD toxicity of the agent tested. However, an in vivo study with 20 CD patients on a GFD challenged with 3.0 or 7.5 g gluten/day for 14 days did not show any significant change in the lactulose-to-mannitol ratio, whereas biopsy morphology, antibody titers, and gastrointestinal symptoms changed in the majority of patients [41]. Thus, the degree of correlation between abnormal intestinal permeability to sugars and proteins/peptides remains to be established.

Regarding blood tests, patients with confirmed CD undergo a 3-day oral challenge with the agent to be tested. Peripheral blood mononuclear cells (PBMCs) are isolated after several days and incubated with the agent (peptide or protein) [42]. Interferon-γ (IFN-γ) responses are then measured by a cytokine-specific assay.

As the rectum provides a site of easy access for obtaining mucosal tissues, the response to local gluten challenge has been investigated [43]. The rectal mucosa of CD patients challenged with 2 g of a gluten digest showed a significant swelling of the lamina propria, a rapid fall in mast cells, a marked rise of IELs, and a substantial infiltration of lymphocytes in the lamina propria. These observations demonstrate that the rectal mucosa is sensitized to gluten and, thus, offers a convenient approach for investigative and diagnostic purposes.

3.1.3 In vitro Testing

The development of in vitro systems for testing toxicity was a key step in the studies on pure proteins and peptides because small amounts (≈1 mg or even less) can be tested. The organ culture of intestinal tissue of CD

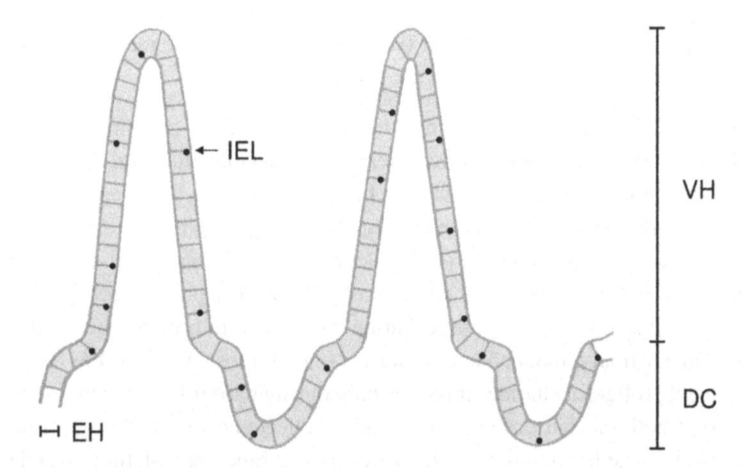

■ **FIGURE 2.15** Schematic drawing of the intestinal epithelium and indication of the factors used for the measurement of in vivo toxicity (IEL, intraepithelial lymphocyte; EH, enterocyte height; VH, villous height; DC, depth of crypt).

patients has been proposed to be the most reliable in vitro model and may mirror the in vivo situation. The test was originally introduced by Browning and Trier in 1969 [44]. Tissues from CD patients are taken as part of the diagnostic procedure and incubated in a culture medium containing the protein or peptide to be tested [45]. The biopsies can be kept viable in the culture system for 24–48 h or even longer, although there is no guarantee of quality of mucosal morphology after a long-term culture [31]. Originally, biopsies of active CD patients were taken, and the tissues showed improvement of enzyme activity, signs of inflammation, and morphology in the culture medium alone but not in the presence of CD-toxic substances. Currently, tissues of patients in remission are incubated with the potentially toxic substance, and markers for CD-specific effects such as cytokines (e.g., IFN-γ, interleukin (IL)-4, and IL-10) and nitric oxide are measured. One of the benefits of this method is that various features characteristic for CD can be reproduced in biopsies from treated patients, thus allowing researchers to find mechanisms related to the development of CD [31]. Because intestinal biopsies contain enterocytes and lamina propria, the model is useful in determining both innate and adaptive responses. A disadvantage is that the organ culture system is not a high-throughput method, and the tissue lacks circulation, nervous system, and connection to lymphatic organs. Although the organ culture system is the best in vitro model for detecting toxic effects, it has been widely replaced by studies on T cells that identify only immunogenic effects.

Since the 1990s, T-cell lines and clones from the small intestinal mucosa or the peripheral blood of CD patients have been used to measure immunogenic effects of proteins and peptides and to test potential novel treatment forms [46]. T-cell lines and clones raised against gluten are useful for performing a large number of experiments and readily demonstrate the T-cell response to stimuli. Gluten-sensitive T cells can be isolated from intestinal biopsies cultured and stimulated in vitro [46] or can be found in the blood of treated CD patients on day 6 after a 3-day oral gluten challenge [42]. A frequently used test is the T-cell proliferation assay performed by incubation of intestinal CD-sensitive T cells with the putative antigen (≈100–200 µg/ml) treated with TG2 in the presence of antigen-presenting cells (APCs) (e.g., B cells) and tritiated thymidine. The proliferation of T cells determined by scintillation measurements is a parameter for immunogenic effects. Additionally, the production of IFN-γ or ILs can be measured. T-cell tests have been used widely to compare the level of immunogenic effects. For example, the proliferation assay was applied to measure the stimulation index (counts per minute for antigen divided by counts per minute without antigen) and IFN-γ concentration after incubation with different gliadin peptides [47] and oat cultivars [48] (Table 2.8). Because the sensitivity of T cells is strongly variable and depends on the patient they were taken from and on the procedure of stimulation, only relative values can be determined when taking a reference gluten protein or peptide for comparison. The use of gluten-sensitive T-cell lines from multiple CD patients rather than from gluten-sensitive clones has been recommended [49].

Because T cells sensitive for gluten are rare in the intestinal tissue, they cannot be directly evaluated. The only known source of fresh polyclonal gluten-sensitive T cells at a sufficiently high frequency is the peripheral blood from CD donors, taken directly after a short-term oral gluten challenge [42]. Peripheral blood mononuclear cells of CD patients, collected after several days of gluten challenge, are incubated with the potential antigen using 96-well plates. The release of IFN-γ is counted by an automated reader and allows the comprehensive mapping of immunogenic T-cell epitopes in gluten proteins [50].

In general, it should be mentioned that T cells do not necessarily reflect the small intestine in vivo because they lack any connection to other cell types present in the intestine. In addition, T cells frequently differ in their reaction to antigens, which is why the application of several simultaneous T-cell lines from different patients is needed. Moreover, immunogenicity does not always correspond to the toxicity demonstrated by in vivo or organ culture tests. For example, avenin, the prolamin fraction of oats, was shown to be immunogenic in T-cell tests but nontoxic in organ culture tests [51,52].

Less difficult screening assays such as skin test, agglutination test with human K562(S) cells, leukocyte migration inhibition test, or macrophage

Table 2.8 Reactivity of Gluten-Sensitive T Cells Toward Gliadin Digests, Gliadin Peptides, and Avenin Digests from Different Cultivars [47,48][a]

Sample	SI	IFN-γ (pg/ml)
PT-gliadin	7	9
Peptide G9 (α56–75/E65)	37	180
Peptide G5 (α56–68/E65)	2	23
Peptide G4 (α62–75/E65)	12	55
PTC-gliadin	1.8	9.4
PTC-avenin OF 720	0.7	3.4
PTC-avenin OH 727	1.0	4.8
PTC-avenin OM 719	1.3	7.9

[a] *SI, stimulation index; IFN-γ, interferon-γ; PT, peptic-tryptic; PTC, peptic-tryptic-chymotryptic.*

procoagulant activity test have not gained common acceptance. Since the 1990s, two epithelial cell culture models, T84 cells and Caco-2 cells, have been used as models for testing CD-specific effects [31]. T84 cells are derived from a lung metastasis of colon cancer. This cell line, although of colonic origin, is widely used in studying intestinal epithelial permeability to macromolecules and ions. T84 cells also have been applied in research into CD pathogenesis, for instance, studying the innate immune reactions [53] and effects on intestinal permeability [54]. Caco-2 cells originate from a relatively well-differentiated human colon adenocarcinoma. When reaching confluence, cells differentiate spontaneously and possess an ultrastructural morphology of differentiated enterocytes with an apical surface covered by microvilli. Caco-2 cells contain tight junctions and a number of enzymes and transporters that are characteristic of cells lining the intestine [55]. Owing to these characteristics, Caco-2 cells are widely used as models for the intestinal epithelial barrier, as well as in studies related to CD. For instance, they have been used to clarify how individual peptides are processed [56] and how antibodies of CD patients participate in disease pathogenesis [57].

3.1.4 Animal Models

Apart from human intestinal material, cultures of the immature intestine of rat or chick fetus have been used to demonstrate the cytotoxic activity of gliadin fractions [58,59]. CD-active compounds inhibit development and morphogenesis of the very immature small intestine, showing that gliadin peptides may have a direct damaging activity against the small intestinal mucosa during the early phase of its morphogenesis. Another approach has been to study the disruption of rat liver lysosomes caused by active gliadin peptides [60].

To better understand the immunologic pathways and mechanisms of CD, a number of attempts have been made to create an animal model for various purposes. Currently, there are three models that spontaneously generate gluten-dependent diarrhea: (1) the dog, (2) the rhesus macaque, and (3) the horse model [32,61]. In the dog model, Irish setters develop partial villous atrophy and IEL infiltration in response to the consumption of gluten [62]. Gluten-dependent, small intestinal mucosal damage has been described in rhesus macaques [63], and gluten-dependent increased levels of antibodies have been observed in horses with inflammatory small bowel disease [64]. Common to all three of these spontaneous models is the lack of association with HLA-DQ2/8 alleles. Other models (e.g., with mice, rats, or rabbits) are not spontaneous and need gluten sensitization, chemical and/or drug treatment, and genetic alterations to develop features of CD. The mouse model has a big advantage over the other models because transgenes can be introduced to evaluate the contribution of specific genes to the development of CD. For example, transgenic mice were generated expressing human HLA-DQ2 or -DQ8, but none of the animals used developed full-blown villous atrophy [65,66]. De Paolo and coworkers reported that gliadin-fed humanized HLA-DQ8 mice overexpress IL-15 in the lamina propria, a condition resembling early developing CD; however, the mucosal architecture remains normal [67]. Numerous studies used transgenic mice to investigate different elements of CD pathogenesis (e.g., the role of $CD4^+$ T cells, TG2, IL-15, and intestinal microbiota) [32,61]. Specific mouse models also were used to test novel therapies for CD [32,61] (see Chapter 3, Section 2). Examples targeting pathogenic steps are modification of gluten peptides, suppression of the innate response, the blocking of Zonulin-1, suppression of inflammatory T-cell response, and the blocking of IL-15 or receptors of IL-15. Regardless of all these attempts, the animal model for CD that reproduces all the aspects of this disorder still awaits development.

3.1.5 Level of Toxicity

A number of publications provide speculations on the level of CD toxicity of cereals, protein fractions and types, and peptides. For example, hexaploid common wheat has frequently been described as the most toxic cereal. Diploid and tetraploid wheat species were suggested to be less toxic than hexaploid common wheat [68–70]. Gliadins tend to be more toxic than glutenins [36]; within gliadins, α-gliadins were proposed to be most toxic, with γ- and ω-gliadins having lower toxicity [71–73]. D- and C-hordeins were found to be most immunogenic among hordeins [74]. Numerous reports have emphasized that the 33-mer peptide from α2-gliadin is the most important immunogenic agent within gluten peptides. Are all these assumptions justified, and is it possible at all to determine the level of CD toxicity and immunogenicity?

In vivo challenge cannot be considered for a statistically significant evaluation of the level of toxicity owing to the limited number of willing patients, the relatively high amounts of agents necessary to produce toxic effects, and the high experimental effort. In contrast, the organ culture of small intestinal biopsies derived from CD patients (see Section 3.1.3) offers the possibility for measuring differences in toxic effects. Tissues of patients in remission are incubated with the potentially toxic substance, and markers for CD-specific effects, such as enzyme activities, morphologic characteristics, and cytokine concentrations, can be measured. Positive and negative control substances should be included into the experiments. As an example, the examination of peptide α31–49 and five alanine-substituted variants tested with specimens of 10 CD patients is shown in Table 2.9 [75]. Frazer's fraction FIII (the water-soluble part of a peptic-tryptic digest of wheat gluten) and ovalbumin were used as positive and negative controls, respectively, and changes of the enterocyte height (Figure 2.15), compared to the medium alone, were used as markers for toxicity. The results demonstrated that the unmodified peptide α31–49 was as toxic as the positive control; peptides α31–49/A31 and α31–49/A36 were less toxic; and peptides α31–49/A38, α31–49/A39, and α31–49/A42 were nontoxic. Considering that the organ culture system contains a wide variety of cell types and mirrors the in vivo situation, it is surprising that the method has been used only in a few studies.

In contrast, tests with gluten-sensitive T cells (see Section 3.1.3) obtained from the small intestinal mucosa and peripheral blood of CD patients have been used widely for the evaluation of CD-specific immunogenic effects. Examples are shown in Table 2.8, and Figures 1.18 and 1.19. The sensitivity and specificity of T-cell lines and clones, however, are strongly dependent on several parameters (e.g., the patients they were taken from and the agent used for stimulation). Some T cells are highly specific for particular gluten peptides, but others cross-react with homologous peptides, and the ratio between these T cells may vary from patient to patient [76]. To overcome these limitations, the application of several simultaneous T-cell lines from different patients rather than T-cell clones has been recommended [49].

Table 2.9 Changes of Enterocyte Height (μm) of Specimens Cultured with Peptide α31–49 and Five Alanine (A)-Substituted Peptide Variants, Frazer's Fraction FIII (FFIII), and Ovalbumin (OVA) [75]

	Peptide							
Patient	**FFIII**	**α31–49**	**A31**	**A36**	**A38**	**A39**	**A42**	**OVA**
1	−7.9	−6.7	−6.3	−11.5	4.4	−1.6	3.8	0.7
2	−9.5	−6.5	1.8	9.0	−6.2	6.0	10.6	4.2
3	−13.3	−9.6	−13.7	−8.4	−1.4	−0.8	−2.5	−0.2
4	−12.3	−18.6	−5.8	−9.4	1.5	−0.4	−1.3	−1.9
5	−7.5	2.0	−3.7	−1.6	13.1	10.5	6.0	2.7
6	−12.5	−15.5	−1.2	−1.6	0.7	−2.4	−7.3	−6.9
7	−11.8	−10.9	−3.0	−2.4	1.1	1.2	0.9	−1.6
8	−17.7	−9.7	−12.1	−18.8	−5.4	−1.8	−3.8	−3.2
9	−6.6	n.t.	−0.1	6.7	n.t.	9.0	7.3	−1.6
10	−4.1	n.t.	n.t.	n.t.	−1.7	n.t.	n.t.	2.8
Mean	−10.3	−9.4	−4.9	−3.9	0.7	2.2	1.5	−0.5

n.t. = not tested.

3.2 Toxicity of Cereals

Early investigations, beginning in 1950 with Dicke's thesis, indicated that wheat, rye, and barley were harmful to CD patients, whereas rice and corn were not [36]. Plants outside of the *Poaceae* family, such as buckwheat and potatoes, were regarded as safe. Because the technique of intestinal biopsy was not available at that time, research relied on feeding tests and the subsequent appearance of symptoms and fat or xylose malabsorption. Later, histological studies on intestinal biopsies and immunogenic responses were used for toxicity judgment. Only wheat and oats have been extensively studied, resulting in an undoubted toxicity of wheat, although there is still disagreement about the toxicity of oats (see following discussion). Testing of rye and barley has been rather minimal, but their strong similarities with wheat, deduced from the structures of storage proteins, support their CD toxicity (see Section 2.2). Corn, rice, sorghum, millet, and all noncereal plants have come to be regarded as safe, presumably because no contradictory evidence from diets including these crops has been encountered over decades. The safety of wheat-free sorghum food products was confirmed by in vitro and in vivo tests as well as by genomic, biochemical, and immunochemical analyses [77,78].

According to Kasarda, the taxonomy of plants might provide useful guidance in classifying them as safe or unsafe [79,80]. All definitely toxic grains (wheat, rye, barley) are found in a single tribe, the *Triticeae*, within the grass family (Figure 2.2). Owing to this botanical relationship and similar protein patterns [81,82], all wheat species, triticale, and all botanical forms of rye and barley should be avoided by CD patients. Oats, controversially judged with regard to toxicity, belong to the same subfamily (*Pooideae*) but to another tribe (*Aveneae*). All nontoxic common cereals (rice, corn, sorghum, millet) and rarely used cereals (Teff®, ragi, Job's tears) are more distant from the *Triticeae* and show separate evolutionary lines within the grass family. Seeds outside the grass family, such as buckwheat, amaranth, and quinoa, are assumed to be safe.

Tetraploid (durum, emmer) and diploid (einkorn) wheat species were proposed to contain fewer protein epitopes toxic for CD patients than hexaploid (common, spelt) wheat because of the absence of the D-genome [83]. Indeed, they have fewer gluten protein components; however, protein amounts in flour are even higher, and all gluten protein types are present [82]. Moreover, N-terminal sequencing of α-gliadins showed a high degree of concordance among the different wheat species [84]. Nevertheless, differences in the level of stimulatory epitopes may exist. Molberg and coworkers found that the protein fragments identical or equivalent to the immunogenic 33-mer peptide (see Section 3.5) are encoded by α-gliadin genes on wheat chromosome 6D and, thus, are absent from gluten of diploid einkorn (genome AA) and tetraploid durum wheat (genome AABB) [85]. A lack of toxicity of *Triticum monococcum* gliadin was also shown in an in vitro organ culture system [86]. Other findings, however, based on gluten-sensitive T-cell and organ culture tests provided evidence for CD toxicity of ancient wheat species [49,87].

The incorporation of oats into a GFD could provide high fiber, vitamin B, magnesium, zinc and iron contents, increased palatability, and beneficial effects on cardiovascular health [88]. However, the necessity of excluding oats from the diet for CD patients remains controversial. An overview on toxicity tests including number of individuals challenged, amount of oats given daily, duration of the challenge, and clinical measurement has been presented by the groups of Sontag-Strohm [89] and Pawloska [90]. Reports on oat toxicity during 1953–1976 revealed different effects after oat in vivo challenge: effects were either harmful, as indicated by malabsorption tests, or harmless, as indicated by intestinal biopsies. These studies, however, were based on a small number of patients, the challenge duration was brief, and oat samples were not tested for contamination with wheat, rye, or barley. Studies afterward were more comprehensive, and a larger number of patients were challenged with oats proven to be pure. Different cohorts, including up to 92 CD patients and controls, were challenged with 10–93 g oats per day over 3–60 months. The types of tests and measurements used were mainly duodenal biopsy with histological judgment and serological tests. The results revealed that oats were tolerated clinically and caused neither histological damage nor induced cellular or humoral immune responses. Even long-term studies over 1–5 years, respectively, demonstrated that patients tolerated oats without any adverse effects [91,92]. Another study described that children with CD tolerated oats in their GFD for 2 years, during which they were regularly monitored [93]. Similar findings were made in patients with dermatitis herpetiformis, another gluten-related disorder (see Chapter 1, Section 4.5.1) [94,95]. Two studies, however, showed harmful effects of oats on a small number of patients [96,97]. Owing to the limited number of cases sensitive to oats, no numeral estimate of the size of this subgroup is available. Most likely, this subgroup may constitute less than 1% of CD patients [98].

Despite the predominantly good clinical evidence, the inclusion of oats in the GFD has been continuously debated. It was argued that the relatively low content of avenins, the prolamin fraction of oats, explained the apparent safety for most patients. Thereupon, tests with pure avenins isolated from oat flours were performed (see Section 3.3). Again, clear results were not obtained. For example, T-cell tests showed immune responses equivalent to the prolamin fractions of wheat (gliadins), rye (secalins), and barley (hordeins), whereas organ culture tests were negative [51,52,99].

In conclusion, clinical studies provide limited results in favor of a general harmlessness of oats for CD patients. It has been recommended that those who continuously consume oats (20–25 g/day for children, 50–70 g/day for adults) need proper clinical follow-ups [100]. In addition, oat products should be tested for contaminations with wheat, rye, or barley because the commercial oat supply may be heavily contaminated with these grains [101]. Several research groups are currently studying the diversity in oat potential immunogenicity as a basis for the selection of oat varieties with no toxicity in CD. Differences in the two known immunogenic avenin epitopes (see Table 1.5) among oat varieties indicate that selection and breeding of completely safe oat varieties for all CD patients may be a realistic possibility [102]. Studies on T cells isolated from CD patients showed that oat cultivars may have a different immunogenic potential, either nonimmunogenic, medium immunogenic, or highly immunogenic [48]. The degree of immunogenicity was related to the presence of specific glutamine- and proline-rich peptides [103]. However, the evaluation of avenin genes in 13 diploid, tetraploid, and hexaploid oat species revealed that all contained the two CD-specific avenin epitopes [104]. The authors concluded that it is very unlikely that oat cultivars devoid of these epitopes can be found.

3.3 Toxicity of Protein Fractions

Early investigations led to the conclusion that wheat, rye, barley, and, possibly, oats are harmful to CD patients, whereas corn, rice, sorghum, and millet have been considered harmless (see Section 3.2). Among toxic cereals, investigations have been focused on wheat proteins from the beginning and later on oat proteins. Early workers established toxicity using feeding tests based on the production of symptoms, such as steatorrhea, and on measurements of xylose or fat malabsorption [36]. The pioneering studies of Dicke's group demonstrated that gluten, the rubber-like protein fraction of wheat dough, not the water-soluble fraction (albumins), bore the toxic factor [105]. Fractionation of wheat gluten led to the conclusion that the alcohol-soluble gliadin fraction was the most toxic factor, whereas the effect of the insoluble glutenin fraction was described controversially as either nontoxic, weakly toxic, or as toxic as the gliadin fraction. It should be mentioned that the glutenin fraction is generally contaminated by modified ω-, α-, and γ-gliadins having odd numbers of cysteines, which are covalently bound to glutenin aggregates via interchain disulfide bonds

[106,107]. Therefore, statements on glutenin toxicity should not be based on studies on the whole glutenin fraction but on purified glutenin subunits (see Section 3.4).

Further elementary studies were performed with either the gliadin fraction or wheat gluten. Important results include the following [36]: heating of gliadins as well as the cleavage of disulfide bonds by oxidation did not diminish toxicity. In consequence, the three-dimensional structure of gliadins is not important for their toxic effect. In contrast, the complete degradation of gliadins into amino acids by acid hydrolysis renders them harmless. Glutamine, the most frequent amino acid of cereal storage proteins, also can be tolerated by CD patients. The extensive deamidation of glutamine side chains into glutamic acid side chains by diluted hydrochloric acid accompanied by limited cleavage of peptide bonds provokes detoxification of gliadins, showing that glutamine residues are important for CD-toxic effects. In accordance with the in vivo situation, the in vitro digestion of wheat gluten or gliadins with pepsin and trypsin alone or followed by pancreatin results in the retention of toxicity. Such enzymatic hydrolyzates of CD-toxic proteins have been used frequently as positive controls for toxicity tests because they are soluble in water or salt solution in contrast to intact gliadins and gluten. The most cited example is the so-called Frazer's fraction III, the water-soluble portion of a peptic-tryptic (PT-) digest of wheat gluten [108].

As equivalents to the gliadin fraction, the prolamin fractions of rye and barley are associated with CD toxicity; however, this finding has been reached without intensive testing. A comparative study on 22 patients revealed that PT-digests of gliadins, secalins, and hordeins elicit similar toxic effects on cultured biopsies [109]. The glutelin fractions of rye and barley have not been investigated to this day. Due to the contradictory results on oats, the oat prolamin fraction (avenins) has been isolated and extensively tested for CD toxicity by in vivo challenge, organ culture, and T-cell tests. Two patients with CD and dermatitis herpetiformis, respectively, were challenged with 2.5 g of pure avenins daily for 5 days and then with 2.5 g 9 days later [99]. Subsequent examination of intestinal biopsy specimens and skin biopsy samples did not show any toxic effect of avenin. CD-specific effects of PT-digests of gliadins and avenins were compared in organ culture tests on CD and non-CD biopsies; IFN-γ and IL-2 were used as markers for an immunogenic response [51]. After culturing with PT-gliadin ($n=9$), a significant increase of markers was observed. In contrast, there was no response when CD biopsies ($n=8$) were cultured with PT-avenin.

In another study, PT-gliadin, PT-secalin, PT-hordein, and PT-avenin were comparatively tested using proliferation assays with five different intestinal

T-cell lines of CD patients [52]. The results demonstrated immune reactivity of all T-cell lines to all PT-digests. However, there was a remarkable difference between PT-avenin and the other digests: Treatment with TG2 enhanced the response to gliadins, secalins, and hordeins, whereas this enzyme caused little or no enhancement of avenin responsiveness. The authors of both studies concluded that antigen immunogenicity shown by T-cell experiments does not equate with toxicity, which has to be confirmed by organ culture tests or in vivo challenge. Recently, the immunogenicity of avenin digests from three oat cultivars and of a gliadin digest (positive control) and an oryzin digest (negative control) was determined with isolated peripheral blood mononuclear T cells from 10 CD patients. The measurement of T-cell proliferation and IFN-γ release indicated different cultivar-dependent responses to the avenin digests, which were either high-immunogenic, medium-immunogenic, or nonimmunogenic (Table 2.8) [48]. Differences in the degree of immunogenicity of avenins were ascribed to the presence of different immunogenic epitopes within the avenin sequences [103].

3.4 Toxicity of Protein Types

The prolamin and glutelin fractions of wheat, rye, and barley consist of several protein types (see Section 2.2). Detailed studies on their CD toxicity are incomplete and restricted to the gliadin and glutenin types of wheat. Hekkens and coworkers were the first to demonstrate the toxicity of the well-defined gliadin subfraction A-gliadin, a group of aggregable α-type gliadins, by instillation into the small intestine of a CD patient, followed by biopsy [110]. The toxicity of A-gliadin was then confirmed by in vitro tests, such as organ culture tests [111]. At that time, carbohydrates that could possibly be covalently bound to gliadins (glycoproteins) were suspected to contribute to CD-toxic effects (lectin-like reactions) [112]. The analysis of A-gliadin, however, demonstrated that covalently bound carbohydrates were absent and, therefore, not involved in activating CD [113]. Subsequent in vivo and in vitro studies indicated that all gliadin subfractions (α-, β-, γ-, and ω-gliadins, in terms of electrophoretic mobilities) induce CD-toxic effects [114,115]. The results favored the viewpoint of a decreasing toxicity from α- to ω-gliadins [116,117]. However, the subfractions investigated were not necessarily pure with respect to the protein type, and the ω-fraction was not differentiated into the ω5- and ω1,2-types. Highly purified ω-gliadins (probably a mixture of ω5- and ω1,2-gliadins) were used to challenge two CD patients by rectal introduction [118]. Characteristic responses by mucosal $CD3^+$ and $\gamma\delta^+$ lymphocytes indicated a specific response of rectal mucosa to this gliadin type.

Afterward, in vivo and organ culture studies on the toxicity of proteins were strongly reduced because of the availability of synthetic peptides and T-cell tests (see Section 3.1.3). Molberg and colleagues isolated from wheat flour a subfraction of HMW-GS consisting of five components (subunits 1Ax2, 1Dx5, 1Bx7, 1By9, and 1Dy10) and used recombinant single subunits 1Dx5 or 1Dy10 expressed in *Escherichia coli* [119]. Both the subfraction and the single subunits were tested by a series of T cells sensitive for HMW-GS, either in the native form or deamidated by TG2. The results indicated that the intestinal T cells of 9 of 22 CD patients responded to deamidated HMW-GS but not to the native proteins. For in vivo challenge and T-cell tests, a mixture of HMW-GS (1Dx5, 1Bx7, 1By9, 1Dy10) was isolated from wheat flour and carefully purified by precipitation and HPLC [120]. T-cell lines from 11 of 17 CD patients were significantly stimulated. The differences in response to native and TG2-deamidated subunits were not significant. Three CD patients were challenged with 500 mg of subunits each, and 4 h after commencing infusions, a significant change in small intestinal morphology (e.g., ratio of villous height to crypt depth) was observed. Moreover, the expression of IL-15 in the small intestine increased beginning 2 h after the infusion. Consecutively, in vitro studies on toxicity were performed with single recombinant HMW-GS 1Dx5 and 1Dy10 purified from transgenic yeast and transgenic corn, respectively [121]. Gluten-sensitive T cells from 4 of 13 CD patients responded to subunit 1Dx5 and 3 of 11 to subunit 1Dy10. Both subunits 1Dx5 and 1Dy10 tested by in vivo challenge in one patient induced significant changes in the ratio of villous height to crypt depth and enterocyte height. Increased staining for IL-15 was seen from 2 h after challenge with both subunits. Summing up, the three studies described show clearly that HMW-GS can exacerbate CD just as gliadins can. Subsequent studies demonstrated that patients with untreated CD have raised antibody levels to HMW-GS 1Dy10, indicating the participation of this type of proteins in the adaptive immune response [122].

In contrast to gliadins and HMW-GS, LMW-GS and single protein types of rye (see Section 2.2) have not been tested for CD toxicity up to now. Their potential toxicity has been derived from studies on corresponding peptides (see Section 3.5). Hordein-sensitive T cells induced by oral barley challenge were used to test different hordein types for CD-specific immunogenicity [74]. All fractions were immunogenic, but D- and C-hordeins were most active.

3.5 Toxicity of Peptides

The introduction of organ culture tests (see Section 3.1.3) opened a new area in the study on gluten peptide toxicity because small amounts could be tested. Nevertheless, only few attempts have been made to isolate and characterize pure gluten peptides. The problems included the following: the gluten protein fractions consist of numerous components, and the required enzymatic digestion results in hundreds of different peptides. Moreover, the efficiency of methods for preparative separation of peptides was limited and amino acid sequences of gluten proteins were not known until the 1980s. At that time, promising studies were possible only through the cooperation of hospitals doing research on CD with laboratories experienced in cereal protein chemistry. Three partner groups were successful in isolating and testing peptides from digests of different gliadin preparations, either from total gliadins [123–125], β-gliadins [126], or α-gliadins [127]. Congruently, their results indicated that glutamine- and proline-rich sequences of α-gliadins (α1–55) within section I (Figure 2.8) were involved in activating CD, whereas other sequences (α56–68, α247–266) were negative (Table 2.10). The tetrapeptide sequences PSQQ and QQQP, common for active peptides, were considered to be key sequences for further investigations. Conformation studies showed that β-turns were the dominant structural feature of active peptides [132].

In 1991, a panel of synthetic peptides containing sequences of α-gliadins was tested by instillation into the small intestine or organ culture of intestinal mucosa. The dodecapeptide α206–217 (including PSQQ) showed a toxic effect in vivo [128]. Three synthetic peptides from α-gliadins were tested in vivo and in vitro [39,45]. Consistently, peptide α31–49 was shown to be toxic, whereas peptides α3–21 and α202–220 were not toxic—the latter results contrasting those on peptides α1–30 [127], α3–24 [125], and α206–217 [128]. Furthermore, in vivo tests presented evidence that the synthetic peptides α31–43 and α44–55 were toxic, whereas peptide α56–68 was inactive [129]. Organ culture testing of peptides α31–55 and α31–43 revealed activity at a low concentration, whereas peptide α44–55 turned out to be active only at a high concentration [130]. Variants of peptide α31–49, in which single amino acid residues were substituted with alanine, remained active in the organ culture test when residues L31 and P36 were substituted, but lost toxicity when residues P38, P39, and P42 were substituted [75]. Four CD patients in remission underwent challenges with peptide α56–75 and a negative control peptide from β-casein [35]. The gliadin peptide caused intestinal damage in all patients, whereas the casein peptide elicited no response. The toxicity of gliadin peptide α51–70 was assessed using an organ culture system [131].

Even if the investigations described may be partly unsatisfactory with regard to the number of tests, purity of peptides, and accordance of results, it can be concluded that most of the toxic sequences occur in the

Table 2.10 Amino Acid Sequences of Peptides Tested for CD Toxicity by Instillation and Organ Culture Tests

Sequence	Source	Position	Toxicity[a]	Reference
VPVPQLQPQNPSQQQPQEQVPL	Gliadin	α3–24	+(OC)	[125]
VQQQQFPGQQQPFPQQPYPQPQPFPSQQPY	Gliadin	α25–55	+(OC)	[125]
VRVPVPQLQPQNPSQQQPQEQVPLVQQQQF	A-gliadin	α1–30	+(OC)	[127]
LGQQQPFPPQQPYPQPQPFPSQQPY	A-gliadin	α31–55	+(OC)	[127]
LQLQPFPQPQLPY	A-gliadin	α56–68	−(OC)	[127]
CNVYIAPYCTIAPFGIFGTN	A-gliadin	α247–266	−(OC)	[127]
LGQGSFRPSQQN	Synthetic	α206–217	+(IN)	[128]
LGQQQPFPPQQPYPQPQPF	Synthetic	α31–49	+(IN, OC)	[39,45]
QQYPLGQGSFRPSQQNPQA	Synthetic	α202–220	−(IN, OC)	[39,45]
VPVPQLQPQNPSQQQPQEQ	Synthetic	α3–21	−(IN, OC)	[39,45]
AGQQQPFPPQQPYPQPQPF	Synthetic	α31–49, A31	+(OC)	[75]
LGQQQAFPPQQPYPQPQPF	Synthetic	α31–49, A36	+(OC)	[75]
LGQQQPFAPQQPYPQPQPF	Synthetic	α31–49, A38	−(OC)	[75]
LGQQQPFPAQQPYPQPQPF	Synthetic	α31–49, A39	−(OC)	[75]
LGQQQPFPPQQAYPQPQPF	Synthetic	α31–49, A42	−(OC)	[75]
LGQQQPFPPQQPY	Synthetic	α31–43	+(IN)	[129,130]
PQPQPFPSQQPY	Synthetic	α44–55	+(IN)	[129]
LQLQPFPQPQLPY	Synthetic	α56–68	−(IN)	[129]
LQLQPFPQPQLPYPQPQLPY	Synthetic	α56–75	+(IN)	[35]
SQQPYLQLQPFPQPQLPYSQ	Synthetic	α51–70	+(OC)	[131]

[a]*IN, instillation; OC, organ culture.*

N-terminal domain of α-gliadins and mainly consist of glutamine, proline, and hydrophobic amino acids (leucine, phenylalanine, tyrosine). Corresponding sequences of γ- and ω-gliadins, glutenin subunits, secalins, hordeins, and avenins have not been tested yet by in vivo challenge and organ culture tests.

The search for CD-active peptides has shifted toward epitopes that stimulate intestinal gluten-sensitive T-cell lines and clones of CD patients. A small selection of the first generation (1999–2005) of immunogenic peptides reported by the groups of van de Wal [133], Vader [134,135], Arentz-Hansen [136], and Shan et al. [137,138] is presented in Table 2.11. More immunogenic peptides identified by intestinal T-cell assays are mentioned in the paper of Camarca and colleagues [139]. Given the heterogeneity of wheat, rye, and barley proteins, it is not surprising that a large number of T-cell epitopes exist. The major part of peptides is HLA-DQ2 restricted and derives from the glutamine- and proline-rich sequence domains (see Section 2.2). A number of studies have shown that patients respond heterogeneously to

Table 2.11 Amino Acid Sequences of Selected Gluten Peptides Stimulatory for Intestinal T Cells of CD Patients

Origin	Sequence[a]	Reference
α2	LQLQPFPQP**Q**LPYPQP**Q**LPYPQP**Q** LPYPQPQPF	[136]
α20	PFRP**Q**QPYPQPQPQ	[134]
γ5	FLQP**Q**QPFP**Q**QP**Q**QPYP**Q**QP**Q**QPFPQ	[138]
γ5	QFSQP**QQ**QFPQPQ	[136]
LMW 156	QQQQPPFS**Q**QQ**Q**SPFSQQQQ	[134]
LMW 17	QQPPFS**QQ**Q**Q**QPLPQ	[134]
HMW 2	GQ**Q**GYYPTSP**Q**QS	[133]
HMW 2	**Q**GYYPTSP**Q**QSG	[133]
Sec α2	QPFPQP**Q**QPFPQSQ	[135]
Sec α9	P**Q**QPFPQP**Q**QPFPQ	[135]
Hor α2	Q**Q**FPQP**Q**QPFPQQP	[135]
Hor α9	P**Q**QPFPQP**Q**QPFRQ	[135]
Av α9[A]	QYQPYPEQ**Q**EPFVQ	[135]
Av α9[B]	QYQPYPEQ**Q**QPFVQ	[135]

[a]*Glutamine (Q) residues targeted by TG2 are in bold.*

different epitopes and that there also are differences between children and adults [134].

Another approach to detect immunogenic gluten peptides was used by Tye-Din and coworkers [50]. PBMCs were freshly isolated from CD patients, who were challenged with wheat, rye, or barley over 3 days. A library of synthetic peptides derived from gliadins, glutenins, secalins, and hordeins were treated with TG2, incubated with the PBMCs, and screened with an IFN-γ ELISpot assay. The results revealed a high number of immunogenic peptides from all types of the gluten proteins investigated. Interestingly, the peptides that stimulated T cells were the same among patients who ate the same cereal: Gliadin and glutenin peptides were stimulatory only after wheat challenge, secalin peptides only after rye challenge, and hordein peptides only after barley challenge. Only one common peptide of ω-gliadin and C-hordein (QPFPQPEQPFPW) was immunodominant regardless of the grain consumed. Comparative studies using both intestinal $CD4^+$ T cells and PBMCs identified several common immunogenic sequences revealing a convergence between the two approaches.

The Food Allergy Research and Resource Program of the Department of Food Science and Technology, University of Nebraska–Lincoln, USA, has compiled a database of CD-active gluten peptides [140]. It includes more than 1000 native or deamidated peptides described in more than 60 publications. These peptides have their origins in all types of wheat gliadins and glutenins and also in rye secalins, barley hordeins, and oat avenins. Some authors have subdivided CD-active peptides into "toxic" peptides generating an innate immune response and "immunogenic" peptides generating an adaptive immune response [31,141,142]. The discrepancy between the numbers of immunogenic peptides identified by T-cell tests and of toxic peptides identified by in vivo or organ culture tests is extraordinary: 1014 peptides have been classified as immunogenic, nine peptides as toxic, and five peptides as both toxic and immunogenic. The question of whether immunogenicity corresponds to toxicity in any case remains to be answered [143]. In summary, a common feature among toxic/immunogenic peptides is the presence of multiple proline and glutamine residues, which gives rise to four unique structural and functional properties [138,144]:

1. These peptides are exceptionally resistant to proteolysis by gastric, pancreatic, and intestinal digestive proteases because of their high proline content. As a result, a high intestinal concentration of potentially immunogenic peptides is maintained following a gluten-containing diet.
2. Selected glutamine residues in these gluten peptides are deamidated or transamidated by TG2 under physiological conditions, leading to enhanced immunogenicity (see Chapter 1, Section 6.3.1).
3. The proline-rich gluten peptides naturally adopt a left-handed polyproline II helical conformation, which is the preferred conformation of all bound major histocompatibility complex class II ligands.
4. Large peptides that contain multiple HLA-DQ–binding epitopes have a greater T-cell stimulatory activity than small peptides containing only one epitope.

REFERENCES

[1] Food and Agriculture Organization of the United Nations. http://faostat3.fao.org [accessed December 2013].

[2] Bouchenak-Khelladi Y, Salamin N, Savolainen V, Forest F, van der Bank M, Chase MW, et al. Large multi-gene phylogenetic trees of the grasses (Poaceae): progress towards complete tribal and generic level sampling. Mol Phylogenet Evol 2008;47:488–505.

[3] Koehler P, Wieser H. Chemistry of cereal grains. In: Gobbetti M, Gaenzle M, editors. Handbook of sourdough biotechnology. New York: Springer; 2013. pp. 11–45.

[4] Dupont FM, Vensel WH, Tanaka CK, Hurkman WJ, Altenbach SB. Deciphering the complexities of the wheat flour proteome using quantitative two-dimensional electrophoresis, three proteases and tandem mass spectrometry. Proteome Sci 2011;9:10.

[5] Osborne TB. Vegetable proteins. London: Longmans Green; 1924.

[6] Wieser H, Bushuk W, MacRitchie F. The polymeric glutenins. In: Wrigley C, Bekes F, Bushuk W, editors. Gliadin and glutenin: the unique balance of wheat quality. St. Paul (USA): AACC International; 2006. pp. 213–40.

[7] Wieser H, Seilmeier W, Eggert M, Belitz HD. Tryptophangehalt von Getreideproteinen. Z Lebensm Unters Forsch 1983;177:457–60.

[8] Wieser H, Seilmeier W, Belitz HD. Vergleichende Untersuchungen über partielle Aminosäuresequenzen von Prolaminen und Glutelinen verschiedener Getreidearten. I. Proteinfraktionierung nach Osborne. Z Lebensm Unters Forsch 1980;170:17–26.

[9] Wieser H, Kieffer R. Correlations of the amount of gluten protein types to the technological properties of wheat flours determined on a micro-scale. J Cereal Sci 2001;34:19–27.

[10] Gellrich C, Schieberle P, Wieser H. Biochemical characterization and quantification of the storage protein (secalin) types in rye flour. Cereal Chem 2003;80:102–9.

[11] Lange M, Vincze E, Wieser H, Schjoerring JK, Holm PB. Suppression of C-hordein synthesis in barley by antisense constructs results in a more balanced amino acid composition. J Agric Food Chem 2007;55:6074–81.

[12] Wieser H. Cereal protein chemistry. In: Feighery C, O'Farelly C, editors. Gastrointestinal immunology and gluten-sensitive disease. Dublin (Ireland): Oak Tree Press; 1994. pp. 191–202.

[13] Payne PI, Nightingale MA, Krattinger AF, Holt LM. The relationship between HMW glutenin subunit composition and the bread-making quality of British-grown wheat varieties. J Sci Food Agric 1987;40:51–65.

[14] Tatham AS, Miflin BJ, Shewry PR. The β-turn conformation in wheat gluten proteins: relationship to gluten elasticity. Cereal Chem 1985;62:405–12.

[15] Bailey CH. A translation of Beccari's lecture "concerning grain" (1728). Cereal Chem 1941;18:555–61.

[16] Wieser H. Chemistry of gluten proteins. Food Microbiol 2007;24:115–9.

[17] Grosch W, Wieser H. Redox reactions in wheat dough as affected by ascorbic acid. J Cereal Sci 1999;29:1–16.

[18] Mueller S, Wieser H. The location of disulfide bonds in α-type gliadins. J Cereal Sci 1995;22:21–7.

[19] Mueller S, Wieser H. The location of disulfide bonds in monomeric γ-type gliadins. J Cereal Sci 1997;26:169–76.

[20] Wrigley CW. Biopolymers: giant proteins with flour power. Nature 1996;381:738–9.

[21] Koehler P, Wieser H. Comparative studies of high Mr subunits of rye and wheat. III. Localisation of cysteine residues. J Cereal Sci 2000;32:189–97.

[22] Eckert B, Amend T, Belitz HD. What is unique about wheat gluten? Microscopic observations on flour particles of various cereals. In: Gluten proteins 1993. Detmold (Germany): Association of Cereal Proteins; 1994. pp. 498–504.

[23] Bushuk W, Wadhawan C. Wheat gluten is good not only for breadmaking. In: Pomeranz Y, editor. Wheat is unique. St. Paul (MN, USA): AACC; 1989. pp. 263–75.

[24] Day L, Augustin MA, Batey IL, Wrigley CW. Wheat-gluten uses and industry needs. Trends Food Sci Technol 2006;17:82–90.

[25] Esen A. A proposed nomenclature for the alcohol-soluble proteins (zeins) of maize (*Zea mays* L.). J Cereal Sci 1987;5:117–28.

[26] Shull JM, Watterson JJ, Kirleis AW. Proposed nomenclature for the alcohol-soluble proteins (kafirins) of *Sorghum bicolor* (L. Moench) based on molecular weight, solubility, and structure. J Agric Food Chem 1991;39:83–7.

[27] Juliano BO. Polysaccharides, proteins, and lipids. In: Juliano BO, editor. Rice chemistry and technology. 2nd ed. St. Paul (USA): AACC; 1985. pp. 98–142.

[28] Rubenstein I, Geraghti DE. The genetic organization of zein. In: Pomeranz Y, editor. Advances in cereal science and technology, vol. VIII. St. Paul (USA): AACC; 1986. pp. 297–315.

[29] Cabrera-Chavez F, Iametti S, Miriani M, de la Barca AMC, Mamone G, Bonomi F. Maize prolamins resistant to peptic-tryptic digestion maintain immune-recognition by IgA from some celiac disease patients. Plant Foods Hum Nutr 2012;67:24–30.

[30] Ortiz-Sanchez JP, Cabrera-Chavez F, de la Barca AMC. Maize prolamins could induce a gluten-like cellular immune response in some celiac disease patients. Nutrients 2013;5:4174–83.

[31] Lindfors K, Rauhavirta T, Stenman S, Maeki M, Kaukinen K. In vitro models for gluten toxicity: relevance for celiac disease pathogenesis and development of novel treatment options. Exp Biol Med 2012;237:119–25.

[32] Stoven S, Murray JA, Marietta EV. Latest in vitro and in vivo models of celiac disease. Expert Opin Drug Discov 2013;8:445–57.

[33] Wieser H, Antes S, Seilmeier W. Quantitative determination of gluten protein types in wheat flour by reversed-phase high-performance liquid chromatography. Cereal Chem 1998;75:644–50.

[34] van Eckert R, Berghofer E, Ciclitira PJ, Chirdo F, Denery-Papini S, Ellis HJ, et al. Towards a new gliadin reference material – isolation and characterisation. J Cereal Sci 2006;43:331–41.

[35] Fraser JS, Engel W, Ellis HJ, Moodie SJ, Pollock EL, Wieser H, et al. Coeliac disease: in vivo toxicity of the putative immunodominant epitope. Gut 2003;52:1698–702.

[36] Shewry PR, Tatham AS, Kasarda DD. Cereal proteins and coeliac disease. In: Marsh MN, editor. Coeliac disease. Oxford (UK): Blackwell Scientific Publications; 1992. pp. 305–48.

[37] Janatuinen EK, Pikkarainen PH, Kemppainen TA, Kosma VM, Jarvinen RM, Uusitupa MI, et al. A comparison of diets with and without oats in adults with celiac disease. N Engl J Med 1995;333:1033–7.

[38] Hekkens WTJM, Haex AJC, Willighagen RGJ. Some aspects of gliadin fractionation and testing by a histochemical method. In: Booth CC, editor. Coeliac disease. Edinburgh, London (UK): Churchill Livingstone; 1970. pp. 11–9.

[39] Sturgess R, Day P, Ellis HJ, Lundin KEA, Gjertsen HA, Kontakou M, et al. Wheat peptide challenge in coeliac disease. Lancet 1994;343:758–61.

[40] Grootjans J, Thuijls G, Verdam F, Derikx JP, Lenaerts K, Buurman WA. Non-invasive assessment of barrier integrity and function of the human gut. World J Gastrointest Surg 2010;2:61–9.

[41] Leffler D, Schuppan D, Pallav K, Najarian R, Goldsmith JD, Hansen J, et al. Kinetics of the histological, serological and symptomatic responses to gluten challenge in adults with coeliac disease. Gut 2013;62:996–1004.

[42] Anderson RP, van Heel DA, Tye-Din JA, Barnardo M, Salio M, Jewell DP, et al. T cells in peripheral blood after gluten challenge in coeliac disease. Gut 2005;54:1217–23.

[43] Loft DE, Marsh MN, Sandle GI, Crowe PT, Garner V, Gordon D, et al. Studies of intestinal lymphoid tissue. XII. Epithelial lymphocyte and mucosal responses to rectal gluten challenge in celiac sprue. Gastroenterology 1989;97:29–37.

[44] Browning TH, Trier JS. Organ culture of mucosal biopsies of human small intestine. J Clin Invest 1969;48:1423–32.

[45] Shidrawi RG, Day P, Przemioslo R, Ellis HJ, Nelufer JM, Ciclitira PJ. In vitro toxicity of gluten peptides in celiac disease assessed by organ culture. Scand J Gastroenterol 1995;30:758–63.

[46] van de Wal Y, Kooy YMC, van Veelen PA, Pena SA, Mearin LM, Molberg O, et al. Small intestinal T cells of celiac disease patients recognize a natural pepsin fragment of gliadin. Proc Natl Acad Sci USA 1998;95:10050–4.

[47] Ellis HJ, Pollock EL, Engel W, Fraser JS, Rosen-Bronson S, Wieser H, et al. Investigation of the putative immunodominant T cell epitopes in coeliac disease. Gut 2003;52:212–7.

[48] Comino I, Real A, de Lorenzo L, Cornell H, Lopez-Casado MA, Barro F, et al. Diversity in oat potential immunogenicity: basis for the selection of oat varieties with no toxicity in coeliac disease. Gut 2011;60:915–22.

[49] Suligoj T, Gregorini A, Colomba M, Ellis HJ, Ciclitira PJ. Evaluation of the safety of ancient strains of wheat in coeliac disease reveals heterogeneous small intestinal T cell responses suggestive of coeliac toxicity. Clin Nutr 2013;32:1043–9.

[50] Tye-Din JA, Stewart JA, Dromey JA, Beissbarth T, van Heel DA, Tatham A, et al. Comprehensive, quantitative mapping of T cell epitopes in gluten in celiac disease. Sci Transl Med 2010;2:41–51.

[51] Kilmartin C, Lynch S, Abuzakouk M, Wieser H, Feighery C. Avenin fails to induce a Th1 response in coeliac tissue following in vitro culture. Gut 2003;52: 47–52.

[52] Kilmartin C, Wieser H, Abuzakouk M, Kelly J, Jackson J, Feighery C. Intestinal T cell responses to cereal proteins in celiac disease. Dig Dis Sci 2006;51:202–9.

[53] Maiuri L, Luciani A, Villella VR, Vasaturo A, Giardino I, Pettoello-Mantovani M, et al. Lysosomal accumulation of gliadin p31–43 peptide induces oxidative stress and tissue transglutaminase-mediated PPARγ downregulation in intestinal epithelial cells and coeliac mucosa. Gut 2010;59:311–9.

[54] Bethune MT, Siegel M, Howles-Banerji S, Khosla C. Interferon-γ released by gluten-stimulated celiac disease-specific intestinal T cells enhances the transepithelial flux of gluten peptides. J Pharmacol Exp Ther 2009;329:657–68.

[55] Lammers KM, Lu R, Brownley J, Lu B, Gerard C, Thomas K, et al. Gliadin induces an increase in intestinal permeability and zonulin release by binding to the chemokine receptor CXCR3. Gastroenterology 2008;135:194–204.

[56] Barone MV, Nanayakkara M, Paolella G, Maglio M, Vitale V, Troiano R, et al. Gliadin peptide P31–43 localises to endocytic vesicles and interferes with their maturation. PLoS One 2010;5:e12246.

[57] Luebbing N, Barone MV, Rudloff S, Troncone R, Auricchio S, Zimmer KP. Correction of gliadin transport within enterocytes through celiac disease serum. Pediatr Res 2011;70:357–62.

[58] Wood GM, Howdle PD, Losowsky MS. Organ culture of fetal rat small intestine for testing gluten toxicity: a reappraisal. Br J Exp Pathol 1987;68:25–34.

[59] Mothes T, Osman AA, Seilmeier W, Wieser H. The activity of single gliadin components in a fetal chick intestine assay for coeliac disease. Eur Food Res Technol 1999;210:93–6.

[60] Cornell HJ, Townley RRW. Effect of gliadin peptides on rat-liver lysosomes in relation to the pathogenesis of coeliac disease. Clin Chim Acta 1973;49:181–8.

[61] Marietta EV, Murray JA. Animal models to study gluten sensitivity. Semin Immunopathol 2012;34:497–511.

[62] Hall EJ, Batt RM. Dietary modulation of gluten sensitivity in a naturally occurring enteropathy of Irish setter dogs. Gut 1992;33:198–205.

[63] Bethune MT, Borda JT, Ribka E, Liu MX, Phillippi-Falkenstein K, Jandacek RJ, et al. A non-human primate model for gluten sensitivity. PLoS One 2008;3:e1614.

[64] van der Kolk JH, van Putten LA, Mulder CJ, Grinwis GCM, Reijm M, Butler CM, et al. Gluten-dependent antibodies in horses with inflammatory small bowel disease (ISBD). Vet Q 2012;32:3–11.

[65] de Kauwe AL, Chen Z, Anderson RP, Keech CL, Price JD, Wijburg O, et al. Resistance to celiac disease in humanized HLA-DR3-DQ2-transgenic mice expressing specific anti-gliadin CD4+ T cells. J Immunol 2009;182:7440–50.

[66] D'Arienzo R, Stefanile R, Maurano F, Luongo D, Bergamo P, Mazzarella G, et al. A deregulated immune response to gliadin causes a decreased villous height in DQ8 transgenic mice. Eur J Immunol 2009;39:3552–61.

[67] de Paolo RW, Abadie V, Tang F, Fehlner-Peach H, Hall JA, Wang W, et al. Co-adjuvant effects of retinoic acid and IL-15 induce inflammatory immunity to dietary antigens. Nature 2011;471:220–4.

[68] Auricchio S, de Ritis G, de Vincenzi M, Occorsio P, Silano V. Effects of gliadin-derived peptides from bread and durum wheats on small intestine cultures from rat fetus and coeliac children. Pediatr Res 1982;16:1004–10.

[69] Vincentini O, Maialetti F, Gazza L, Silano M, Dessi M, de Vincenzi M, et al. Environmental factors of celiac disease: cytotoxicity of hulled wheat species *Triticum monococcum*, *T. turgidum* ssp. *dicoccum* and *T. aestivum* ssp. *spelta*. J Gastroenterol Hepatol 2007;22:1816–22.

[70] van den Broeck H, Hongbing C, Lacaze X, Dusautoir JC, Gilissen L, Smulders M, et al. In search of tetraploid wheat accessions reduced in celiac disease-related gluten epitopes. Mol Biosyst 2010;6:2206–13.

[71] Frisoni M, Corazza GR, Lafiandra D, de Ambrogio E, Filipponi C, Bonvicini F, et al. Wheat deficient in gliadins: promising tool for treatment of coeliac disease. Gut 1995;36:375–8.

[72] Spaenij-Dekking L, Kooy-Winkelaar Y, van Veelen P, Drijfhout JW, Jonker H, van Soest L, et al. Natural variation in toxicity of wheat: potential for selection of nontoxic varieties for celiac disease patients. Gastroenterology 2005; 129:797–806.

[73] Carroccio A, di Prima L, Noto D, Fayer F, Ambrosiano G, Villanacci V, et al. Searching for wheat plants with low toxicity in celiac disease: between direct toxicity and immunologic activation. Dig Liver Dis 2011;43:34–9.

[74] Tanner GJ, Howitt CA, Forrester RI, Campbell PM, Tye-Din JA, Anderson RP. Dissecting the T-cell response to hordeins in coeliac disease can develop barley with reduced immunotoxicity. Aliment Pharmacol Ther 2010;32:1184–91.

[75] Biagi F, Ellis HJ, Parnell ND, Shidrawi RG, Thomas PD, O'Reilly N, et al. A non-toxic analogue of a coeliac-activating gliadin peptide: a basis for immunomodulation? Aliment Pharmacol Ther 1999;13:945–50.

[76] Koning F. Celiac disease: quantity matters. Semin Immunopathol 2012;34:541–9.

[77] Ciacci C, Maiuri L, Caporaso N, Bucci C, del Giudice L, Rita-Massardo D, et al. Celiac disease: in vitro and in vivo safety and palatability of wheat-free sorghum food products. Clin Nutr 2007;26:799–805.

[78] Pontieri P, Mamone G, de Caro S, Tuinstra MR, Roemer E, Okot J, et al. Sorghum, a healthy and gluten-free food for celiac patients as demonstrated by genome, biochemical, and immunochemical analyses. J Agric Food Chem 2013;61:2565–71.

[79] Kasarda DD. Toxic cereals in coeliac disease. In: Feighery C, O'Farrelly C, editors. Gastrointestinal immunology and gluten-sensitive disease. Dublin (Ireland): Oak Tree Press; 1994. pp. 203–20.

[80] Kasarda DD. Grains in relation to celiac disease. Cereal Foods World 2001;46:209–10.

[81] Forssell F, Wieser H. Dinkel und Zöliakie. Z Lebensm Unters Forsch 1995;201:35–9.

[82] Wieser H. Comparative investigations of gluten proteins from different wheat species. I. Qualitative and quantitative composition of gluten protein types. Eur Food Res Technol 2000;211:262–8.

[83] van den Broeck HC, Smulders MJM, Hamer RJ, Gilissen LJWJ, van der Meer I. Coeliac-safe wheat. A novel wheat to decrease the prevalence and symptoms of coeliac disease. Agro Food Ind Hi-Tech 2011;22:18–21.

[84] Wieser H. Comparative investigations of gluten proteins from different wheat species. III. N-terminal amino acid sequences of α-gliadins potentially toxic for coeliac patients. Eur Food Res Technol 2001;213:183–6.

[85] Molberg O, Uhlen AK, Jensen T, Solheim-Flaete N, Fleckenstein B, Arentz-Hansen H, et al. Mapping of gluten T-cell epitopes in the bread wheat ancestors: implications for celiac disease. Gastroenterology 2005;128:393–401.

[86] Pizzuti D, Buda A, D'Odorico A, D'Inca R, Chiarelli S, Curioni A, et al. Lack of intestinal mucosal toxicity of *Triticum monococcum* in celiac disease patients. Scand J Gastroenterol 2006;41:1305–11.

[87] Gianfrani C, Maglio M, Rotondi-Aufiero V, Camarca A, Vocca I, Iaquinto G, et al. Immunogenicity of monococcum wheat in celiac patients. Am J Clin Nutr 2012;96:1339–45.

[88] Pulido OM, Gillespie Z, Zarkadas M, Dubois S, Vavasour E, Rashid M, et al. Introduction of oats in the diet of individuals with celiac disease: a systematic review. Adv Food Nutr Res 2009;57:235–85.

[89] Sontag-Strohm T, Lehtinen P, Kaukovirta-Norja A. Oat products and their current status in the celiac diet. In: Arendt EK, dal Bello F, editors. Gluten-free cereal products and beverages. New York (USA): Academic Press; 2008. pp. 191–202.

[90] Pawlowska P, Diowksz A, Kordialik-Bogacka E. State-of-the-art incorporation of oats into a gluten-free diet. Food Rev Int 2012;28:330–42.

[91] Cooper SEJ, Kennedy NP, Mohamed BM, Abuzakouk M, Dunne J, Byrne G, et al. Immunological indicators of coeliac disease activity are not altered by long-term oats challenge. Clin Exp Immunol 2013;171:313–8.

[92] Janatuinen EK, Kemppainen TA, Julkunen RJK, Kosma VM, Maeki M, Heikkinen M, et al. No harm from five years ingestion of oats in coeliac disease. Gut 2002;50:332–5.

[93] Koskinen O, Villanen M, Korponay-Szabo I, Lindfors K, Maeki M, Kaukinen K. Oats do not induce systemic or mucosal autoantibody response in children with coeliac disease. J Pediatr Gastroenterol Nutr 2009;48:559–65.

[94] Hardman CM, Garioch JJ, Leonard JN, Thomas HJ, Walker MM, Lortan JE, et al. Absence of toxicity of oats in patients with dermatitis herpetiformis. N Engl J Med 1997;337:1884–7.

[95] Reunala T, Collin P, Holm K, Pikkarainen P, Miettinen A, Vuolteenaho N, et al. Tolerance to oats in dermatitis herpetiformis. Gut 1998;43:490–3.

[96] Lundin KEA, Nilsen EM, Scott HG, Loberg EM, Gjoen A, Bratlie J, et al. Oats induced villous atrophy in coeliac disease. Gut 2003;52:1649–52.

[97] Arentz-Hansen H, Fleckenstein B, Molberg O, Scott H, Koning F, Jung G, et al. The molecular basis for oat intolerance in patients with celiac disease. PLoS Med 2004;1:84–92.

[98] Salovaara H, Kanerva P, Kaukinen K, Sontag-Strohm T. Oats – an overview from celiac disease point of view. In: Arendt EK, Dal Bello F, editors. The science of gluten-free foods and beverages. St. Paul (USA): AACC International; 2009. pp. 69–82.

[99] Hardman C, Fry L, Tatham A, Thomas HJ. Absence of toxicity of avenin in patients with dermatitis herpetiformis. N Engl J Med 1999;340:321.

[100] Zimmer KP. Nutrition and celiac disease. Curr Probl Pediatr Adolesc Health Care 2011;41:244–7.

[101] Koerner TB, Cleroux C, Poirier C, Cantin I, Alimkulov A, Elamparo H. Gluten contamination in the Canadian commercial oat supply. Food Addit Contam 2011; 28:705–10.

[102] Mujico JR, Mitea C, Gilissen LJWJ, de Ru A, van Veelen P, Smulders MJM, et al. Natural variation in avenin epitopes among oat varieties: implications for celiac disease. J Cereal Sci 2011;54:8–12.

[103] Real A, Comino I, de Lorenzo F, Merchan F, Gil-Humanes J, Gimenez MJ, et al. Molecular and immunological characterization of gluten proteins isolated from oat cultivars that differ in toxicity for celiac disease. PLoS One 2012;7:e48365.

[104] Londono DM, van´t Westende WPC, Goryunova S, Salentijn EMJ, van den Broeck HC, van der Meer IM, et al. Avenin diversity analysis of the genus *Avena* (oat). Relevance for people with celiac disease. J Cereal Sci 2013;58:170–7.

[105] van de Kamer JH, Weijers HA, Dicke WK. Coeliac disease. IV. An investigation into the injurious constituents of wheat in connection with their action on patients with coeliac disease. Acta Paediatr 1953;42:223–31.

[106] Lew EJL, Kuzmicky DD, Kasarda DD. Characterization of low-molecular-weight glutenin subunits by reversed-phase high-performance liquid chromatography, sodium dodecyl sulfate-polyacrylamide gel electrophoresis, and N-terminal amino acid sequencing. Cereal Chem 1992;69:508–15.

[107] Wieser H, Seilmeier W, Belitz HD. Characterization of ethanol-extractable reduced subunits of glutenin separated by reversed-phase high-performance liquid chromatography. J Cereal Sci 1990;12:63–71.

[108] Frazer AC, Fletcher RF, Ross CA, Shaw B, Sammons HG, Schneider R. Gluten-induced enteropathy: the effect of partially digested gluten. Lancet 1959;2:252–5.

[109] Bracken SC, Kilmartin C, Wieser H, Jackson J, Feighery C. Barley and rye prolamins induce an mRNA interferon-γ response in coeliac mucosa. Aliment Pharmacol Ther 2006;23:1307–14.

[110] Hekkens WTJM. The toxicity of gliadin, a review. In: McNicholl B, McCarthy CF, Fottrell PF, editors. Perspectives in coeliac disease. Lancaster (UK): MTP Press; 1978. pp. 3–15.

[111] Falchuk ZM, Nelson DL, Katz AJ, Bernardin JE, Kasarda DD, Hague NE, et al. Gluten-sensitive enteropathy: influence of histocompatibility type on gluten sensitivity in vitro. J Clin Invest 1980;66:227–33.

[112] Koettgen E, Volk B, Mueller M, Gerok W. Studies on the lectin properties of gluten and on the pathomechanism of celiac disease. Fresenius Z Anal Chem 1984;317:702–3.

[113] Bernardin JE, Saunders RM, Kasarda DD. Absence of carbohydrate in celiac-toxic A-gliadin. Cereal Chem 1976;53:612–4.

[114] Ciclitira PJ, Evans DJ, Fagg NL, Lennox ES, Dowling RH. Clinical testing of gliadin fractions in coeliac patients. Clin Sci 1984;66:357–64.

[115] Howdle PD, Ciclitira PJ, Simpson FG, Losowsky MS. Are all gliadins toxic in coeliac disease? an in vitro study of alpha, beta, gamma and omega gliadins. Scand J Gastroenterol 1984;19:41–7.

[116] Jos J, Charbonnier L, Mougenot JF, Mosse J, Rey J. Isolation and characterization of the toxic fraction of wheat gliadin in celiac disease. In: McNicholl B, McCarthy CF, Fottrell PE, editors. Perspectives in coeliac disease. Lancaster (UK): MTP Press; 1978. pp. 75–90.

[117] Sinclair TS, Ohannesian AD, Jones D. Which gliadin fraction is toxic? Gut 1983;24:A492.

[118] Ensari A, Marsh MN, Moriarty KJ, Moore CM, Fido RJ, Tatham AS. Studies in vivo of ω-gliadins in gluten sensitivity (coeliac sprue disease). Clin Sci 1998;95:419–24.

[119] Molberg O, Solheim-Flaete N, Jensen T, Lundin KEA, Arentz-Hansen H, Anderson OD, et al. Intestinal T-cell responses to high-molecular-weight glutenins in celiac disease. Gastroenterology 2003;125:337–44.

[120] Dewar DH, Amato M, Ellis HJ, Pollock EL, Gonzalez-Cinca N, Wieser H, et al. The toxicity of high molecular weight glutenin subunits of wheat to patients with coeliac disease. Eur J Gastroenterol Hepatol 2006;18:483–91.

[121] Ellis HJ, Dewar DH, Gonzales-Cinca N, Pollock EL, Wieser H, Ciclitira PJ. The toxicity of recombinant high-molecular-weight glutenin subunits of wheat to patients with coeliac disease. In: Stern M, editor. Proceedings of the 20th meeting of the working group on prolamin analysis and toxicity. Zwickau (Germany): Verlag Wissenschaftliche Scripten; 2006. pp. 83–5.

[122] Ellis HJ, Lozano-Sanchez P, Bermudo-Redondo C, Suligoj T, Biagi F, Bianchi PI, et al. Antibodies to wheat high-molecular-weight glutenin subunits in patients with celiac disease. Int Arch Allergy Immunol 2012;159:428–34.

[123] Wieser H, Belitz HD, Ashkenazi A, Idar D. Isolation of coeliac active peptide fractions from gliadin. Z Lebensm Unters Forsch 1983;176:85–94.

[124] Wieser H, Belitz HD, Ashkenazi A. Amino acid sequence of the coeliac active peptide B3142. Z Lebensm Unters Forsch 1984;179:371–6.

[125] Wieser H, Belitz HD, Idar D, Ashkenazi A. Coeliac activity of the gliadin peptides CT-1 and CT-2. Z Lebensm Unters Forsch 1986;182:115–7.

[126] Jos J, de Tand MF, Arnaud-Battandier F, Boissel JP, Popineau Y, Wajcman H. Separation of pure toxic peptides from a β-gliadin subfraction using high-performance liquid chromatography. Clin Chim Acta 1983;134:189–98.

[127] de Ritis G, Auricchio S, Jones HW, Lew EJL, Bernardin JE, Kasarda DD. In vitro (organ culture) studies of the toxicity of specific A-gliadin peptides in celiac disease. Gastroenterology 1988;94:41–9.

[128] Mantzaris G, Jewell DP. In vivo toxicity of a synthetic dodecapeptide from A gliadin in patients with coeliac disease. Scand J Gastroenterol 1991;26:392–8.

[129] Marsh MN, Morgan S, Ensari A, Wardle T, Lobley R, Mills C, et al. In vivo activity of peptides 31-43, 44–55, 56-68 of α-gliadin in gluten sensitive enteropathy (GSE). Gastroenterology 1995;108:A871.

[130] Maiuri L, Troncone R, Mayer M, Coletta S, Picarelli A, de Vincenzi M, et al. In vitro activities of A-gliadin related synthetic peptides. Damaging effect on the atrophic coeliac mucosa and activation of mucosal immune response in treated coeliac mucosa. Scand J Gastroenterol 1996;31:247–53.

[131] Martucci S, Fraser JS, Biagi F, Corazza GR, Ciclitira PJ, Ellis HJ. Characterizing one of the DQ2 candidate epitopes in coeliac disease: A-gliadin 51–70 toxicity assessed using an organ culture system. Eur J Gastroenterol Hepatol 2003;15:1293–8.

[132] Tatham AS, Marsh MN, Wieser H, Shewry PR. Conformational studies of peptides corresponding to the coeliac-activating regions of wheat α-gliadins. Biochem J 1990;270:313–8.

[133] van de Wal Y, Kooy YMC, van Veelen P, Vader W, August SA, Drijfhout JW, et al. Glutenin is involved in the gluten-driven mucosal T cell response. Eur J Immunol 1999;29:3133–9.

[134] Vader W, Kooy Y, van Veelen P, de Ru A, Harris D, Benckhuijsen W, et al. The gluten response in children with celiac disease is directed toward multiple gliadin and glutenin peptides. Gastroenterology 2002;122:1729–37.

[135] Vader LW, Stepniak DT, Bunnick EM, Kooy YMC, de Haan W, Drijfhout JW, et al. Characterization of cereal toxicity for celiac patients based on protein homology in grains. Gastroenterology 2003;125:1105–13.

[136] Arentz-Hansen H, McAdam SN, Molberg O, Fleckenstein B, Lundin KEA, Joergensen TJD, et al. Celiac lesion T cells recognize epitopes that cluster in regions of gliadins rich in proline residues. Gastroenterology 2002;123:803–9.

[137] Shan L, Molberg O, Parrot I, Hausch F, Filiz F, Gray GM, et al. Structural basis for gluten intolerance in celiac sprue. Science 2002;297:2275–9.

[138] Shan L, Qiao SW, Arentz-Hansen H, Molberg O, Gray GM, Sollid LM, et al. Identification and analysis of multivalent proteolytically resistant peptides from gluten: implications for celiac sprue. J Proteome Res 2005;4:1732–41.

[139] Camarca A, del Mastro A, Gianfrani C. Repertoire of gluten peptides active in celiac disease patients: perspectives for translational therapeutic applications. Endocr Metab Immune Disord Drug Targets 2012;12:207–19.

[140] http://www.allergenonline.org.

[141] Ciccocioppo R, di Sabatino A, Corazza GR. The immune recognition of gluten in coeliac disease. Clin Exp Immunol 2005;140:408–16.

[142] Fasano A. Zonulin and its regulation of intestinal barrier function: the biological door to inflammation, autoimmunity, and cancer. Physiol Rev 2011;91:151–76.

[143] Stern M, Ciclitira PJ, van Eckert R, Feighery C, Janssen FW, Mendez E, et al. Analysis and clinical effects of gluten in coeliac disease. Eur J Gastroenterol Hepatol 2001;13:741–7.

[144] Kim CY, Quarsten H, Bergseng E, Khosla C, Sollid LM. Structural basis for HLA-DQ2-mediated presentation of gluten epitopes in celiac disease. Proc Natl Acad Sci USA 2004;101:4175–9.

Chapter 3

Treatment of Celiac Disease

CHAPTER OUTLINE

1. CONVENTIONAL THERAPY

1.1 Gluten-Free Diet

Permanent lifelong adherence to a gluten-free diet (GFD) is the current essential treatment of celiac disease (CD). Even after many years of gluten avoidance, CD patients never acquire tolerance to gluten, and re-exposure to gluten reactivates the disease. The introduction of a GFD must be based on the diagnostic spectrum of CD (see Chapter 1, Section 5). As a rule, a GFD is currently indicated in all cases of symptomatic CD, dermatitis herpetiformis, non-celiac gluten sensitivity, gluten ataxia, and diarrhea-predominant irritable bowel syndrome [1] (see Chapter 1, Section 4). In

Celiac Disease and Gluten. http://dx.doi.org/10.1016/B978-0-12-420220-7.00003-1

cases of wheat-dependent exercise-induced anaphylaxis, a GFD is indicated; however, patients do not need to restrict rye, barley, and oat consumption. It is unclear whether individuals with asymptomatic CD would benefit from a GFD in view of the decreased quality of life that can result from it (see Section 1.5). It is believed that patients with untreated CD—even patients with positive serology but normal small intestinal histology—have an increased mortality risk. However, increased mortality has also been described in treated CD patients. Therefore, the true effect of the GFD on mortality is uncertain [2]. Similarly, early studies indicated that untreated patients had a higher risk of malignancy than the general population. In treated patients, this risk was smaller than the risk in untreated patients, but still higher than in the general population. However, later studies showed the risk to be more modest, especially from the viewpoint of absolute risk [3]. Other risk conditions, such as osteoporosis and fractures, should be evaluated in future studies to obtain an overall picture of the entity of unrecognized CD. Whether asymptomatic patients detected by screening in at-risk groups should follow a GFD remains doubtful [4]. A GFD has been recommended for silent CD cases but not for potential cases [5].

The GFD appears to be an increasing "fad" diet; its popularity has shown a steady increase since 2008 and is expected to increase further. Gluten-free foods are now ubiquitous; supplying gluten-free products online, to supermarkets, and to health food stores is a multibillion- (US) dollar industry. However, no current data suggest that the general population should maintain a gluten-free life style. A recent popular notion—that the consumption of wheat makes one fat and ill and should be avoided by the general population [6]—is scientifically unfounded [7]. It should be taken into consideration that wheat is an important provider of carbohydrates, B vitamins, minerals, and trace elements and constitutes one of the main bases for the alimentation of the world population.

A strict GFD means that the daily intake of gluten should be less than 20 mg. This corresponds to around one-hundredth of a slice of bread. Comparatively, normal people in the Western population ingest about 20,000 mg (factor 1000!) of gluten on average. CD patients may consume gluten-free foods from two categories. First, they are allowed to eat a wide range of common foods such as meat, fish, milk products, vegetables, and fruits. The ingestion of wheat-based starch hydrolysates, glucose syrup, and maltodextrins does not have harmful effects on histology or inflammation in CD patients in remission as compared with a placebo [8]. However, patients should be aware of numerous composite foods that contain "hidden" sources of gluten, such as thickened sauces and soups, puddings, and sausages (see Chapter 2, Section 2.3).

Second, according to the Codex Standard for Gluten-Free Foods, CD patients may consume dietetic foods that are gluten-free (see Chapter 4, Section 3.1). Most dietetic gluten-free foods are alternatives to traditional cereal-based goods such as bread and other baked products, pasta, breakfast cereals, and beer. They are made from nontoxic grains and flours such as rice and corn or pseudocereals (e.g., amaranth, buckwheat, and quinoa) (see Chapter 4, Section 1). CD patients should be careful with products that are not certified gluten-free because these products may have been contaminated by CD-toxic cereals along the production line (i.e., in the field, during transport, storage, or processing). It is estimated that patients who are strictly adherent to a GFD will consume 5–50 mg of gluten every day on average as a result of gluten contamination [9]. If patients have any doubt as to whether a product may contain gluten, they should not use it. Because of the possible risk of cross-contamination, the Academy of Nutrition and Dietetics Celiac Disease Toolkit recommends that individuals with CD buy naturally gluten-free grains and flours that are labeled gluten-free [10]. At home, gluten-free food should always be prepared, stored, and handled separately from gluten-containing food. If separate areas are not available, preparing the gluten-free meal before other meals is recommended.

Dietetic gluten-free foods used to be niche market products, available almost exclusively in health food shops, pharmacies, and through mail-order companies. Over the past decade, the market for gluten-free products has grown enormously owing to the increased number not only of diagnosed CD patients but also of non-CD individuals who wish to exclude gluten from their diet. Nowadays, gluten-free products also are offered in many supermarkets, restaurants, and hotels, and the assortment of goods has increased rapidly. Studies on commercially available gluten-free products in four European countries show that most products (99.5%) meet the gluten threshold of 20 mg/kg [11]. Unfortunately, commercially available products labeled gluten-free are significantly more expensive than corresponding conventional foods. For this reason, CD patients in some countries receive financial assistance to compensate for this higher cost.

1.2 Follow-up Management

Follow-up is necessary to confirm the diagnosis by making an objective assessment of the patient's response and compliance to a GFD (see Chapter 1, Section 5). From a medical perspective, the benefits of a GFD in symptomatic CD patients are obvious. Most patients show rapid clinical improvement, with their symptoms disappearing around 2 weeks after commencing the GFD. CD-specific serum antibody titers can take from 6–12 weeks to normalize, and, finally, complete histological resolution may not occur until a GFD has been followed for 2 years [12]. Approximately 5% of CD patients do not respond to a GFD. The primary cause of failure is continued ingestion of gluten, either unintentional or intentional [13]. Other reasons are conditions that complicate or coexist with CD. The most feared cause of nonresponsive CD is refractory CD (see Chapter 1, Section 4.4). If the reasons for nonresponsiveness cannot be clarified, looking into whether the diagnosis of CD was accurate should be considered.

Newly diagnosed patients should be referred to a health-care team, including a physician and an expert dietitian, as soon as possible. Patients should be evaluated at regular intervals, and a lifelong follow-up is recommended. Before the start of their GFD, patients may have had nutrient deficiencies, particularly folic acid and iron, that require correction with supplements for a certain period [12]. After beginning the diet, it may be necessary to limit patient consumption of lactose (e.g., in milk products) because of low lactase activities in the small intestine. In such cases, calcium and vitamin D supplementation should be considered. When there is intense diarrhea, electrolyte supplements may be required during the first days of treatment. Most patients can be followed up based on symptom resolution, improved laboratory abnormalities, and declining levels of serum antibodies. Analysis of the latter can be done by measuring serum antibodies to transglutaminase 2 (TG2) and deamidated gliadin peptides (see Chapter 1, Section 5.1). If antibodies remain elevated or become positive again, an endoscopy with biopsies should be considered. Recovery and adherence to a GFD should be controlled, possibly at 6–12 months after diagnosis and then annually.

CD patients should be monitored by a registered dietitian who has expertise in CD and GFD. The education of patients and their families is central to the management of CD [13]. They should understand the causes of CD, the medical complications of insufficiently controlled disease, the risk of family members developing CD, and the importance of maintaining a strict GFD lifelong. Topics of dietary counseling include identifying hidden sources of gluten, ensuring adequate nutrition, and labeling of gluten-free products.

Celiac societies (see Section 1.6) can provide CD patients with accurate and useful information and can recommend local support groups that are compliant with a GFD. Meetings may present medical advice and the opportunity to exchange information and problems. They also give people the chance to help those who are just starting a GFD. Specific websites include helpful information, for example, on the availability of gluten-free foods, general patient information, clinical and quality-of-care guidelines, and diagnostic tests.

1.3 Compliance to the Gluten-Free Diet

Serology, dietitian interviews, and rebiopsy are usually utilized for the assessment of adherence to a GFD (see Section 1.2). Leffler and coworkers developed the clinically relevant and easy "Celiac Dietary Adherence Test" (CDAT) that allows the standardized evaluation of adherence with a superior performance to the TG2 antibody test [14]. The CDAT is a 7-question survey relying on general questions on symptoms, self-efficacy, and gluten avoidance habits. Answer scores on a 5-point scale each are additive, with higher scores denoting worse GFD adherence. Another study has proven that patient interview for monitoring dietary compliance is more sensitive than serology in identifying patients who do not adhere to the GFD [15].

The degree of strict adherence to a GFD is strongly variable. A systematic review reported a range from 42% to 91%, depending on the definition and method of assessment [16]. Intentional nonadherence to the GFD was found to be less frequent than inadvertent lapses [17]. Compliance is lowest among ethnic minorities, adolescents, and adults diagnosed in childhood. Reasons include lack of knowledge, poor availability and labeling of gluten-free products, and difficulties in identifying gluten-free food when dining out [18]. Some patients in remission incorrectly believe that the absence of classical symptoms indicates that gluten can be tolerated, when gluten-containing food is occasionally eaten. To increase adherence, CD patients require improved doctor–patient communication, more detailed counseling, and better availability and labeling of gluten-free products. Patients should be informed that noncompliance with a GFD may be associated with an increased risk for certain types of cancer and death [19]. Moreover, they should be told that the absence of apparent symptoms does not reduce health risks. Permanent follow-up management is important to strengthen adherence to the diet.

1.4 Nutritional Status

The biological value of gluten proteins is rather low due to the lack of essential amino acids (see Tables 2.2 and 2.3). From a nutritional point of view, a diet free of gluten may, therefore, not be disadvantageous for CD patients. Nevertheless, a GFD does not guarantee adequate nutrient intake, and some nutritional deficiencies have been described after treatment with a long-term GFD for about 8–12 years [13]. A number of studies indicate an unbalanced intake of carbohydrates, protein, and fat as well as limited intake of certain essential nutrients. For example, dietary fiber intake is insufficient among CD patients [20,21]. It has been proposed that this imbalance is due to the fact that gluten-free breads are often made from starches and/or refined flours poor in fiber. Pseudocereals are usually consumed as whole grains or whole grain flours, and thus, have a higher nutritional value and fiber content than common cereals; the incorporation of these seeds (see Chapter 4, Section 1) into the diet of CD patients is recommended [22]. Moreover, numerous adult CD patients carefully treated with a GFD for several years show signs of poor status of vitamins (folate, vitamins B_6, and B_{12}) and minerals (iron, calcium) [21,23,24]. The results suggest that when following up adults with CD, the vitamin status should be reviewed. A double-blind, placebo-controlled multicenter trial showed a significant improvement in patients' general well-being after 6 months of supplementation with B vitamins [25]. A study of de Palma and coworkers has reported a reduction in beneficial gut bacteria in subjects on a GFD, which may have unknown pathophysiological consequences in the host [26]. Generally, CD patients are advised to increase their consumption of naturally gluten-free foods that are rich in fiber and vitamins, such as fruits, vegetables, legumes, and nuts [20].

1.5 Quality of Life

A lifelong GFD is difficult to sustain owing to the restricted availability and higher cost (factor 2 and higher) of gluten-free food alternatives, their poorer quality of taste, flavor, texture and mouthfeel, small levels of unexpected gluten contaminations, and cultural practices, leading to a substantial social burden. CD can severely impact patients in their health-related quality of life (HRQOL). Several studies on HRQOL in CD have been conducted in Europe and North America. One hundred forty-seven CD patients who had been on a GFD for at least 12 months gave the following responses to questionnaires [27]: 68% reported that their dietary restrictions reduced their enjoyment of food, 46% believed their foods cost them more than that of people without restrictions, and 21% said these higher costs were a problem for them. About half the patients reported doing things they enjoyed less often because of their restrictions; and the most common activity sacrificed was dining out. Fifty-two percent felt different from other people, 65% reported frequent feelings of frustration, and 56% were more worried about their health because of their diagnosis. Despite these findings, most patients reported being pleased with having been diagnosed, as they noticed improvement of their physical and psychological conditions. However, 27% of patients without classical symptoms regretted being diagnosed with the disease. The results of questionnaires to 387 US patients, all diagnosed by a physician and on a GFD, are presented in Table 3.1 [28]. The questionnaires had 20 items across four relevant subscales (limitations, dysphoria, health concerns, and inadequate treatment).

Table 3.1 Factor Analysis of Quality of Life of Celiac Disease (CD) Patients on a Gluten-Free Diet (GFD) [28]

Quality Parameters	Factor[a]
Limitations	
▪ Trouble socializing because of my disease	0.73
▪ Limited in eating meals with coworkers	0.65
▪ Difficulties during travel and long trips	0.63
▪ Socially stigmatized	0.58
▪ Afraid to eat out	0.58
▪ Thinking about food all the time	0.54
▪ Unable to have special food, e.g., birthday cake	0.51
▪ Cannot live normal life	0.51
Dysphoria	
▪ Overwhelmed about having CD	0.73
▪ Frightened by having CD	0.71
▪ Depressed because of CD	0.70
▪ Don't know enough about CD	0.61
Health Concerns	
▪ Concerned that CD will cause other health problems	0.80
▪ Concerned that my long-term health will be affected	0.79
▪ Worried about increased risk of cancer	0.78
▪ Worried about increased risk of family members	0.55
Inadequate Treatment	
▪ Diet is an insufficient treatment	0.72
▪ Not enough treatment	0.67
▪ CD is incurable	0.62

[a]*Factors higher than 0.5 are meaningful.*

The factor analysis (factors >0.5 are meaningful) demonstrated that all four subscales are relevant for patients on a GFD. Health concerns appear to be most important. A Swedish study on middle-aged CD patients on a GFD revealed that men reported a level of quality of life that was clearly superior to that of women [29]. The additional diagnosis of type 1 diabetes in adult CD patients has an even more pronounced negative effect on quality of life, particularly in women [30].

When patients were asked about their wishes, they usually wished that their stores would carry more gluten-free foods and their restaurants would offer more gluten-free options. Other frequently mentioned issues include more research on CD, intensified screening, earlier diagnosis, more knowledge on the GFD provided to physicians, and diagnosis without endoscopy [18]. Patients' most pronounced desire is the development of a pill or vaccine that would allow them to eat gluten-containing foods [31,32].

1.6 Celiac Societies

Interests of CD patients are represented by more than 100 national celiac societies worldwide. They are volunteer organizations that aim to help people with CD. Celiac societies play a very important role particularly in the first stage of the disease. Patients need advice on practical, social, and legal problems and contact with other patients. Many of the societies publish handbooks listing gluten-free foods and pharmaceuticals that are available on the market. They provide access to current information on dining out and traveling. Another mission of celiac societies is to raise public awareness of CD and take a stand on legal and political issues. Some societies support different research projects. Moreover, they give companies that produce gluten-free products the license to use the "gluten-free" symbol (see Chapter 4, Section 3.3).

The Association of European Coeliac Societies (AOECS), an independent nonprofit organization, is the umbrella organization of 39 national societies from 33 countries across Europe [33]. The AOECS was founded in 1988 and cooperates with scientists and gastroenterologists to provide CD patients with information and any help to maintain their GFD. Since 1992, AOECS has had the status of "Observer" in the world-wide Codex Alimentarius Commission and has participated in all sessions of the Commission and some Codex Committees. The AOECS has assisted very actively in the elaboration of all Codex Standards and Guidelines for labeling of foods for normal consumption, genetically modified foods, and special dietary foods. In addition to working on subjects of international importance involving CD and the GFD, AOECS coordinates international activities and matters of common interest to its members, disseminates information among members, gives any necessary advice and assistance to small or recently formed celiac societies, and lobbies for awareness of gluten intolerance. Recently, a registration system for licensing the "Crossed Grain" symbol was developed to avoid any prohibited use.

2. ALTERNATIVE THERAPIES

The conventional treatment of CD, a lifelong strict GFD, is a big challenge for CD patients (see Section 1), which may lead to poor compliance and inadvertent intake of gluten. Thus, there is an urgent need to develop safe and effective alternatives. However, any alternative treatment should have a safety profile competitive with the GFD [34]. Novel therapies are still in the early stages of development, and before any effective substance or treatment is used in humans, extensive toxicological testing will be necessary.

Owing to the enormous increase of knowledge about the pathomechanism of CD during the last decades (see Chapter 1, Section 6), a number of novel strategies for the prevention and treatment of CD have been developed. Most of them consist of interventions in the digestive process and mucosa permeability, inhibition of enzymes and cytokines, and blockage of receptors. Lists of new nondietary therapies for CD have been presented in several review articles [35–38]. A simplified scheme of pathogenic targets for possible treatments is shown in Figure 3.1. Phase II clinical trials to test the efficacy of novel alternative treatments for CD are already ongoing. However, before they admit any treatment candidates into phase III trials, researchers must develop novel reliable noninvasive surrogate markers for

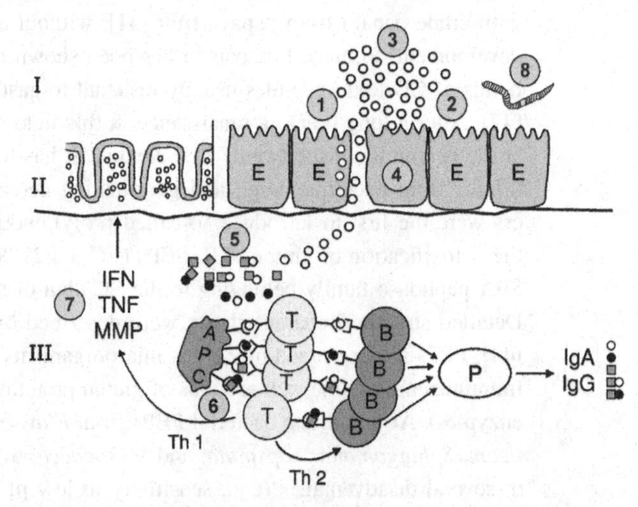

■ FIGURE 3.1 Scheme of the immune response in the pathomechanism of celiac disease (CD) and indication of possible future treatments of CD. (1) Oral enzyme therapy; (2) gluten-sequestering polymers; (3) probiotic bacteria; (4) permeability inhibitors; (5) inhibition of transglutaminase 2 (TG2); (6) human leukocyte antigen (HLA)-DQ blocking; (7) modulation of inflammation; and (8) hookworm therapy. I = intestinal lumen; II = epithelium; III = lamina propria; APC = antigen-presenting cell; B = B cell; E = enterocyte; IFN = interferon-γ; Ig = immunoglobulin; MMP = matrix metalloproteinase; P = plasma cell; T = CD4+ T cell; TG = tissue transglutaminase; Th = T helper; TNF = tumor necrosis factor. (Please see color plate at the back of the book.)

intestinal injury and disease activity, which accurately reflect patient-related outcomes [38].

2.1 Oral Enzyme Therapy

Usually, food proteins are degraded into small peptides and free amino acids by gastric, pancreatic, and brushborder enzymes. However, the high proline content (see Tables 2.5–2.7), particularly in the repetitive sections of the amino acid sequences, renders gluten proteins highly resistant to complete proteolytic digestion (see Chapter 1, Section 6.1). Enzymatic degradation of gluten proteins that abolishes their immunogenic and toxic activities is an attractive approach to oral therapy (no. 1 in Figure 3.1). Strategies for the detoxification of gluten have been based on oral treatment with special peptidases that hydrolyze CD-toxic proteins to nontoxic fragments that should contain less than nine amino acid residues (see Chapter 1, Section 6). The advantage of oral enzyme therapy, when compared to other therapies, is that the exogenous gluten is targeted by the treatment and not by endogenous effectors [39].

First attempts to detoxify gluten with enzymes were performed by incubation with a fresh extract of pig intestinal mucosa membrane [40] or with crude papain from papaya fruit [41], without any progress in further development. Remarkably, papain has been shown to cleave Q–Q peptide bonds of CD-toxic peptides usually resistant to gastrointestinal peptidases [42]. After a long break, a renaissance in this field of CD research started at the beginning of the twenty-first century. It has focused mainly on peptidases from bacteria, fungi, and germinating cereals. Shan and coworkers were the first to introduce so-called prolyl endopeptidases (PEPs) for the detoxification of gluten [43]. PEPs (EC 3.4.21.26) are classified in the S9A peptidase family belonging to the SC clan of serine-type peptidases. Detailed structural characteristics were described by the group of Osorio [44]. PEPs are expressed in various microorganisms and are able to cleave immunogenic proline-rich sections of gluten proteins (postproline cleaving enzymes). At first, three bacterial PEPs from *Flavobacterium meningosepticum, Sphingomonas capsulata,* and *Myxococcus xanthus* were used. Due to several disadvantages (e.g., sensitivity to low pH and pepsin, need for additional enzymes to degrade intact proteins, long reaction time), a PEP from *S. capsulata* was combined with a glutamine-specific cysteine endoprotease (EP-B2) from green barley grains [45]. This two-enzyme cocktail is active in both neutral and acidic medium, resistant to pepsin, and degrades gluten within a few minutes of simulated duodenal conditions. A combined PEP and EP-B2 preparation, called ALV003, was evaluated in three phase

I and IIa clinical studies. In general, it was found to be safe and well tolerated, with no dose-limiting toxicities. Moreover, the preparation is highly effective in degrading gluten primarily in the stomach before it reaches the duodenal compartment. ALV003 is currently being investigated in further phase II studies involving 20 patients.

Gordon and coworkers identified an endopeptidase named kumamolisin-As from the acidophilic bacterium *Alicyclobacillus sendaiensis* that is highly active under acidic conditions [46]. The initial enzyme specificity was modified by computational design toward the peptide bond P–Q, which occurs frequently in peptides immunogenic in CD (Table 2.11). The engineered enzyme (KumaMax) exhibited a 116-fold greater proteolytic activity in a model gluten tetrapeptide (PQLP) than the wildtype enzyme, as well as a more than 800-fold switch in substrate specificity toward immunogenic portions of gluten peptides. The half-life time of the gliadin peptide α9/57–68 (QLQPFPQPQLPY) incubated with KumaMax was calculated to be 8.5 min. The enzyme is highly active under acidic conditions and resistant to pepsin (pH 4) and trypsin (pH 7). These combined properties make the engineered peptidase a promising candidate as an oral therapeutic for CD.

Lactic acid bacteria (lactobacilli) are also known to possess a complex peptidase system. Wheat and rye sourdoughs are particularly rich in lactobacilli, and some of them have specific peptidases capable of hydrolyzing proline-rich proteins and peptides. Studies using a mixture—not a single strain—of sourdough lactobacilli and bifidobacteria (preparation VSL#3) have shown that a complex pattern of peptidases is necessary to degrade proline-rich proteins and peptides [47]. The combination of lactobacilli and fungal peptidases (see following discussion) has been proposed as bringing new perspectives to the elimination of gluten toxicity [48]. Moreover, the ability of distinct probiotic *Bifidobacteria* species to reduce the toxic effects of gluten was shown using cell culture assays [49]. The first clinical trial addressing these effects has been announced. Microbial enzymes derived from dental plaque in the human oral cavity were also shown to hydrolyze gluten-derived proline-rich peptides [50].

Among fungal peptidases, the PEP from *Aspergillus niger* (AN-PEP) has been shown to degrade gluten proteins and peptides highly efficiently [51]. The enzyme works optimally at pH 4–5, remains stable at pH 2, and is completely resistant to digestion with pepsin. It degrades intact gluten proteins as well as T-cell stimulatory peptides much faster than bacterial PEPs. Another advantage is that strains of the genus *Aspergillus* have a food grade status, and recombinant AN-PEP can be produced at low costs in an industrial setting. AN-PEP has been shown to digest gluten in a slice of bread and in a whole meal using a dynamic gastrointestinal model mimicking conditions found in the stomach and small intestine. The digestion of gluten already occurs in the stomach, and hardly any immunogenic epitopes reach the small intestine [52]. Clinical trials of AN-PEP preparations are widely advanced. The combination of two other food-grade peptidases from *A. niger* (aspergillo pepsin) and *A. oryzae* (dipeptidyl peptidase IV) also are able to detoxify moderate amounts of gluten [53]. The enzyme preparation consisting of both enzymes (STAN 1) is currently in clinical trials with CD patients.

Endogenous peptidases of germinating cereals have been known for a long time to be capable of extensively degrading storage proteins. Peptidases extracted from germinated rye bran were shown to degrade intact wheat, rye and barley prolamins and glutelins, as well as CD-toxic gliadin peptides to a high degree [54]. The enzymes, a complex combination of endo- and exopeptidases, are active between pH 3 and 9, reaching an optimum at pH 4.5 and 50 °C, and at pH 6.5, between 50 °C and 60 °C. CD-toxic gliadin peptides are cleaved into fragments of less than nine amino acid residues. Treatment of a peptic-tryptic digest from gliadin with isolated peptidases from germinated wheat grains results in the loss of CD toxicity, as shown by T-cell proliferation and organ culture tests [55]. Although no human in vivo studies have yet been undertaken with germinated cereal peptidases, this potential type of therapy could be developed further because of distinct advantages: the enzymes are derived from a naturally safe food source, and no genetic engineering is necessary. Their production is part of well-established technological processes (malting of cereal grains, brewing of beer) and is, therefore, simple and cheap.

As a continuation of previous studies [40], enzyme therapy using peptidases from porcine duodenal mucosa has been proposed [56]. CD patients were challenged with modest amounts of gluten daily; the enzyme preparation (capsules of "Glutenen") was administered to half of the group and a placebo to the other half. CD symptoms, serum antibodies, and histology of duodenal mucosa were found to be ameliorated during enzyme therapy compared with the placebo group. Peptidases from wheat-bug (*Eurygaster* ssp.) were also shown to have the potential for an extensive degradation of gluten proteins [57].

A key question that must be addressed regarding all these enzyme therapies is the gluten dose that can be effectively detoxified in vivo by a given enzyme dose [37]. Oral enzyme therapy probably will not be able to sufficiently degrade grams of gluten, the normal daily ingestion, but it could eliminate the damaging effect of gluten contaminations present in the GFD. A second point that needs to be addressed is the impact of other potentially competing dietary proteins on the efficiency of enzyme therapy. Finally, alternatives to enzyme delivery (once per meal via oral capsule) may be investigated using improved dosage schedules and delivery routes.

2.2 Gluten-Sequestering Polymers

An alternative strategy for detoxifying gluten in vivo is based on the binding of gluten to a polymeric resin (no. 2 in Figure 3.1). In in vitro studies, a linear high-molecular-weight copolymer of hydroxyethyl methacrylate and sodium 4-styrene sulfonate, P(HEMA-co-SS), has been shown to bind gluten proteins under simulated gastric and intestinal conditions. It also abolished the deleterious effects of gliadin on cells in culture [58]. However, many other nutrient proteins apart from gluten will interact with the polymer and limit its activity in CD patients. Future clinical trials have to establish the safety of the polymers in vivo and the gluten dose that can be effectively detoxified by a given dose of polymers.

2.3 Probiotic Bacteria

CD has been associated with changes in gut microbiota that contribute to the proinflammatory milieu of the disease (see Chapter 1, Section 3.2). Distinct *Bifidobacteria* have been found to reduce the toxic effects of gluten [59]. These findings, together with the known immune regulatory properties of *Bifidobacteria*, have opened up prospects of developing these probiotes into an alternative therapy for CD (no. 3 in Figure 3.1). Although the exact mode of action of these bacteria remains obscure, the first clinical trial addressing the effects of *Bifidobacteria* in untreated CD has been announced.

2.4 Permeability Inhibitors

Patients with active CD have increased intestinal permeability as measured by tight junction structural analysis (see Chapter 1, Section 6.2). Zonulin has been identified as an important regulator of epithelial permeability. After binding of gluten peptides to the chemokine receptor CXCR3, zonulin is released and subsequently increases intestinal permeability. This observation has led to a novel treatment option for CD based on the inhibition of zonulin (no. 4 in Figure 3.1). The purpose is to prevent the passage of immunogenic peptides through the intestinal cell layer by decreasing paracellular permeability. One of the candidates is larazotide acetate (AT-1001), an octapeptide that contains amino acid sequences shared by the receptor binding-motif of zonulin. AT-1001 antagonizes zonulin action via receptor blockade and, therefore, prevents mucosal impairment. This therapeutic agent was tested in 14 CD patients in remission, all of whom had intact intestinal permeability without increased cytokine production even after gluten challenge [60]. A follow-up randomized, double-blinded, placebo-controlled, phase II trial showed that AT-1001, when compared with a placebo, was safe and well tolerated, reduced proinflammatory cytokine production, and reduced gastrointestinal symptoms in patients receiving a daily 2.5 g-dose of gluten [61]. However, the impact of AT-1001 on the transcellular pathway of gluten-derived peptides has not been explored.

2.5 Inhibition of Transglutaminase 2

TG2 plays a critical role in the adaptive immune response of CD (see Chapter 1, Section 6.3.1). Conversion of specific glutamine residues to glutamate residues catalyzed by TG2 results in an increased affinity of gluten peptides to human leukocyte antigen (HLA)-DQ molecules, and thus, in increased T-cell stimulation. Therefore, selective inhibition of TG2 could be an effective therapeutic approach for CD (no. 5 in Figure 3.1). Several types of competitive, reversible and irreversible inhibitors of TG2 have been suggested as potential agents for the treatment of CD and other diseases (e.g., cancer) [62–64]. These include irreversible inhibitors, such as thiodiazoles, epoxides, α,β-unsaturated amides, and dihydroisooxazoles, as well as reversible inhibitors, such as thienopyrimidines, cinnamoyl compounds, β-aminoethylketones, and acylidene oxindoles. Some of them have been studied for CD specificity using animal and human biopsy testing. For example, cystamine leads to reduced T-cell response after gluten challenge of small intestinal biopsies from CD patients [65]. 2-[(2-oxopropyl)thio]imidazolium derivatives (L-682777, R-283) inhibit human TG2 and block the activation of pathogenic gluten-sensitive T cells [66]. A proof-of-concept study investigated whether two TG2 inhibitors, cell-impermeable R281 and cell-permeable R283, can prevent the toxic effects of gliadin in vitro [67]. The results suggested that the inhibitors are able to reduce certain gliadin-induced effects. Dihydroisoxazole compounds (e.g., KCC009) have been shown to be well tolerated and to inhibit TG2 effectively [68]. They have a short serum half-life, which would limit the exposure of other organs to them. Thioredoxin, which irreversibly blocks TG2 activation in a dose-dependent fashion, could represent another intriguing therapeutic option [69]. However, TG2 inhibition will not completely eliminate all immunogenic epitopes active in the adaptive response, and the innate response is not prevented at all. Moreover, because TG2 is ubiquitously expressed in the body, any novel drug based on TG2 inhibition has to be designed to work selectively in the small intestine. Today, clinical trials are in the planning stages.

2.6 HLA-DQ Blocking

Immunogenic gluten peptides bind to HLA-DQ molecules on the surface of antigen-presenting cells and drive the activation of T cells and, subsequently, the adaptive immune response (see Chapter 1, Section 6.3.1). Blocking the binding site of HLA-DQ2/8 could suppress the presenting process and provides another approach to CD treatment (no. 6 in Figure 3.1) [70]. A decapeptide from durum wheat (QQPQDAVQPF) was shown to have an antagonistic effect on gliadin in vitro using small intestinal mucosa from CD patients [71]. Studies on peripheral blood mononuclear cells proposed that the effect of the peptide is based on a shift of the T-cell response from the immunostimulant T-helper (Th)1 to the Th2 phenotype [72]. Based on gliadin peptides that activate the adaptive immunity, different types of peptide blockers have been developed. They have a much higher affinity (up to 200-fold) to DQ molecules than native gliadin peptides but are not recognized by T-cell receptors. These antagonists include cyclic and dimeric peptide analogs, peptides in which proline residues have been replaced by azidoproline residues, and nonapeptide analogs flanked by N- and C-terminal sequences that enhance binding [73,74]. Aldehyde-bearing gluten peptide analogs also were designed as tight-binding HLA-DQ2 ligands [75]. The aldehyde group can block the active lysine in the DQ2-binding pocket through Schiff's base formation. DQ2 blocking also was achieved by a 33-mer peptide analog, in which the residues L11 and L18 were replaced with sterically bulky groups [76]. The use of a positional scanning nonapeptide library has resulted in the design of new high-affinity peptide ligands by the combination of optimal amino acid residues in each position of the DQ2-binding frame [77]. A new peptide library-based method was presented, and it allows the identification of high-affinity ligands binding to HLA-DQ2.5 and the refined definition of peptide binding motifs [78]. Whether these compounds are nontoxic, nonimmunogenic, and able to completely suppress the immune response remains to be established. Also, concerns exist about how the modified peptides would reach their target cells in the lamina propria while competing with the luminal immunogenic gluten peptides. Moreover, the chances of success of using peptide analogs to modulate specific immune responses could be hampered by the wide heterogeneity of the gluten-sensitive T-cell epitopes [79,80].

2.7 Modulation of Inflammation

T-cell activation is regarded as one of the cornerstones in CD pathogenesis. The migration of the gluten-sensitive effector T cells from the blood to the small intestinal mucosa is guided by chemokine CCL25 and its receptor CCR9. Blockage of the CCL25/CCR9 interaction by a selective antagonist would prevent the migration of T cells to the intestinal lamina propria and has been regarded as a therapeutic strategy in CD. The antagonists CCX2282B (Traficet-EN®) and CCX025 inhibiting the CCR9 receptor of T cells have been developed for Crohn's disease and CD, and clinical trials are currently being performed or planned.

It also has been suggested that antibodies against cytokines might be a future approach to treating CD (no. 7 in Figure 3.1). It is well known that the activation of gluten-sensitive T cells leads to the secretion of many different cytokines. In turn, a cascade of inflammatory reactions is triggered, which results in mucosal injury and villous atrophy. Therefore, blocking of cytokines by specific monoclonal antibodies may prevent their activation. Several antibodies (e.g., against interferon (IFN-)γ (Fontolizumab), CD3 (Visilizumab, Teplizumab, Otelixizumab), CD20 (Rituximab, Tositumomab, Ibritumomab), and interleukin (IL-)15 (AMG 714)), are undergoing clinical evaluation for the treatment of different autoimmune diseases and CD [36,37]. The use of antibodies against tumor necrosis factor (TNF)-α (Infliximab) has been shown to be beneficial for patients with irritable bowel syndrome and refractory CD. Blocking IL-15 or its signaling pathway might help particularly to control refractory CD II and prevent the evolution toward aggressive T-cell lymphoma.

2.8 Vaccination

One of the most sought after goals of alternative therapy of CD is the development of a therapeutic vaccination constructed with a panel of most immunodominant gluten epitopes. This strategy is currently being evaluated—with encouraging results—for both allergy and autoimmune diseases [81,82]. With the goal of inducing a "tolerogenic" response in CD patients, a desensitizing or therapeutic vaccine (NexVax2) has been developed based on a mixture of three selected immunogenic 16-mer peptides from α- and γ-gliadins and hordeins. The vaccine is suited only for patients with the HLA-DQ2 haplotype because the peptides are presented only by HLA-DQ2. Subcutaneous immunization with this method was shown to be well tolerated and fairly safe, and it has not had any serious adverse effects in patient volunteers [83]. Further clinical trials will evaluate the efficacy of this vaccination approach in view of the high number of different immunogenic epitopes in wheat, rye, and barley proteins. It should be noted that vaccine therapy could be associated with the risk of immune system activation and consequent flare of the disease.

2.9 Hookworm Therapy

Infestation with the hookworm *Necator americanus* has been suggested as a possible treatment for autoimmune diseases and CD (no. 8 in Figure 3.1). This parasite is thought to play an important role in modulating the host's immune system—for example, by skewing the proinflammatory Th1 response to a less aggressive Th2 response. In a placebo-controlled clinical trial, CD patients were inoculated with *N. americanus* and then challenged with a high dose of gluten [84]. Unfortunately, the infection failed to prevent intestinal mucosa deterioration or immune response to gluten. Future trials might show whether this treatment can protect better against lower amounts of gluten than past treatments.

2.10 Monitoring the Treatment Effect

Specific and sensitive methods are necessary to assess the efficacy of alternative treatments for CD [37]. A bona fide animal model for CD has not been discovered or engineered. Assays for treatment efficacy are, therefore, conducted by in vivo and in vitro tests, and in surrogate animal models [39]. Histological changes in intestinal biopsies after gluten challenge would be the "gold standard" for assessing CD toxicity (see Chapter 2, Section 3.1.2). However, this procedure is extremely challenging to implement in clinical trials because it is subjective and requires invasive and expensive endoscopic examination. Symptom scores also will be unsuitable for this purpose because of the extreme variability of symptoms associated with CD. Possibly, the measurement of CD-specific T cells that enter the bloodstream after a short-term gluten challenge [85,86] can be adopted for early clinical trials of new drug candidates [87]. Considering that the small intestinal organ culture method has been widely used in studies aiming to clarify the pathogenesis of CD, it is surprising that the method has been used only in a few studies related to novel treatment forms [88]. Serum antibodies have inadequate sensitivity, and the measurement of intestinal permeability is not specific—in particular, in monitoring the effects of low-to-moderate gluten challenge. Better availability of animal models would be highly appreciated by researchers developing novel treatment strategies. However, the most conspicuous limitation is the lack of a functional CD-specific animal model [88]. Thus, drug development is currently hampered by the lack of specific and sensitive methods for measuring disease activity.

2.11 Concluding Remarks

Currently, the only treatment for CD is a lifelong strict adherence to a GFD, which clearly prevents the illness without causing any harmful side effects. However, a GFD is difficult to maintain and expensive, and compliance to the diet is sometimes poor. Therefore, CD patients have expressed a desire for alternative or complementary treatments that are less burdensome than a strict GFD. Improved knowledge of CD pathogenesis has enabled researchers to develop alternative strategies to treat the disorder; phase II clinical trials to test the efficacy of novel treatments already are ongoing. A number of current clinical studies have shown promising results, but these studies have been of short duration and low significance [89]. Therefore, studies with longer duration periods and greater significance will be needed to assess both the efficacy and long-term safety of every approach. Before allowing any treatment candidates to enter phase III trials, researchers must develop novel, reliable, noninvasive surrogate markers for intestinal injury and disease activity, which accurately reflect clinical trial outcomes [38]. An important point to address is the amount of gluten that can be detoxified in vivo. This will determine whether each treatment will enable patients to consume gluten ad libitum, to ingest sparing quantities only, or simply to avert inflammation when trace gluten is inadvertently encountered [39]. The first medications to become available most likely will be marketed as a supplement to the GFD rather than a substitute. One must carefully weigh the risks, benefits, and costs of alternatives and define under what conditions and indications such novel therapies might be warranted [34].

REFERENCES

[1] Pietzak M. Celiac disease, wheat allergy, and gluten sensitivity: when gluten free is not a fad. J Parenter Enteral Nutr 2012;36:68S–75S.

[2] West J, Logan RFA, Smith CJ, Hubbard RB, Card TR. Malignancy and mortality in people with coeliac disease: population based cohort study. BMJ 2004;329:716–9.

[3] Goldacre MJ, Wotton CJ, Yeates D, Seagroatt V, Jewell D. Cancer in patients with ulcerative colitis, Crohn's disease and coeliac disease: record linkage study. Eur J Gastroenterol Hepatol 2008;20:297–304.

[4] Mubarak A, Houwen RHJ, Wolters VM. Celiac disease: an overview from pathophysiology to treatment. Minerva Pediatr 2012;64:271–87.

[5] Stern M. Current therapy. In: Fasano A, Troncone R, Branski D, editors. Frontiers in celiac disease. Basel (Switzerland): Karger; 2008. pp. 114–22.

[6] Davis W. Wheat belly. Emmaus (USA): Rodale Press; 2011.

[7] Jones J. Wheat belly – an analysis of selected statements and basis theses from the book. Cereal Foods World 2012;57:177–89.

[8] Kaukinen K, Salmi T, Collin P, Huhtala H, Kaerjae-Lahdensuu T, Maeki M. Clinical trial: gluten microchallenge with wheat-based starch hydrolysates in coeliac disease patients - a randomized, double-blind, placebo-controlled study to evaluate safety. Aliment Pharmacol Ther 2008;28:1240–8.

[9] Catassi C, Fabiani E, Iacono G, D'Agate C, Francavilla R, Biagi F, et al. A prospective, double-blind, placebo-controlled trial to establish a safe gluten threshold for patients with celiac disease. Am J Clin Nutr 2007;85:160–6.

[10] Academy of Nutrition and Dietetics. Celiac disease toolkit. Chicago: American Dietetic Association; 2011.

[11] Gibert A, Kruizinga AG, Neuhold S, Houben GF, Canela MA, Fasano A, et al. Might gluten traces in wheat substitutes pose a risk in patients with celiac disease? A population-based probabilistic approach to risk estimation. Am J Clin Nutr 2013;97:109–16.

[12] Garcia-Manzanares A, Lucendo AJ. Nutritional and dietary aspects of celiac disease. Nutr Clin Pract 2011;26:163–73.

[13] Saturni L, Ferretti G, Bacchetti T. The gluten-free diet: safety and nutritional quality. Nutrients 2010;2:16–34.

[14] Leffler DA, Dennis M, Edwards-George JB, Jamma S, Magge S, Cook EF, et al. A simple validated gluten-free diet adherence survey for adults with celiac disease. Clin Gastroenterol Hepatol 2009;7:530–6.

[15] Zanchi C, Ventura A, Martelossi S, di Leo G, di Toro N, Not T. Rapid anti-transglutaminase assay and patient interview for monitoring dietary compliance in celiac disease. Scand J Gastroenterol 2013;48:764–6.

[16] Hall NJ, Rubin G, Charnock A. Systematic review: adherence to a gluten-free diet in adult patients with coeliac disease. Aliment Pharmacol Ther 2009;30:315–30.

[17] Hall NJ, Rubin GP, Charnock A. Intentional and inadvertent non-adherence in adult coeliac disease. A cross-sectional survey. Appetite 2013;68:56–62.

[18] Ukkola A, Maeki M, Kurppa K, Collin P, Huhtala H, Kekkonen L, et al. Patients' experiences and perceptions of living with coeliac disease – implications for optimizing care. J Gastrointestin Liver Dis 2012;21:17–22.

[19] Cotton D, Taichman D, Williams S, Crowe SE. Celiac disease. Ann Intern Med 2011. ITC5-1-16.

[20] Hager AS, Axel C, Arendt EK. Status of carbohydrates and dietary fiber in gluten-free diet. Cereal Foods World 2011;56:109–14.

[21] Shepherd SJ, Gibson PR. Nutritional inadequacies of the gluten-free diet in both recently-diagnosed and long-term patients with coeliac disease. J Hum Nutr Diet 2013;26:349–58.

[22] Alvarez-Jubete L, Arendt EK, Gallagher E. Nutritive value and chemical composition of pseudocereals as gluten-free ingredients. Int J Food Sci Nutr 2009;60:240–57.

[23] Hallert C, Grant C, Grehn S, Graennoe C, Hulten S, Midhagen G, et al. Evidence of poor vitamin status in coeliac patients on a gluten-free diet for 10 years. Aliment Pharmacol Ther 2002;16:1333–9.

[24] Thompson T, Dennis M, Higgins LA, Lee AR, Sharrett MK. Gluten-free diet survey: are Americans with coeliac disease consuming recommended amounts of fibre, iron, calcium and grain foods? J Hum Nutrit Diet 2005;18:163–9.

[25] Hallert C, Svensson M, Tholstrup J, Hultberg B. Clinical trial: B vitamins improve health in patients with coeliac disease living on a gluten-free diet. Aliment Pharmacol Ther 2009;29:811–6.

[26] de Palma G, Nadal I, Collado MC, Sanz Y. Effects of a gluten-free diet on gut microbiota and immune function in healthy adult human subjects. Br J Nutr 2009;102:1154–60.

[27] Hallert C, Graennoe C, Hulten S, Midhagen G, Stroem M, Svensson H, et al. Quality of life of adult coeliac patients treated for 10 years. Scand J Gastroenterol 1998;33:933–8.

[28] Whitaker JKH, West J, Holmes GKT, Logan RFA. Patient perceptions of the burden of coeliac disease and its treatment in the UK. Aliment Pharmacol Ther 2009;29:1131–6.

[29] Dorn SD, Hernandez L, Minaya MT, Morris CB, Hu Y, Leserman J, et al. The development and validation of a new coeliac disease quality of life survey (CD-QQL). Aliment Pharmacol Ther 2010;31:666–75.

[30] Bakker SF, Pouwer F, Tushuizen ME, Hoogma RP, Mulder CJ, Simsek S. Compromised quality of life in patients with both Type 1 diabetes mellitus and coeliac disease. Diabet Med 2013:835–9.
[31] Aziz I, Evans KE, Papageorgiou V, Sanders DS. Are patients with coeliac disease seeking alternative therapies to a gluten-free diet? J Gastrointestin Liver Dis 2011;20:27–31.
[32] Tennyson CA, Simpson S, Lebwohl B, Lewis S, Green PHR. Interest in medical therapy for celiac disease. Ther Adv Gastroenterol 2013;6:358–64.
[33] Deutsch H. 20 years AOECS. In: Stern M, editor. Proceedings of the 23nd meeting working group on prolamin analysis and toxicity. Zwickau (Germany): Verlag Wissenschaftliche Scripten; 2009. pp. 125–37.
[34] Kagnoff MF. Celiac disease: pathogenesis of a model immunogenetic disease. J Clin Invest 2007;117:41–9.
[35] McAllister C, Kagnoff MF. The immunopathogenesis of celiac disease reveals possible therapies beyond the gluten-free diet. Semin Immunopathol 2012;34:581–600.
[36] Rashtak S, Murray JA. Review article: coeliac disease, new approaches to therapy. Aliment Pharmacol Ther 2012;35:768–81.
[37] Sollid LM, Khosla C. Novel therapies for coeliac disease. J Intern Med 2011;269:604–13.
[38] Lindfors K, Laehdeaho ML, Kalliokoski S, Kurppa K, Collin P, Maeki M, et al. Future treatment strategies for celiac disease. Expert Opin Ther Targets 2012;16:665–75.
[39] Bethune MT, Khosla C. Oral enzyme therapy for celiac disease. Methods Enzymol 2012;502:241–71.
[40] Frazer AC, Fletcher RF, Ross CA, Shaw B, Sammons HG, Schneider R. Gluten-induced enteropathy: the effect of partially digested gluten. Lancet 1959;2:252–5.
[41] Messer M, Anderson CM, Hubbard L. Studies on the mechanism of destruction of the toxic action of wheat gluten in coeliac disease by crude papain. Gut 1964;5:295–303.
[42] Wieser H, Belitz HD. Isolation and enzymatic fragmentation of the coeliac-active gliadin peptide CT-1. Z Lebensm Unters Forsch 1992;195:22–6.
[43] Shan L, Molberg O, Parrot I, Hausch F, Filiz F, Gray GM, et al. Structural basis for gluten intolerance in celiac sprue. Science 2002;297:2275–9.
[44] Osorio C, Wen N, Gemini R, Zemetra R, Wettstein D, Rustgi S. Targeted modification of wheat grain protein to reduce the content of celiac causing epitopes. Funct Integr Genomics 2012;12:417–38.
[45] Gass J, Bethune MT, Siegel M, Spencer A, Khosla C. Combination enzyme therapy for gastric digestion of dietary gluten in patients with celiac sprue. Gastroenterology 2007;133:472–80.
[46] Gordon SR, Stanley EJ, Wolf S, Toland A, Wu SJ, Hadidi D, et al. Computational design of an α-gliadin peptidase. J Am Chem Soc 2012;134:20513–20.
[47] de Angelis M, Rizzello CG, Fasano A, Clemente MG, de Simone C, Silano M, et al. VSL#3 probiotic preparation has the capacity to hydrolyze gliadin polypeptides responsible for celiac sprue. Biochim Biophys Acta 2006;1762:80–93.
[48] Rizzello CG, de Angelis M, di Cagno R, Camarca A, Silano M, Losito I, et al. Highly efficient gluten degradation by Lactobacilli and fungal proteases during food processing: new perspectives for celiac disease. Appl Environ Microbiol 2007;73:4499–507.

[49] Lindfors K, Blomqvist T, Juuti-Uusitalo K, Stenman S, Venaelaeinen J, Maeki M, et al. Live probiotic *Bifidobacterium lactis* bacteria inhibit the toxic effects induced by wheat gliadin in epithelial cell cultures. Clin Exp Immunol 2008;152:552–8.

[50] Helmerhorst EJ, Zamakhchari M, Schuppan D, Oppenheim FG. Discovery of a novel and rich source of gluten-degrading microbial enzymes in the oral cavity. PLoS One 2010;5:e13264.

[51] Stepniak D, Spaenij-Dekking L, Mitea C, Moester M, de Ru A, Baak-Pablo R, et al. Highly efficient gluten degradation with a newly identified prolyl endoprotease: implications for celiac disease. Am J Physiol 2006;291:G621–9.

[52] Mitea C, Havenaar R, Drijfhout JW, Edens L, Dekking L, Koning F. Efficient degradation of gluten by a prolyl endoprotease in a gastrointestinal model: implications for coeliac disease. Gut 2008;57:25–32.

[53] Ehren J, Moron B, Martin E, Bethune MT, Gray GM, Khosla C. A food-grade enzyme preparation with modest gluten detoxification properties. PLoS One 2009;4:e6313.

[54] Hartmann G, Koehler P, Wieser H. Rapid degradation of gliadin peptides toxic for coeliac disease patients by proteases from germinating cereals. J Cereal Sci 2006;44:368–71.

[55] Stenman SM, Lindfors K, Venalainen JI, Hautala A, Maennistoe PT, Garcia-Horsman JA, et al. Degradation of coeliac disease – inducing rye secalin by germinating cereal enzymes: diminishing toxic effects in intestinal epithelial cells. Clin Exp Immunol 2010;161:242–9.

[56] Cornell HJ, MacRae FA, Melny J, Pizzey CJ, Cook F, Mason S, et al. Enzyme therapy for management of coeliac disease. Scand J Gastroenterol 2005;40:1304–12.

[57] Olanca B, Oezay DS. Preparation and functional properties of gluten hydrolysates with wheat-bug (Eurygaster spp.) protease. Cereal Chem 2010;87:518–23.

[58] Pinier M, Fuhrmann G, Galipeau H, Rivard N, Murray JA, David CS, et al. The copolymer P(HEMA-co-SS) binds gluten and reduces immune response in gluten-sensitized mice and human tissue. Gastroenterology 2012;142:316–25.

[59] Medina M, de Palma G, Ribes-Koninckx C, Calabuig M, Sanz Y. Bifidobacterium strains suppress in vitro the pro-inflammatory milieu triggered by the large intestinal microbiota of coeliac patients. J Inflamm 2008;5:19.

[60] Paterson BM, Lammers KM, Arrieta MC, Fasano A, Meddings JB. The safety, tolerance, pharmacokinetic and pharmacodynamic effects of single doses of AT-1001 in coeliac disease subjects: a proof of concept study. Aliment Pharmacol Ther 2007;26:757–66.

[61] Kelly CP, Green PHR, Murray JA, di Marino A, Colatrella A, Leffler DA, et al. Larazotide acetate in patients with coeliac disease undergoing a gluten challenge: a randomised placebo-controlled study. Aliment Pharmacol Ther 2013;37:252–62.

[62] Siegel M, Khosla C. Transglutaminase 2 inhibitors and their therapeutic role in disease states. Pharmacol Ther 2007;115:232–45.

[63] Caccamo D, Curro M, Ientile R. Potential of transglutaminase 2 as a therapeutic target. Expert Opin Ther Targets 2010;14:989–1003.

[64] Badarau E, Collighan RJ, Griffin M. Recent advances in the development of tissue transglutaminase (TG2) inhibitors. Amino Acids 2013;44:119–27.

[65] Molberg O, McAdam S, Lundin KEA, Kristiansen C, Arentz-Hansen H, Kett K, et al. T cells from celiac disease lesions recognize gliadin epitopes deamidated in situ by endogenous tissue transglutaminase. Eur J Immunol 2001;31:1317–23.

[66] Freund KF, Doshi KP, Gaul SL, Claremon DA, Remy DC, Baldwin JJ, et al. Transglutaminase inhibition by 2-[(2-oxopropyl)thio]imidazolium derivatives: mechanism of factor XIIIa inactivation. Biochemistry 1994;33:10109–19.

[67] Rauhavirta T, Oittinen M, Kivistoe R, Maennistoe PT, Garcia-Horsman JA, Wang Z, et al. Are transglutaminase 2 inhibitors able to reduce gliadin-induced toxicity related to celiac disease? A proof-of-concept study. J Clin Immunol 2013;33:134–42.

[68] Watts RE, Siegel M, Khosla C. Structure-activity relationship analysis of the selective inhibition of transglutaminase 2 by dihydroisoxazoles. J Med Chem 2006;49:7493–501.

[69] Jin X, Stamnaes J, Kloeck C, di Raimondo TR, Sollid LM, Khosla C. Activation of extracellular transglutaminase 2 by thioredoxin. J Biol Chem 2011;286:37866–73.

[70] Anderson RP, van Heel DA, Tye-Din JA, Jewell DP, Hill AVS. Antagonists and non-toxic variants of the dominant wheat gliadin T cell epitope in coeliac disease. Gut 2006;55:485–91.

[71] Silano M, Leonardi F, Trecca A, Mancini E, di Benedetto R, de Vincenzi M. Prevention by a decapeptide from durum wheat of in vitro gliadin peptide-induced apoptosis in small-bowel mucosa from coeliac patients. Scand J Gastroenterol 2007;42:786–7.

[72] Silano M, di Benedetto R, Maialetti F, de Vincenzi A, Calcaterra R, Trecca A, et al. 10-residue peptide from durum wheat promotes a shift from a Th1-type response towards a Th2-type response in celiac disease. Am J Clin Nutr 2008;87:415–23.

[73] Xia J, Bergseng E, Fleckenstein B, Siegel M, Kim CY, Khosla C, et al. Cyclic and dimeric gluten peptide analogues inhibiting DQ2-mediated antigen presentation in celiac disease. Bioorg Med Chem 2007;15:6565–73.

[74] Kapoerchan VV, Wiesner M, Overhand M, van der Marel GA, Koning F, Overkleeft HS. Design of azidoproline containing gluten peptides to suppress CD4$^+$ T-cell responses associated with celiac disease. Bioorg Med Chem 2008;16:2053–62.

[75] Siegel M, Xia J, Khosla C. Structure-based design of α-amido aldehyde containing gluten peptide analogues as modulators of HLA-DQ2 and transglutaminase 2. Bioorg Med Chem 2007;15:6253–61.

[76] Xia J, Siegel M, Bergseng E, Sollid LM, Khosla C. Inhibition of HLA-DQ2-mediated antigen presentation by analogues of a high affinity 33-residue peptide from α2-gliadin. J Am Chem Soc 2006;128:1859–67.

[77] Juese U, van de Wal Y, Koning F, Sollid LM, Fleckenstein B. Design of new high-affinity peptide ligands for human leukocyte antigen-DQ2 using a positional scanning peptide library. Hum Immunol 2010;71:475–81.

[78] Juese U, Arntzen M, Hojrup P, Fleckenstein B, Sollid LM. Assessing high affinity binding to HLA-DQ2.5 by a novel peptide library based approach. Bioorg Med Chem 2011;19:2470–7.

[79] Caputo I, Lepretti M, Martucciello S, Esposito C. Enzymatic strategies to detoxify gluten: implications for celiac disease. Enzyme Res 2010. Article ID 174354.

[80] Camarca A, Anderson RP, Mamone G, Fierro O, Facchiano A, Costantini S, et al. Intestinal T cell responses to gluten peptides are largely heterogeneous: implications for a peptide-based therapy in celiac disease. J Immunol 2009;182:4158–66.

[81] Larche M, Wraith DC. Peptide-based therapeutic vaccines for allergic and autoimmune diseases. Nat Med 2005;11:S69–76.

[82] Larche M. Immunotheraphy with allergen peptides. Allergy Asthma Clin Immunol 2007;3:53–9.

[83] Brown GJ, Daveson J, Marjason JK, Ffrench RA, Smith D, Sullivan M, et al. A phase I study to determine safety, tolerability and bioactivity of Nexvax2® in HLA DQ2+ volunteers with celiac disease following a long-term, strict gluten-free diet. Gastroenterology 2011;140:S437–8.

[84] Daveson AJ, Jones DM, Gaze S, McSorley H, Clouston A, Pascoe A, et al. Effect of hookworm infection on wheat challenge in celiac disease – a randomised double-blinded placebo controlled trial. PLoS One 2011;6:e17366.

[85] Anderson RP, van Heel DA, Tye-Din JA, Barnardo M, Salio M, Jewell DP, et al. T cells in peripheral blood after gluten challenge in coeliac disease. Gut 2005;54:1217–23.

[86] Raki M, Fallang LE, Brottveit M, Bergseng E, Quarsten H, Lundin KEA, et al. Tetramer visualization of gut-homing gluten-specific T cells in the peripheral blood of celiac patients. Proc Natl Acad Sci USA 2007;104:2831–6.

[87] Tye-Din JA, Anderson RP, French RA, Brown GJ, Hodsman P, Siegel M, et al. The effects of ALV003 pre-digestion of gluten on immune response and symptoms in celiac disease in vivo. Clin Immunol 2010;134:289–95.

[88] Lindfors K, Rauhavirta T, Stenman S, Maeki M, Kaukinen K. In vitro models for gluten toxicity: relevance for celiac disease pathogenesis and development of novel treatment options. Exp Biol Med 2012;237:119–25.

[89] Stoven S, Murray JA, Marietta E. Celiac disease: advances in treatment via gluten modification. Clin Gastroenterol Hepatol 2012;10:859–62.

Chapter 4

Gluten-Free Products

CHAPTER OUTLINE

Celiac Disease and Gluten. http://dx.doi.org/10.1016/B978-0-12-420220-7.00004-3

Strict lifelong adherence to a gluten-free diet (GFD) is currently the only effective treatment of celiac disease (CD) (see Chapter 3, Section 1.1). Therefore, all gluten-containing foods produced from wheat, rye, barley, and oats such as bread, other baked products, pasta, and beer have to be avoided. This can be managed either by substituting these products with gluten-free alternatives or by consuming products from wheat, rye, barley, and oats that have been rendered gluten-free.

1. PRODUCTS FROM GLUTEN-FREE RAW MATERIALS

According to Codex Stan 118–1979 (see Section 3.1), dietetic gluten-free foods must not contain more than 20 mg gluten/kg as consumed. The raw materials used for the production of dietetic gluten-free products are mainly nontoxic cereals (e.g., corn, rice, sorghum, millet) and pseudocereals (e.g., amaranth, buckwheat, quinoa). Dietary surveys documented that patients on GFDs often consume less than the recommended amounts of B vitamins, iron, calcium, and fiber [1,2]. The reason for this is that traditionally, mostly refined flours from rice and corn, whose germ and bran fractions have been removed, or even pure starches are used as base materials for gluten-free foods. This suggests that more emphasis should be placed on the nutritional quality of GFDs to encourage patients to consume enriched and fortified products whenever possible.

Pseudocereals such as amaranth, quinoa, and buckwheat have been recommended as nutritious ingredients in gluten-free formulations owing to their high protein quality and abundant quantities of fiber and minerals such as calcium and iron [3]. Incorporation of these gluten-free grains in an unrefined form into the GFD could not only add variety but also improve its nutritional value. Several studies have reported the successful formulation of pseudocereal-containing gluten-free products such as bread, pasta, and confectionery products. However, commercialization of these products still is quite limited, and only a small number of products containing pseudocereals are available. More research is necessary to fully exploit the functionality of these seeds as gluten-free ingredients in the production of palatable products, which also are nutritionally balanced [3]. The inclusion of oats into the GFD is still controversial (see Chapter 2, Section 3.2). Obviously, most people suffering from CD tolerate oats. The consumption of uncontaminated oats can considerably improve the nutritional quality of a GFD and expand the range of foods suitable for CD patients [4,5]. Some celiac societies recommend the inclusion of oats into the GFD, but not without special caution.

Today, formulations of gluten-free products are strongly variable and can involve different flours (e.g., from nontoxic cereals, pseudocereals, chestnut), starches (e.g., from rice, corn, potato, cassava), proteins (e.g., from milk, egg, soy), and hydrocolloids (e.g., hydroxypropylmethyl-cellulose, carrageenan, xanthan gum) [6]. A possibility for improving the nutritional profiles of gluten-free cereals and pseudocereals is the germination of the seeds before inclusion as ingredients into the GFD [7]. However, this practice may negatively affect the texture and taste of the products. For the improvement of texture and aroma of gluten-free products, microbial fermentation (e.g., in form of a sourdough) has been recommended [8]. To improve fiber uptake, gluten-free products can be enriched by the addition of psyllium husk, cellulose, or fiber from sugar beets, citrus, peas, vegetables, apples, or bamboo [9].

In general, the quality and availability of dietetic gluten-free products on the market have continuously improved during the past decades. Different formulations that improve the quality of gluten-free biscuits, cookies, cakes, pasta, and pizza have been presented by Gallagher [10]. Nevertheless, numerous CD patients are still unsatisfied, for example because of poor flavor, texture, and mouthfeel compared with gluten-containing counterparts. As described in the following section, the replacement of wheat bread and barley beer is one of the most critical aspects of a GFD and a challenge for food technologists, bakers, and brewers.

1.1 Gluten-Free Bread

The unique quality of wheat bread is the result of the special properties of gluten proteins (gliadins and glutenins) (see Chapter 2, Section 2.3). They provide flour with a high water absorption capacity; dough with cohesiveness, viscosity, elasticity, and gas-holding ability; and bread with high volume and a porous crumb [11]. In short, wheat gluten is considered by many to be the heart and soul of bakery products [12]. All other cereal flours yield breads of poor quality with low volume and small-pored, unelastic crumb when baked under standardized conditions (Figure 4.1). It is extremely difficult to mimic all of the desired gluten properties. Replacing gluten requires employing a mix of allowed flours, proteins, hydrocolloids, and special technologies in an attempt to replace the numerous functions of gluten [11,13]. Usually, starch-containing flours or starches from safe sources (e.g., corn, rice, potatoes) are the base materials used in the production of gluten-free bread. Wheat starch may be allowed at a national level provided that its gluten content is lower than 100 mg/kg, and the gluten content of the final product does not exceed 20 mg/kg. To mimic the water absorption capacity and dough viscosity contributed by gluten proteins, several hydrocolloids are recommended. These compounds are hydrophilic carbohydrate polymers that act as water binders, improve rheological dough properties and bread texture, and slow down the retrogradation of starch [11]. Hydroxypropylmethyl-cellulose, carboxymethyl-cellulose, carrageenan, xanthan gum, guar gum, and sodium alginate are

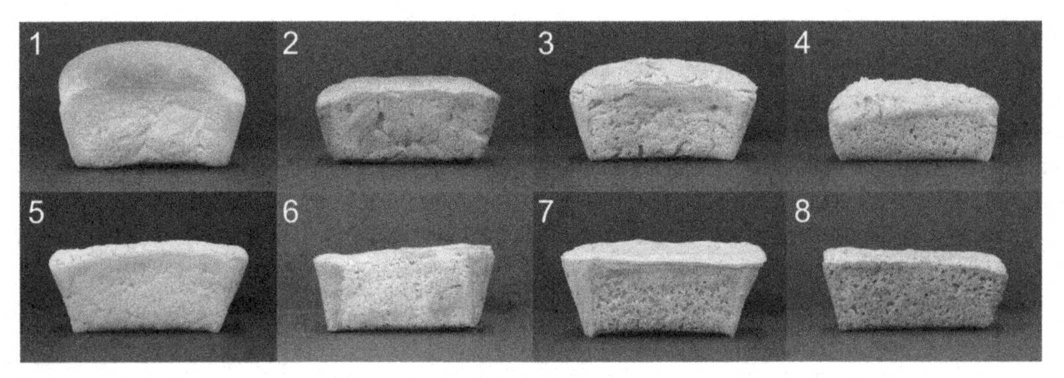

■ **FIGURE 4.1** Appearance of breads from different cereal and pseudocereal flours baked under standardized conditions (1, wheat; 2, rye; 3, barley; 4, oats; 5, rice; 6, corn; 7, buckwheat; 8, sorghum). (Please see color plate at the back of the book.)

examples of such compounds used in gluten-free bread production. Instead of gluten proteins, other protein sources have to be added. Dairy ingredients such as caseinates, skim milk powder, or whey protein concentrate and soy products, egg proteins, or corn protein (zein) have been recommended [11]. In addition to enhancing texture, these proteins improve the nutritional properties of gluten-free breads. However, lactose intolerance (milk) and allergenic potential (soy, egg, milk) are limiting factors for the use of these gluten substitutes. The use of lactic acid bacteria and gluten-free sourdough, enzymes such as transglutaminase, peptidases, laccase, or glucose oxidase, and treatment at high hydrostatic pressure are further possibilities for improving gluten-free bread quality [4,11]. Recently, psyllium has been described as gluten replacement with the least effect on aroma and texture of bread [14,15]. Sensory analysis showed a high acceptance rate among both CD patients and healthy controls. Altogether, the various methods show that one single ingredient in gluten-free bread production cannot replace gluten and its functionality [13].

The process of gluten-free bread-making differs significantly from that of standard wheat breads. Gluten-free doughs are much less cohesive and elastic than wheat doughs [13]. They are highly smooth, more sticky, less pasty, and difficult to handle. Most gluten-free doughs tend to contain higher water levels and have a more fluid-like structure comparable to the batter of a cake. They require shorter mixing, proofing, and baking times than wheat doughs. The volumes of the breads are mostly smaller, their crumbs firmer, and their crusts softer [13]. A short shelf life, rapid staling, a dry mouthfeel, and a dissatisfactory taste are also some of the disadvantages of gluten-free breads. Despite countless efforts to improve gluten-free bread quality [8], ongoing studies on optimized formulations and processes are still necessary.

1.2 Gluten-Free Beer

Brewing of beer can be traced back almost 5000 years in many parts of the world. Beer, together with bread, was an important part of the diet of ancient cultures. Barley and, in parts, wheat have been traditionally used as main ingredients of beer. Usually, conventional beer based on barley and wheat malt contains gluten far over the allowed threshold level for gluten-free products [16]. With regard to gluten-free beer, investigations have focused on the production of malt and beer from safe cereals, such as rice, corn, and millet, and pseudocereals, such as buckwheat, quinoa, and amaranth [17]. A number of studies indicates that the processes of malting and brewing have to be adapted to the applied raw material to get a product similar to conventional beer. Currently, only sorghum, millet, and buckwheat beers appear to be successful and are available on the market. However, the flavor of products made with alternative ingredients may not yet be acceptable to many CD patients. Further intensive research work is necessary to develop products comparable to conventional beer. Significant differences in the immunogenicity of different barley varieties raise the prospect of breeding barley cultivars with low levels of gluten [18].

2. PRODUCTS RENDERED GLUTEN-FREE

Products made from gluten-containing cereals may be rendered gluten-free by special processing. The gluten content of these products has to be reduced to a level below 20 mg/kg, and in some countries, to a level between 20 and 100 mg/kg in total [19] (see Section 3.1). Cereal-based products rendered gluten-free are mainly wheat starch, wheat flour and dough, and beverages.

2.1 Wheat Starch

Starch from wheat was the first ingredient of gluten-free foods that was "rendered" gluten-free. It has been frequently used as base material for the production of gluten-free baked foods since the introduction of the GFD as the essential treatment of CD. Wheat starch still is appreciated as ingredient for gluten-free baked products because of its favorable properties. It absorbs up to 45% water during dough preparation, acts as an inert filler in the continuous network of the dough, and creates a gas-permeable structure. In baking, the highest dough density is reached by the use of wheat starch due to its favorable composition of large and small granules. All other starches create doughs with higher incorporation of air [13]. Also, the highest bread volume is reached by the use of wheat starch. However, wheat starch may contain residual gluten that can vary widely in concentrations from below 20 mg/kg to more than 500 mg/kg because its level depends on the process of starch production (e.g., washing steps).

The widespread use of wheat starch for the production of gluten-free baked goods was the background for the first Draft Revised Codex Standard for Gluten-Free Foods (Codex Stan 118-1979) established in 1981 and amended in 1983 [20]. At that time, the analytical method, determination of nitrogen (N), was limited to wheat starch, and the threshold was set at N=0.05% on dry matter base (see Section 3.1). However, only a part of N in wheat starch is protein-N; another part belongs to nonprotein N-containing compounds, such as phospholipids. The protein fraction contains numerous nongluten proteins, such as surface associated proteins (e.g., purothionins, histones, and friabilin), in addition to gluten proteins [21]. In consequence, the N content of wheat starch is only weakly correlated with the gluten content and does not reflect the true gluten content [22]. The same is true for wheat starch derivatives, such as maltodextrin, glucose syrup, and dextrose. As an example, the poor correlation (r=0.232) between N content determined by the Kjeldahl method and the gliadin content determined by gel permeation liquid chromatography [22] (see Section 4.4.3) is shown in Figure 4.2. Further Draft Revised Standards eliminated the threshold based on the N content

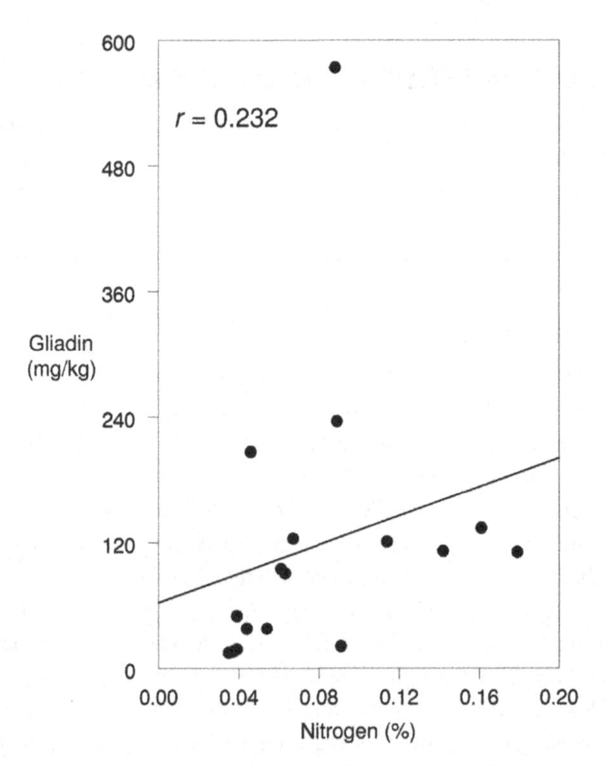

■ **FIGURE 4.2** Correlation between the nitrogen and gliadin contents in different wheat starches.

and substituted it with the threshold for the gluten content determined by an immunochemical method. Wheat starch-based gluten-free products, which meet the current Codex Standard, were shown to be as safe for CD patients as a naturally GFD by a prospective and randomized study [23]. Equivalent results were obtained with wheat starch derivatives [24].

2.2 Enzyme-Treated Products

A number of suggestions have been made to detoxify gluten in raw materials and foods by enzymatic treatment [25]. Lactic acid bacteria (lactobacilli) are known to possess a very complex peptidase system. Sourdough is particularly rich in lactobacilli, and some of them have specific peptidases capable of hydrolyzing proline-rich proteins and peptides [26]. Four sourdough strains: (1) *Lactobacillus alimentarius*, (2) *Lactobacillus brevis*, (3) *Lactobacillus sanfranciscensis*, and (4) *Lactobacillus hilgardii* are known to possess the entire combination of peptidases needed to hydrolyze proline-rich proteins and peptides [27]. These lactobacilli were used to make a fermented dough containing a mixture of wheat (30%) and nontoxic oat, millet, and buckwheat flours. A long-term fermentation (24 h) achieved an almost complete hydrolysis of gliadins. After baking, the bread was used for in vivo double-blind challenge of CD patients. Bread fermented with baker's yeast and containing approximately 2 g of gluten served as a positive control. Thirteen of the 17 patients showed a marked alteration in intestinal permeability after ingestion of the control bread. When given the sourdough bread to eat, the same 13 patients had values for intestinal permeability that did not differ significantly from the baseline values. The probiotic VSL#3 preparation, a mixture of sourdough lactobacilli and bifidobacteria, also showed the capacity to decrease the toxicity of wheat flour during long fermentation [28]. These results indicate that bread biotechnology using wheat flour, selected lactobacilli, nontoxic flours, and long fermentation time is a novel tool for the production of nontoxic bread from wheat-containing flour. The same approach was successfully adapted for pasta making [29,30] and for the treatment of rye and barley flours [31].

Further efforts were made to increase the hydrolyzing activity of sourdough lactobacilli. Together with fungal prolyl peptidases (see Chapter 3, Section 2.1), a new mixture of selected lactobacilli was used during long-term fermentation of wheat flour dough [32]. Different immunochemical and nonimmunochemical analytical methods revealed an almost complete degradation of gluten proteins, and in vitro testing on CD toxicity was negative. The bread-making quality was similar to that of conventional baker's yeast bread. A 60-day diet of baked goods made from hydrolyzed wheat flour, manufactured with sourdough lactobacilli and fungal peptidases, was not toxic to patients with CD [33]. Sweet baked goods produced from wheat sourdough rendered gluten-free were also shown to be safe for CD patients [34]. An even higher gluten-degrading capacity can be achieved by the use of sourdough prepared from germinated wheat [35]. In summary, the application of sourdough lactobacilli appears to be promising for the elimination of contaminant gluten and the production of gluten-free baked goods. However, sourdough fermentation abolishes the techno-functional properties of gluten, so that the detoxified material may be useful mainly as nutritient- and flavor-rich ingredient in a gluten-free receipe.

Peptidase preparations extracted from germinating cereals are also promising candidates for the degradation of gluten in foods, as was recently shown by its application in cereal-based fermented beverages, such as kwas and malt beer [36]. These were treated with a bran extract of germinated rye that contained a high activity of gluten-degrading peptidases. The incubation of the beverages with 0.1% of the extract for 4 h at 50 °C caused a significant reduction of gluten equivalents determined by the competitive R5 enzyme-linked immunosorbent assay (ELISA) (Figure 4.3). After the beverages were treated with 1% of the extract, gluten could no longer be detected.

Gluten-containing beverages also can be detoxified by treatment with microbial transglutaminase (mTG) [37]. The beverage (e.g., barley-based beer) is incubated with mTG derived from *Streptomyces mobaraensis*. This will lead to crosslinking of residual gluten peptides and formation of insoluble conjugates, which can be removed by filtration (Figure 4.4). If the process has been carried out in a suitable manner, the gluten level in the resulting beer decreases below 20 mg/kg, and it can be labeled gluten-free. The potential of mTG to prevent gluten toxicity was extended to an application in wheat flour.

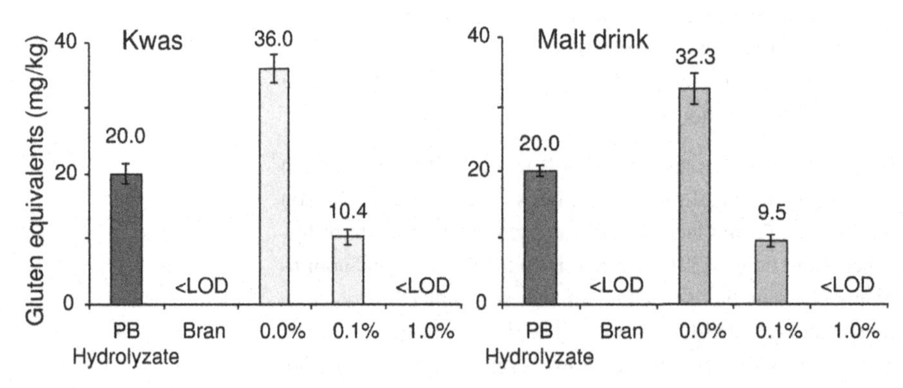

■ **FIGURE 4.3** Reduction of the gluten content of beverages by treatment with peptidases from bran of germinated rye (PB, prolamin barley; LOD, limit of detection). *Adapted from Ref. [36].*

Gianfrani and coworkers discovered that the incubation of the immunogenic gliadin peptide α(56–68) with mTG and lysine or lysine methyl ester inhibits the immune response by the formation of crosslinks [38]. Accordingly, wheat flour was treated with mTG and lysine methyl ester. Gliadin was isolated from the product, digested with pepsin and trypsin, and tested by a T-cell assay exhibiting no T-cell reactivity. In 2012, the effect of such altered wheat in CD patients was studied by a randomized, single-blinded 90-day trial (3.7 g gluten/day) [39]. Clinical relapse (symptoms, intestinal permeability, serology, histology, interferon (IFN)-γ) was diminished in the group receiving the altered wheat in comparison with the CD patients receiving regular flour. Thus, transamidation of gluten-containing food with a food-grade enzyme (mTG) and an appropriate amine (lysine methyl ester) can be used to block gluten toxicity. Although the final functional properties of the modified proteins were not evaluated, their molecular weight distribution was preserved, which is a major advantage over degradation by peptidases.

2.3 Wheat and Barley Deficient in Gluten

Wheat, the most widely grown crop, is immensely diverse with more than 25,000 different cultivars produced by plant breeders worldwide. The hexaploid *Triticum aestivum* (genome AABBDD) is used globally as bread wheat and the tetraploid *Triticum durum* (genome AABB) as pasta wheat. Several hundreds of gluten proteins are in a single wheat cultivar, and most of them contribute to the pathogenesis of CD. Almost all gluten proteins are encoded on chromosomes 1 and 6 of each genome. Gliadins of common wheat are encoded on chromosomes 1A, 1B, 1D, 6A, 6B, and 6D [40]. Six main loci are mapped on the distal ends of the short arms of the chromosomes of the first (Gli-1) and sixth (Gli-2) homologous groups. The specific loci are designated Gli-A1, Gli-B1, Gli-D1, Gli-A2, Gli-B2, and Gli-D2. HMW-glutenin subunits (HMW-GS) are encoded by pairs of paralogous x- and y-type genes present

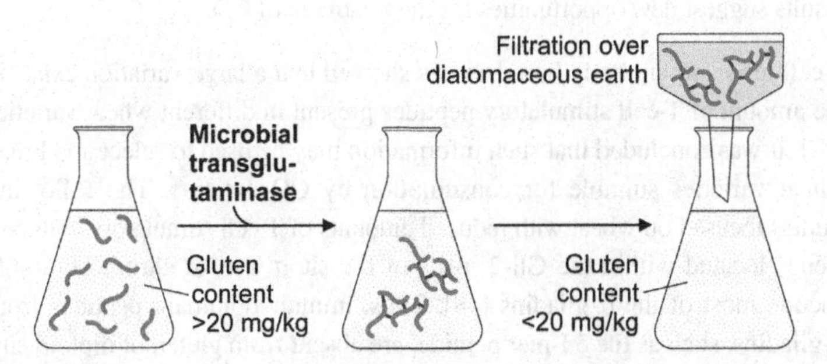

■ **FIGURE 4.4** Schematic representation of the use of microbial transglutaminase to detoxify beverages containing partially hydrolyzed gluten. *Adapted from Ref. [25].*

at loci, designated Glu-1, on the long arms of the homologous group 1 chromosomes (Glu-A1, Glu-B1, and Glu-D1 loci) [41]. LMW-glutenin subunits (LMW-GS) are controlled by genes at the Glu-A3, Glu-B3, and Glu-D3 loci on the short arms of chromosome 1A, 1B, and 1D, respectively [42].

First attempts to look for wheat lines that are not toxic for CD patients were made in the 1970s. Based on the knowledge that toxic A-gliadins (see Chapter 2, Section 3.4) are encoded on chromosome 6A, sufficient amounts of the wheat line Chinese Spring (nullisomic 6A-tetrasomic 6B) were grown for toxicity tests. Two CD patients received 65 g of bread daily from the nullisomic 6A flour, and testing for xylose and fat absorption after 16 days showed no effects [43]. Further studies involved three additional patients challenged with 130 g bread/day; subsequent evaluation of small intestinal mucosa, however, demonstrated that definite tissue damage occurred at the end of the test periods. The group of Ciclitira came to the same conclusion [44]. Consequently, the following questions arose: (1) Is it feasible to construct a new wheat cultivar, from which genes responsible for CD have been deleted, knowing that all gliadins and glutenins can cause mucosal damage in susceptible patients, and (2) would breads from such cultivars be more desirable to CD patients than breads produced without toxic cereals? [44,45]. Today, these are still questions of topical interest.

The next approach to finding nontoxic or less toxic wheat lines was explored in 1995. Frisoni and coworkers compared two wheat lines—one poor in α- and β-gliadins (nomenclature based on electrophoretic mobility) and the other poor in α-, β-, γ-, and ω-gliadins—with the original cultivar [46]. The peptic-tryptic digest of each gliadin fraction was tested for CD toxicity in an in vitro organ culture system with celiac mucosa. A significantly lower toxicity was found for the wheat lines deficient in the different gliadin subfractions compared with wheat containing all gliadin fractions. The differences between the two deficient lines were not significant. According to Frisoni and coworkers, these results suggest new opportunities for the treatment of CD.

T-cell tests and antibody-based assays showed that a large variation exists in the amount of T-cell stimulatory peptides present in different wheat varieties [47]. It was concluded that such information may be used to select and breed wheat varieties suitable for consumption by CD patients. The following studies focused on wheat with reduced amounts of T-cell stimulatory epitopes. Genes located within the Gli-2 locus of the short arm of chromosome 6D encode most of the α-gliadins [48]. Thus, immunodominant peptides from α-gliadins, such as the 33-mer peptide, are absent from gluten of diploid einkorn (AA) and tetraploid (AABB) durum wheat. The effects of deleting individual gluten loci on the levels of epitopes and the technological properties were analyzed using a set of deletion lines of wheat cultivar Chinese Spring [49,50]. The results demonstrated that removing the ω- and γ-gliadin and LMW-GS loci from the short arm of chromosome 1 of the D-genome removed stimulatory epitopes while maintaining technological properties. Studies on numerous tetraploid durum wheat lines were based on the assumption that the dose of exposure to gluten-derived, CD-active epitopes would contribute to a general reduction of the prevalence of CD and symptom severity in the population. The results showed that lines with reduced levels of stimulatory α-gliadin epitopes exist [51,52]. Gliadin derived from *Triticum monococcum* was shown to be unable to induce gluten-sensitive T-cell lines. Thus, the authors concluded that these gliadins also were innocuous in the production of IFN-γ and histological damage [53].

An experimental wheat line (C173) with spontaneous deletions of several gliadins and glutenins, specifically encoded on loci Gli-A2, Gli-D1, and Gli-D3, was tested in vitro by using duodenal mucosal biopsies of CD patients challenged under remission [54]. The results showed that C173 does not decrease the villous-to-crypt ratio but increases the release of the inflammatory cytokines IFN-γ and interleukin-2, as well as the production of anti-transglutaminase (TG) 2 antibodies in the supernatant. Therefore, C173 may not be appropriate for CD patients. Substantial differences in CD-specific epitope profiles among wheat varieties could be attributed to differences in the genetics of the A, B, and D genomes [48,55]. More than 3000 expressed α-gliadin sequences from 11 hexaploid wheat cultivars were analyzed to determine whether they encode for epitopes potentially involved in CD [56]. The results demonstrated that no single α-gliadin exists that lacks all T-cell stimulatory epitopes. Thus, it would be impossible to generate non-toxic wheat by conventional breeding. However, remarkable variations were observed among the three genomes: D-genome α-gliadins were by far the most immunogenic, A-genome α-gliadins had an intermediate immunogenicity profile, and B-genome α-gliadins were the least immunogenic. Mitea and colleagues proposed that it may be possible to generate a new gene that encodes nonimmunogenic α-gliadins by combining the genetic information of the A- and B-genome encoded α-gliadins [56].

RNA interference (RNAi) is one of the most exciting discoveries of the past decades [57]. The discovery won the Nobel Prize in Physiology and Medicine in 2006, and it has become an extremely valuable tool for the specific silencing of genes. Genetic engineering with RNAi led to the successful silencing of α-gliadins in the wheat cultivar Florida without any major effects on the rheological dough properties and baking quality of the resulting line [58]. Van Herpen and colleagues applied a slightly different RNAi strategy: specific α-gliadins harboring the DQ8-restricted epitope α206–217 were targeted in the cultivar Cadenza, leaving the other α-gliadins unaltered [59]. In another study, significant silencing of γ-gliadins was achieved in the wheat cultivar Bobwhite [60], and the expression of gliadins could be strongly downregulated in different transgenic lines [61]. Total gluten proteins were extracted from these lines and tested for their ability to stimulate four different T-cell clones derived from the intestinal lesion of CD patients. The results showed that the downregulation of gliadins can be used to obtain wheat lines with low levels of CD-specific immunogenicity. However, such a strategy may face considerable public opposition to genetically modified wheat, particularly by consumers in European countries.

Altogether, many questions will arise regarding the approach on the development of gluten-deficient wheat. Codex Alimentarius and different national regulations demand a gluten threshold of 20 mg/kg for the product to be labeled gluten-free. This means that the gluten content of wheat grain or flour (≈100,000 mg/kg) has to be reduced by a factor of 1/5000! Studies show that current experimental wheat lines may contain smaller amounts of gluten, but these studies do not provide evidence that this wheat is safe enough for CD patients [62]. If CD-safe wheat can be developed at all, it will have poorer yields and baking characteristics. Thus, the economic efficiency of such an approach is limited, as conventional wheat is a very cheap and robust industrial commodity, and it is unlikely that these specifically modified grains would ever replace commercial wheat strains [63]. They would be grown in alternative, small-scale production systems only, and the higher price might be prohibitive for usage beyond the niche market of products targeted at patients with severe conditions [64]. Last but not least, would baked products from such wheat lines be more desirable in quality than gluten-free products produced without toxic cereals?

Barley is a diploid cereal with pure inbred cultivars available and is, therefore, attractive for use in genetic approaches to detoxification. Tanner and coworkers presented barley lines lacking B- and C-hordeins [65]. Tests with peripheral blood mononuclear cells activated by oral hordein challenge demonstrated that the immunogenicity of these lines was reduced 20-fold compared with that of wild-type barley; therefore, creation of hordein-free barley may be possible.

3. LEGISLATION

3.1 International Regulations—Codex Alimentarius

The Codex Alimentarius describes international food standards, guidelines, and codes that contribute to the safety, quality, and fairness of international food trade. The Commission responsible for the Codex Alimentarius was established by the Food and Agriculture Organization of the United Nations

(FAO) and the World Health Organization (WHO) in 1963. Currently, the Codex Alimentarius Commission has 186 Codex Members made up of 185 member countries and one member organization (EU). It also has 220 Codex Observers including intergovernmental, nongovernmental, and UN organizations. Apart from the functions assigned to the Executive Committee, the tasks of the Codex Alimentarius Commission are divided into those of the General Subject Committees and Commodity Committees. With regard to CD and the GFD, the Codex Committee on Food Labelling (CCFL), the Codex Committee on Methods of Analysis and Sampling (CCMAS), and the Codex Committee on Nutrition and Foods for Special Dietary Uses (CCNFSDU) are of special importance.

3.1.1 CODEX STAN 1-1985

The General Standard for the Labelling of Prepackaged Foods, most recently amended in 2010 [66], states that the following foods and ingredients known to cause hypersensitivity shall always be declared:

- Cereals containing gluten (i.e., wheat, rye, barley, oats, spelt, or their hybridized strains and products of these);
- Crustacea and products of these;
- Eggs and egg products;
- Fish and fish products;
- Peanuts, soybeans, and products of these;
- Milk and milk products (lactose included);
- Tree nuts and nut products; and
- Sulfite in concentrations of 10 mg/kg or more.

3.1.2 CODEX STAN 118-1979

The Codex Standard for Foods for Special Dietary Use for Persons Intolerant to Gluten was established in 1981 and amended in 1983 [67]. Because at that time, no method for measuring gluten was available, the nitrogen content set at a threshold of 0.05% on a dry matter basis was the only methodical point. Kjeldahl and, more recently, Dumas procedures were used for nitrogen determination. However, these methods were limited to wheat starch used in the preparation of gluten-free products.

The latest, currently valid revision was published in 2008 [68]. The products covered by this standard are described as follows:

"Gluten-free foods are dietary foods

a. consisting of or made only from one or more ingredients which do not contain wheat (i.e., all *Triticum* species, such as durum wheat, spelt, and kamut), rye, barley, oats or their crossbred varieties, and the gluten level does not exceed 20 mg/kg in total, based on the food as sold or distributed to the consumer, and/or

b. consisting of one or more ingredients from wheat (i.e., all *Triticum* species, such as durum wheat, spelt, and kamut), rye, barley, oats or their crossbred varieties, which have been specially processed to remove gluten, and the gluten level does not exceed 20 mg/kg in total, based on the food as sold or distributed to the consumer."

With regard to oats, the following footnote was added:

"Oats can be tolerated by most but not all people who are intolerant to gluten. Therefore, the allowance of oats that are not contaminated with wheat, rye or barley in foods covered by this standard may be determined at the national level."

Foods specially processed to reduce gluten content may contain above 20 mg/kg up to 100 mg/kg in total. Decisions on the marketing of these products may be determined at the national level.

In subsidiary definitions "gluten is defined as a protein fraction from wheat, rye, barley, oats or their crossbred varieties and derivatives thereof, to which some persons are intolerant and that is insoluble in water and 0.5 M NaCl." "Prolamins are defined as the fraction from gluten that can be extracted by 40–70% of ethanol. The prolamin from wheat is gliadin, from rye is secalin, from barley hordein and from oats avenin. It is, however, an established custom to speak of gluten sensitivity. The prolamin content of gluten is generally taken as 50%."

All products covered by this standard "should supply approximately the same amount of vitamins and minerals as the original foods they replace" and "be prepared with special care under Good Manufacturing Practice (GMP) to avoid contamination with gluten."

In addition to the general labeling provisions contained in Codex Stan 1-1985 and Codex Stan 146-1985 (General Standard for the Labelling of and Claims for Prepackaged Foods for Special Dietary Uses) [69], some specific requirements were laid down. These include the following: "The term 'gluten-free' shall be printed in the immediate proximity of the name of the product" in case the gluten level of the product does not exceed 20 mg/kg in total. Products containing gluten levels of 20–100 mg/kg total must not be called gluten-free, and the appropriate labeling of such products has to be determined at the national level. "A food which, by its nature, is suitable for use as part of a gluten-free diet, shall not be designated 'special dietary', 'special dietetic' or any equivalent term", but "may bear a statement on the label that 'this food is by its nature gluten-free'".

Regarding methods of analysis and sampling, the following general requirements are stated in the standard:

- "The quantitative determination of gluten in foods and ingredients shall be based on an immunologic method or other method providing at least equal sensitivity and specificity.
- The antibody used should react with the cereal protein fractions that are toxic for persons intolerant to gluten and should not cross-react with other cereal proteins or other constituents of the foods or ingredients.
- Methods used for determination should be validated and calibrated against a certified reference material, if available.
- The detection limit has to be appropriate according to the state of the art and the technical standard. It should be 10 mg gluten/kg or below.
- The qualitative analysis that indicates the presence of gluten shall be based on relevant methods (e.g., ELISA-based methods, DNA methods)."

The Enzyme-Linked Immunoassay R5 Mendez Method is specified as the method for gluten determination. Additionally, the R5 Mendez Method is laid down as a type I method for the analysis of gluten in gluten-free foods in Codex Stan 234-1999, on "Recommended Methods of Analysis and Sampling" [70]. A type I method, also called defining method, is defined as "a method which determines a value that can only be arrived at in terms of the method per se and serves by definition as the only method for establishing the accepted value of the item measured".

3.1.3 CODEX STAN 163-1987

The Codex Standard for Wheat Protein Products Including Wheat Gluten applies to wheat protein products (WWPs) prepared from wheat by various processes [71]. These WWPs are intended for use in the food processing industry and in the production of foods requiring further preparation. To take wheat-related disorders into account, the standard's scope was amended in 2001 by the following sentence:

"Wheat gluten or wheat protein products should not be used for technological reasons, e.g., coating or processing aids for foods which are gluten-free by nature". As stated in the corresponding footnote, this "does not preclude the use of these products as ingredients in composite pre-packaged foods provided that they are properly labelled as ingredients".

3.1.4 CAC/GL 45-2003

The Guideline for the Conduct of Food Safety Assessment of Foods Derived from Recombinat-DNA Plants is important for CD patients because it prevents some research projects that attempt to insert wheat protein genes into

CD-nontoxic cereals such as rice and corn to make them more suitable for baking. As part of the safety assessment of expressed substances, the following three paragraphs deal with the possible allergenicity of proteins [72].

41. "When the protein(s) resulting from the inserted gene is present in the food, it should be assessed for potential allergenicity in all cases. An integrated, stepwise, case-by-case approach used in the assessment of the potential allergenicity of the newly-expressed protein(s) should rely upon various criteria used in combination (since no single criterion is sufficiently predictive on either allergenicity or non-allergenicity)" and be "obtained using sound scientific methods".

42. "The newly expressed proteins in foods derived from recombinant-DNA plants should be evaluated for any possible role in the elicitation of gluten-sensitive enteropathy, if the introduced genetic material is obtained from wheat, rye, barley, oats, or related cereal grains.

43. The transfer of genes from commonly allergenic foods and from foods known to elicit gluten-sensitive enteropathy in sensitive individuals should be avoided unless it is documented that the transferred gene does not code for an allergen or for a protein involved in gluten-sensitive enteropathy."

The assessment strategy of possible allergenicity further specified in Annex 1 is not applicable for assessing whether newly expressed proteins are capable of inducing gluten-sensitive or other enteropathies. Only paragraph 42 is applicable to the issue of enteropathies.

3.2 European Union and National Regulations

3.2.1 European Union

Legislation in the European Union (EU) largely follows the Codex Alimentarius. Definitions, thresholds, and labeling currently specified in the European Commission (EC) Regulation No 41/2009 [73] "concerning the composition and labelling of foodstuffs suitable for people intolerant to gluten" are the same as those in Codex Stan 118-1979 [68]. Foodstuffs "consisting of or containing one or more ingredients made from wheat, rye, barley, oats or their crossbred varieties which have been especially processed to reduce gluten, shall not contain a level of gluten exceeding 100 mg/kg in the food as sold to the final consumer." These products may be labeled with the term 'very low gluten'. If the gluten content does not exceed 20 mg/kg, these products may bear the term 'gluten-free'. Oats consumed by CD patients must have been "specially produced, prepared and/or processed in a way to avoid contamination by wheat, rye, barley, or their crossbred varieties and the gluten content of such oats must not exceed 20 mg/kg." Foodstuffs "consisting of or containing one or more ingredients which substitute wheat, rye, barley, oats or their crossbred varieties shall not contain a level of gluten exceeding 20 mg/kg in the food as sold to the final consumer. The labelling, presentation and advertising of those products shall bear the term 'gluten-free'."

The new Regulation No 609/2013 "on food intended for infants and young children, food for special medical purposes, and total diet replacement for weight control" to be implemented on July 20, 2016 [74], will repeal EC No 41/2009. As stated in article 41 of No 609/2013, the rules on the use of the terms 'gluten-free' and 'very low gluten' should be regulated under Regulation (EU) No 1169/2011 "on the provision of food information to consumers" [75]. EU No 1169/2011 will take effect on December 13, 2014, and aims to provide a high level of consumer protection by establishing requirements for food information and labeling of prepacked and nonprepacked foods. Under this regulation, indication that "any ingredient or processing aid listed in Annex II or derived from a substance or product listed in Annex II causing allergies or intolerances used in the manufacture or preparation of a food and still present in the finished product, even if in an altered form", shall be mandatory. Among the 14 substances or products causing allergies or intolerances listed in Annex II are cereals containing gluten, namely, wheat, rye, barley, oats, spelt, kamut, or their hybridized strains, and their various products. The only exceptions are wheat-based glucose syrups including dextrose, wheat-based maltodextrins, glucose syrups based on barley, and cereals used for making alcoholic distillates including ethyl alcohol of agricultural origin. The indication of gluten-containing ingredients thus will be mandatory for all prepacked and nonprepacked foods. For reasons of clarity and consistency, the rules on the use of the terms 'very low gluten' and 'gluten-free' as contained in EC No 41/2009 will be transferred into EU No 1169/2011. These regulations, to be adopted in EU No 1169/2011, should ensure at least the same level of protection for people who are intolerant to gluten as currently provided by EC No 41/2009. Furthermore, it should be ascertained that CD patients are adequately informed of the difference between a food that is specially treated to reduce the gluten content and another food that is made exclusively from ingredients naturally free of gluten.

3.2.2 Canada

In Canada, the food regulatory framework consists of the Canadian Food and Drugs Act and the Canadian Food and Drug Regulations (FDR) [76]. To enhance the labeling of food allergens and gluten sources in prepackaged foods, the FDR were amended as of August 4, 2012. Under the new rules, subsection B.01.010.1(2) states that if "a food allergen or gluten is present in a prepackaged product, the source of the food allergen or gluten, as the case may be, must be shown on the label of the product", either in the list of ingredients or in a 'Contains' statement. "'Gluten' means

a. any gluten protein from the grain of any of the following cereals or from the grain of a hybridized strain that is created from at least one of the following cereals: (i) barley, (ii) oats, (iii) rye, (iv) triticale, (v) wheat; or
b. any modified gluten protein, including any gluten protein fraction, that is derived from the grain of any of the cereals referred to in paragraph (a) or from the grain of a hybridized strain referred to in that paragraph."

The rules for making a gluten-free claim on foods are specified in division 24 of the FDR that applies to Foods for Special Dietary Use. Section B.24.018 states that it "is prohibited to label, package, sell or advertise a food in a manner likely to create an impression that it is a gluten-free food if the food contains any gluten protein or modified gluten protein, including any gluten protein fraction, referred to in the definition 'gluten' in subsection B.01.010.1(1)." Although no specific threshold is mentioned in the regulations, the purpose of section B.24.018 is to protect the health and safety of CD patients. Based on available scientific evidence, Health Canada considers that gluten-free foods, prepared under "Good Manufacturing Practices", that contain levels of gluten not exceeding 20 mg/kg as a result of cross-contamination meet the health and safety intent of B.24.018 when a gluten-free claim is made [77].

3.2.3 United States of America

Section 343 of the Federal Food, Drug, and Cosmetic Act was amended by the Food Allergen Labeling and Consumer Protection Act (FALCPA) of 2004 [78,79]. FALCPA requires the labeling of eight major food allergens, including wheat, either in a 'Contains' statement or in the list of ingredients. A part of the FALCPA also required the U.S. Food and Drug Administration (FDA) to define and permit use of the term 'gluten-free' on the labeling of foods. The final rule on "Gluten-free labeling of food" was issued under the FALCPA as an amendment to part 101 of Title 21 of the Code of Federal Regulations (21 CFR) and became effective on September 4, 2013 [80,81]. The definitions state that the "term 'gluten-containing grain' means any one of the following grains or their crossbred hybrids":

i. "Wheat, including any species belonging to the genus *Triticum*;
ii. Rye, including any species belonging to the genus *Secale*; or
iii. Barley, including any species belonging to the genus *Hordeum*."

"'Gluten' means the proteins that naturally occur in a gluten-containing grain and that may cause adverse health effects in persons with celiac disease (e.g., prolamins and glutelins)." A food bearing the claim 'gluten-free' in its labeling:

A. "Does not contain any one of the following:
  1. An ingredient that is a gluten-containing grain (e.g., spelt wheat);
  2. An ingredient that is derived from a gluten-containing grain and that has not been processed to remove gluten (e.g., wheat flour); or
  3. An ingredient that is derived from a gluten-containing grain and that has been processed to remove gluten (e.g., wheat starch), if the use of that ingredient results in the presence of 20 parts per million (ppm) or more gluten in the food" or

B. "Inherently does not contain gluten; and
  ii. Any unavoidable presence of gluten in the food bearing the claim in its labeling is below 20 ppm gluten".

To assess compliance, the FDA"will use a scientifically valid method that can reliably detect the presence of 20 ppm gluten in a variety of food matrices, including both raw and cooked or baked products." The FDA takes the view that there are currently no scientifically valid methods for determining gluten in fermented or hydrolyzed products and that a proposed rule on how to address compliance in these cases will be issued. In the meantime, a gluten-free claim is permitted on fermented and hydrolyzed foods that meet all requirements, even though gluten content cannot be reliably measured. Therefore, it is the responsibility of the manufacturer to ensure that fermented and hydrolyzed foods comply with regulations.

For beers, the issue of gluten-free labeling is complicated by the fact that beers made from both malted barley and hops are subject to the labeling requirements under the Federal Alcohol Administration Act issued by the Alcohol and Tobacco Tax and Trade Bureau (TTB). In contrast, beers that are not made from both malted barley and hops (i.e., either without malted barley or hops or without both) are subject to the FDA regulations described above [81]. On August 22, 2013, the TTB issued an announcement that it was reviewing its policy on gluten content statements in light of the recent 21 CFR part 101 amendment [82]. Meanwhile, the Interim Policy on Gluten Content Statements in the Labeling and Advertising of Wines, Distilled Spirits, and Malt Beverages of May 24, 2012, remains in force [83]. This policy allows the use of the term 'gluten-free' for products made from gluten-free raw materials provided that the producer used GMP, took precautions to prevent cross-contamination, and did not use additives, yeast, or storage materials that contain gluten. Products made from gluten-containing materials may bear a statement: "Product fermented from grains containing gluten and (processed *or* treated *or* crafted) to remove gluten. The gluten content of this product cannot be verified, and this product may contain gluten." or "This product was distilled from grains containing gluten, which removed some or all of the gluten. The gluten content of this product cannot be verified, and this product may contain gluten." The TTB will only approve label applications for either statement if a detailed description of the method used to remove gluten from the product and R5 Mendez competitive ELISA results of less than 20 ppm gluten are provided. Similarly, the FDA intends to exercise enforcement discretion for beers that currently make a gluten-free claim and that are (1) made from a non-gluten-containing grain or (2) made from a gluten-containing grain, during which the beer has been subject to processing that the manufacturer has determined will remove gluten. The FDA did not address the use of a universal gluten-free symbol/logo because it does not believe it will necessarily ensure that the gluten-free claim is not false or misleading.

3.2.4 Australia and New Zealand

The binational Food Standards Australia and New Zealand (FSANZ) government agency develops and administers the Food Standards Code (FSC). Regulations related to gluten are laid out in Standards 1.2.7 (Nutrition, Health and Related Claims of January 07, 2013) [84] and 2.9.5 (Food for Special Medical Purposes of February 21, 2013) [85]. According to Standard 1.2.7, "gluten means the main protein in wheat, rye, oats, barley, triticale and spelt relevant to the medical conditions coeliac disease and dermatitis herpetiformis." A nutrient content claim related to gluten may use only the label gluten-free or low gluten or state that a food contains gluten or is high in gluten. For the use of the label gluten-free, a food must not contain "(a) detectable gluten; or (b) oats or their products; or (c) cereals containing gluten that have been malted, or their products." Food with a low gluten content may not contain more than 20 mg gluten/100 g of the food. Standard 2.9.5 prohibits the use of a claim in relation to the gluten content of a food for special medical purposes unless expressly permitted by the clause. A gluten-free claim may be made only "if the food contains (a) no detectable gluten; and (b) no oats or oat products; and (c) no cereals containing gluten that have been malted, or products of such cereals." If a claim is made in relation to the gluten content of a food for special medical purposes, the label on the package must include the average quantity of the gluten in the food. Thus, in Australia and New Zealand, gluten-free means that gluten is not detectable by the most appropriate techniques currently available (<3 mg/kg). This strict interpretation supported by the Australian Competition and Consumer Commission (ACCC) and the New South Wales Food Authority (NSWFA) has been contested by the Australian Food and Grocery Council (AFGC) and the Coeliac Society of Australia that advocate an alteration of the gluten-free definition to the internationally recognized level of less than 20 mg/kg [86].

The major concern is the fact that as analytical testing becomes increasingly sensitive, the level of detection may decrease even further, making it even more difficult for any product to be labeled gluten-free. This also imposes additional costs and constraints for manufacturers to comply with a standard that, based on available scientific evidence, is stricter than required.

3.3 Gluten-Free Symbols

The Crossed Grain symbol (Figure 4.5) is the internationally recognized symbol for gluten-free foods. For CD patients, it is easily recognizable, transcends language barriers, communicates that a product is safe to eat, and acts as a guarantee of quality because all manufacturers using the symbol must conform to high production standards. The intellectual property of the Crossed Grain symbol belongs to Coeliac UK, but it has been registered as a Trademark in the European Union and the United States for use with a broad range of food, drink, and related product categories [87]. The Association of European Coeliac Societies (AOECS) developed the European Licensing System in collaboration with its member societies [88]. Producers or retailers who want to use this symbol should contact their national celiac societies to obtain an annual license and pay a license fee based on their net sales turnover of gluten-free products. The following requirements have to be met:

- The product must be labeled gluten-free or very low gluten, according to standards set by the Codex Alimentarius and EC No 41/2009.

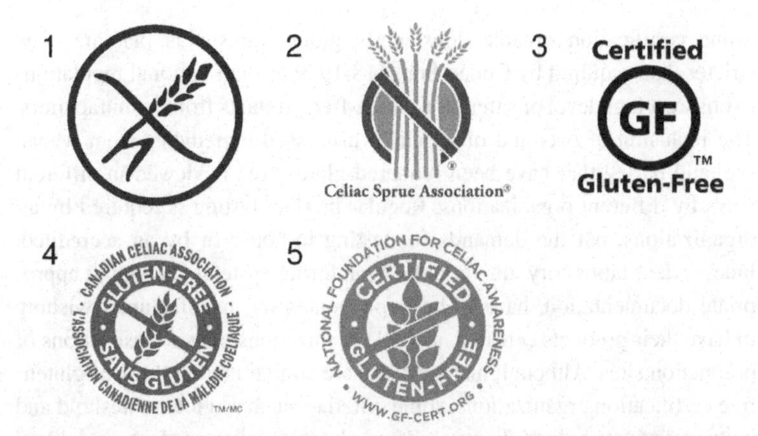

■ **FIGURE 4.5** Gluten-free symbols 1, Crossed Grain symbol, Association of European Coeliac Societies (AOECS); 2, Celiac Sprue Association (CSA) Recognition Seal; 3, Gluten-Free Certification Organization (GFCO) logo; 4, Gluten-Free Certification Program of the Canadian Celiac Association (GFCP-CCA) mark; 5, Gluten-Free Certification Program of the National Foundation for Celiac Awareness (GFCP-NFCA) trademark.

- Test certificates of measured gluten expressed in prolamin content analyzed with the R5 sandwich ELISA for natural and heat-processed foods and the R5 competitive ELISA for hydrolyzed products by an independent, accredited laboratory have to be provided at least once a year.
- Audit certificates for all manufacturing sites in compliance with British Retail Consortium (BRC) standards, International Featured Standards (IFS), or ISO 22,000:2005 have to be presented. A Hazard Analysis and Critical Control Point (HACCP) system must be implemented, and it must include a risk assessment ensuring the avoidance of gluten contamination during all stages of production, storage, transportation, and handling. General Hygienic Practice (GHP) and GMP procedures must be recorded, and a monitoring system including traceability and a nonconformance procedure and corrective actions must be established.

The Crossed Grain symbol may not be used for products that are naturally gluten-free or unprocessed. Nevertheless, some companies simply have created their own gluten-free logos, and a multitude of symbols exist worldwide, creating confusion among consumers about which quality standards apply. Various gluten-free certification programs are offered by different organizations, which apply diverging standards. Table 4.1 provides an overview of selected criteria and shows the differences among four international and national gluten-free certification programs.

Some certification organizations apply gluten thresholds that are even stricter than required by Codex Stan 118-1979 or their national regulations to ensure a high level of safety for gluten-free products from manufacturers. The inclusion of oats and of specially processed ingredients from wheat, rye, and barley that have been rendered gluten-free is viewed in different ways by different organizations. Regular product testing is required by all organizations, but the demands for testing in-house or by an accredited, independent laboratory are variable. Monitoring systems, including appropriate documentation, have to be implemented by manufacturers wishing to have their products certified, and all organizations may do inspections of production sites. Although many criteria are similar among the four gluten-free certification organizations, some criteria—such as gluten threshold and inclusion of oats or ingredients rendered gluten-free in a product—are divergent. This variability in criteria and symbols is likely to be confusing for consumers because they may not be familiar with the underlying requirements for certification associated with a particular symbol. Therefore, establishing an international gluten-free symbol with standardized criteria that is

Table 4.1 Overview of Criteria between the European Licensing System by the Association of European Coeliac Societies (AOECS), Celiac Sprue Association Recognition Seal Program (CSA), Gluten Intolerance Group Gluten-Free Certification Organization (GFCO), and Gluten-Free Certification Program (GFCP) of the Canadian Celiac Association (CCA); also Endorsed by the National Foundation for Celiac Awareness (NFCA) in the United States [88–93]

	AOECS	CSA	GFCO	GFCP
Threshold for gluten in the product (mg/kg)	<20	<5	<10	<20
Can ingredients derived from wheat, rye, and barley that have been processed to remove gluten be included as long as the threshold (mg/kg) is met?	Yes	If toxic fractions are proven absent by MS	Use of such ingredients is not recommended	Meet the requirements of the jurisdiction where the product is sold or the customer demands
Can oats be included as long as the threshold (mg/kg) is met?	Yes	If oat cultivar is void of toxic amino acid sequences by MS	Yes	See above
Is product testing for gluten by an accredited, independent laboratory mandatory prior to licensing?	Yes	Yes	May be done in-house	Highly recommended
Are high-risk raw ingredients (e.g., flour) required to be tested for gluten?	Yes	Yes	Yes	Highly recommended
Is product testing by the manufacturer required throughout the year?	Yes	Highly recommended	Yes	Highly recommended
May this product testing be done in-house by the manufacturer?	Yes	Highly recommended	Yes	Yes, but also external
Is regular product testing by an accredited, independent laboratory mandatory?	Yes, annually	Highly recommended	No	Highly recommended
What antibody shall be used for testing?	R5	R5/G12/best test available	AOAC-based ELISA tests	AOAC-based ELISA tests
Shall a HACCP system be implemented?	Yes	Yes	Yes	Recommended
Are GHP, GMP, risk assessment, staff training, and appropriate documentation required?	Yes	Recommended	Yes	Yes
Is a monitoring system (traceability, nonconformance procedure) required?	Yes, auditor-controlled	Yes	Yes	Yes
Is the use of a dedicated gluten-free line mandatory?	No, but appropriate measures	No, but appropriate measures	No, but appropriate measures	No, but appropriate measures
Are monitoring inspections of production sites done?	Yes	Some, based on risk assessment	Yes, annually	Yes
Duration of the certification period	1 year	1 year	1 year	1 year

AOAC, Association of Official Analytical Chemists International easily recognizable and that guarantees the highest possible level of safety for gluten-free foods is desirable.

4. GLUTEN ANALYSIS

Analytical methods play an important role in the assessment and maintenance of food quality worldwide. In particular, an accurate analysis of food constituents and additives that affect the health of consumers, such as toxic compounds, is essential. Most toxic food constituents are either single compounds such as acrylamide or small groups of compounds such as mycotoxins; the methods for their detection and quantitation can be determined in relation to their special structures. In the case of CD, however, the precipitating factor, gluten, is a complex mixture of proteins with divergent structures. The composition of gluten can vary according to its botanical origin (e.g., cereal species, varieties), agricultural conditions in which the plants were produced (e.g., climate, soil, fertilization), and food processing procedures (e.g., heating, enzymatic degradation). Moreover, knowledge about the toxic epitopes within the proteins in gluten is incomplete. Many laboratories have searched for solutions for accurate gluten determination over the past decades but without coming to a final, widely accepted solution.

Since the 1950s, it has been known that a strict adherence to a GFD is the essential therapy of CD. The daily intake of gluten should be less than 20 mg. All gluten-containing foods from wheat, rye, barley, and oats must be avoided and substituted with gluten-free alternatives (see Section 1). The Codex Alimentarius and other international and national institutions regulate the allowed level of gluten in foods for special dietary use of CD patients (see Section 3). According to the Codex Alimentarius, dietary gluten-free food should not exceed 20 mg gluten/kg; for foods specially processed to reduce gluten content, a threshold of 100 mg/kg can be allowed at the national level.

The detection and accurate quantitation of gluten in foods is essential not only for CD patients but also for the industry producing gluten-free foods and for food control. Minimum requirements for appropriate methods should include sufficient sensitivity, selectivity, and a certified reference material for calibration. Moreover, they should be applicable not only to raw but also to processed materials (heat-treated, fermented, acid-treated). Last but not least, they should be evaluated in collaborative studies and available as commercial assays. Three steps essentially are involved in the analytical procedure:

1. complete extraction of gluten proteins/peptides from the matrix;
2. application of a representative protein/peptide reference for calibration;
3. accurate quantitation of extracted gluten proteins/peptides.

Numerous studies on gluten quantitation have been published during the past decades. Early results were summarized by Denery-Papini and coworkers [94], and completed with more recent results by Wieser [95] and Haraszi and colleagues [96]. Immunological methods, in particular ELISAs, have been the focus for the analysis of gluten proteins and peptides in raw materials and food. Non-immunological methods are equally important as independent control methods; and polymerase chain reaction, mass spectrometry, and column chromatography have been proposed as alternative techniques. Moreover, various analytical procedures such as high-performance liquid chromatography, electrophoresis, and mass spectrometry have decisively contributed to the progress in understanding the pathomechanism of CD.

4.1 Protein Extraction

Gluten-containing materials, raw materials as well as foods, are composed of numerous components. Therefore, the first step in gluten analysis is the extraction of gluten proteins from the matrix, independent of the subsequent quantitation method. Native gluten proteins are not soluble in water or salt solution. The most commonly used solvents for the extraction of gluten proteins are aqueous alcohols: one portion (prolamins) is soluble, whereas the other portion (glutelins) remains in the insoluble residue. Glutelins or total gluten proteins are extractable with aqueous alcohols after the reduction of disulfide bonds. Disaggregating agents such as urea or sodium dodecyl sulfate (SDS) and increased temperature accelerate the dissolving process. The analytical method following extraction determines whether a one-step (direct extraction with aqueous alcohols), a two-step (pre-extraction of albumins and globulins with a salt solution) or even a three-step procedure (subsequent extraction of albumins/globulins, prolamins, and glutelins) is necessary. A one-step procedure for protein extraction would be highly desirable due to simplicity and reproducibility. Gluten peptides, present in fermented foods, for example, are usually soluble in both water/salt solutions and aqueous alcohols.

A previous Draft Revised Codex Standard (document ALINORM 97/26) presented a detailed description of the extraction procedure, whereas the recent Codex Stan 118–1979 (document 08/31/26) refers only to the ELISA R5 Mendez method (see following discussion). According to document ALINORM 97/26, the determination of gluten in foodstuffs or ingredients must be based on the determination of prolamins, defined as the fraction from gluten that can be extracted with 40–70% ethanol. A concentration of 60% is recommended—an earlier study had demonstrated that the optimal extraction of gliadins from wheat flour is achieved with this concentration [97]. Glutelins remain in the insoluble residue and are not included in the analysis. Products with a fat content higher than 10% have to be defatted with n-hexane. The product is then dried at 60°C, milled, and extracted with 60% aqueous ethanol in a volume 10 times its weight. After centrifugation, the supernatant is taken off and stored at 4°C before determination. When a precipitate is formed, it is spun down and discarded. In the case of liquid products, an aliquot is diluted with the volume of pure ethanol, which yields a concentration of 60% ethanol in the resulting mixture. Addition of casein or urea avoids the binding of prolamins to the matrix—for example, to polyphenols, such as those from tea, hops, and cocoa products.

The incomplete extraction of prolamins from heated samples such as baked products is a major problem of gluten analysis when aqueous alcohols are used. Extraction studies on wheat bread spiked with a gliadin standard demonstrated that the extractability of cysteine-containing α- and γ-gliadins was strongly reduced compared to the corresponding flour, whereas that of cysteine-free ω-gliadins was scarcely affected [98]. It has been shown that α- and γ-gliadins are bound to alcohol-insoluble glutenins due to disulfide/sulfhydryl interchain reactions under heat stress. After the reduction of disulfide bonds, however, total gliadins (and glutenin subunits) can be completely recovered in the alcoholic extract from the bread.

The heat-stability of ω-gliadins initiated the development of an immunoassay with monoclonal antibodies (mAbs) against ω-gliadins [99]. Forty percent ethanol was shown to be the most suitable extractant for the quantitative extraction of ω-gliadins from all types of foods (raw, cooked, baked). Another suggestion for improving the extraction of gluten proteins from heated food was limited hydrolysis with pepsin, resulting in yields of about 90% [100]. A two-step extraction protocol (step 1: 50% 2-propanol, room temperature; step 2: 50% 2-propanol + 1% dithiothreitol in Tris/HCl buffer pH 7.5, 60 °C) was recommended for the complete extraction of gluten proteins [101].

The so-called cocktail, the combination of a reducing agent (2-mercaptoethanol) with a disaggregating agent (guanidine), allowed the complete extraction of prolamins (together with glutelins) from both unheated and heat-processed foods in one step [102]. Figure 4.6 compares the recovery of gliadins from wheat flour and corresponding doughs heated from 22 °C to 230 °C and extracted with 60% ethanol (A) or cocktail (B). The recovery of gliadins extracted with 60% ethanol decreased drastically with increasing temperature, whereas the recovery was constantly high when the cocktail was used. With regard to the extraction of both unheated and heat-treated products, incubation with the cocktail for 40 min at 50°C was recommended. The extraction with the cocktail solution is part of the R5 ELISA method

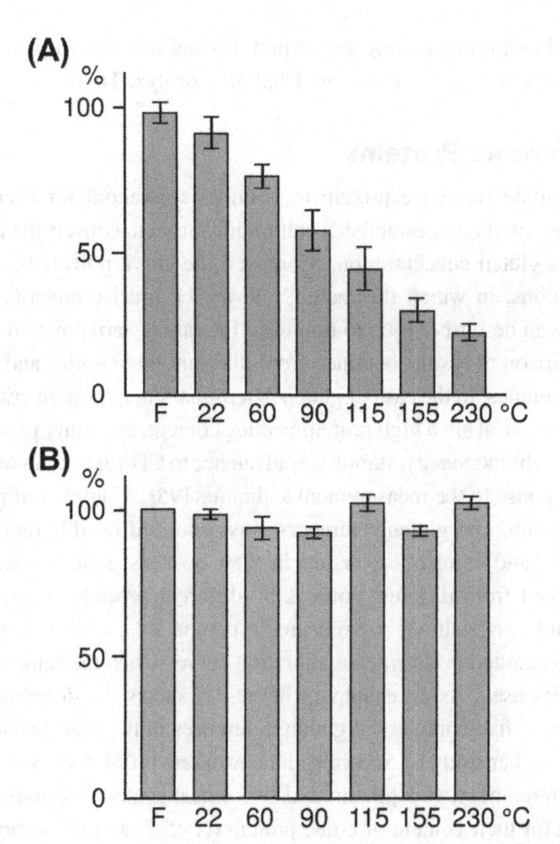

FIGURE 4.6 Recovery of gliadins from wheat flour (F) and doughs heated at different temperatures and extracted with (A) 60% ethanol and (B) cocktail (flour = 100%). *Adapted from Ref. [102].*

recommended by Codex Stan 118–1979 and Codex Stan 234–1999 (Recommended Methods of Analysis and Sampling last revised in 2011) (see Section 3). Because 2-mercaptoethanol is weak in reducing power, toxic, and has an unpleasant stench, protein chemists usually use dithioerythritol or dithiothreitol as an effective and nontoxic agent for reducing polymeric proteins (e.g., [98,101]). However, these agents have to be stored at around −18°C, a temperature that is not suitable for ELISA kits. A promising alternative to replace 2-mercaptoethanol is tris-2-carboxyethyl-phosphine (TCEP) [103]. The combination with guanidine (modified cocktail) revealed similar extraction yields of gliadins compared with the original cocktail. TCEP also was used for an extraction solvent that was compatible with the competitive ELISA [104]. TCEP (5 mmol/l) was combined with the surfactant N-lauroylsarcosine (2%) in phosphate buffer (pH 7), and this extraction system, called UPEX (universal prolamin and glutelin extractant solution), was shown to be a useful tool for extracting gluten proteins and peptides from any kind of food samples, including heat-treated and/or hydrolyzed ones.

4.2 Reference Proteins

An appropriate reference protein or peptide is essential for every gluten quantitation method to establish a calibration curve to convert the measured signal to a gluten concentration. Moreover, the curve reflects the range of concentrations, in which the method allows the precise quantitation. The reference can be further used to minimize interassay variation and to enable the comparison of results obtained from different laboratories and with different techniques. In the case of gluten determination, important criteria for a reference material are a high protein/peptide content, solubility in the extraction solvent, homogeneity, stability, equivalence to CD-toxic compounds, and a good response to the measurement technique [95]. A number of prolamin, mainly gliadin, and gluten references was produced by different research laboratories and companies for use in their own test systems. References were isolated from different sources by different procedures, and protein content and compositions were scarcely comparable. Consequently, most references resulted in divergent calibration curves when the same analytical method was used. As an example, Figure 4.7 shows the different calibration curves of five commercial gliadin references in the same immunoassay [105]. In another study by Schwalb and coworkers [106], four commercially available references, two gliadin and two wheat gluten preparations, were compared for their content of crude protein (N×5.7) and proportions of the

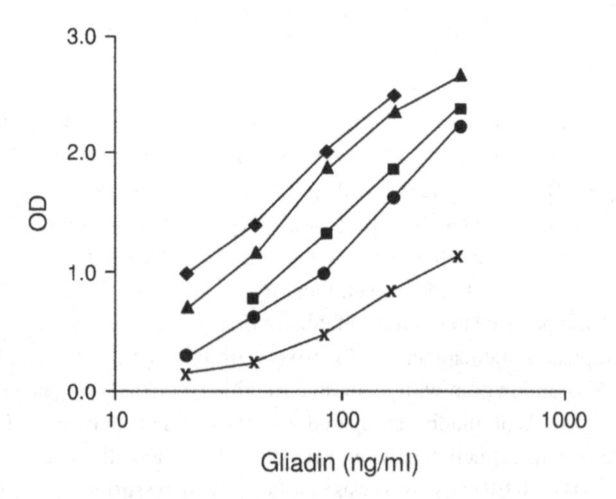

■ **FIGURE 4.7** Calibration curves of different gliadin references determined by the R5 Ridascreen® Gliadin assay. OD, optical density. *Adapted from van Ref. [105].*

Osborne fractions. The contents of crude protein were 78.4% and 91.9% for the gliadin references and 71.0% and 77.0% for the gluten references, respectively. Whereas the proportions of albumins/globulins were rather similar (2.8–8.8%), the proportions of gliadins were extremely divergent, from 30.7% to 71.6% (Figure 4.8). Surprisingly, both gliadin preparations contained high proportions of alcohol-insoluble glutenins (25.4% and 63.8%). The gluten references showed completely different compositions. The first one contained 35.9% gliadins and 61.3% glutenins, but the second one was composed of 56.5% gliadins and 34.7% glutenins. Regarding the gluten content (=gliadins+glutenins) the samples were comparable, with 91.2% and 97.2%. Thus, protein references available on the market show significant differences in crude protein content and proportions of Osborne fractions. References used for calibration should, therefore, be analyzed for the target proteins that will be determined in the subsequent analytical procedure.

The Draft Revised Codex Standard document ALINORM 97/26 (1997) recommended that a gold standard should be prepared by one laboratory under strictly standardized conditions. Considering this advice, the Working Group on Prolamin Analysis and Toxicity (PWG) decided to organize the preparation of a gliadin reference (PWG-gliadin) for collective use [107]. Grains of 28 European wheat cultivars were combined and milled, and the resulting flour was defatted and, stepwise, extracted with 0.4 mol/l NaCl and 60% ethanol. The gliadin extract was desalted, freeze-dried, and homogenized. The reference obtained was homogeneous and completely soluble in 60% ethanol. The crude protein content (N×5.7) was 89.4%, and only 3% albumins and globulins besides gliadins were present.

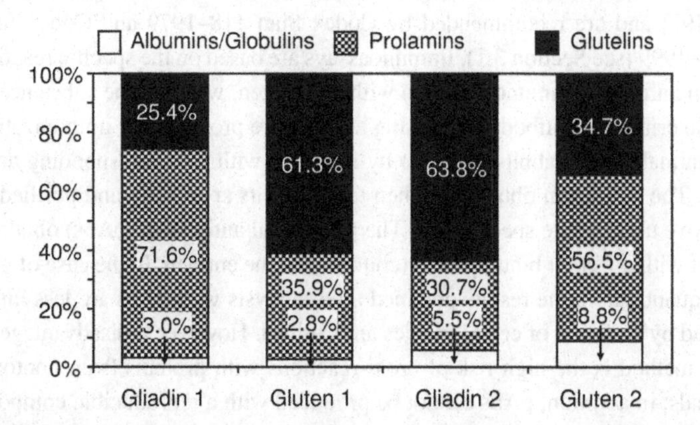

■ **FIGURE 4.8** Proportions of Osborne fractions in four commercially available protein references. *Adapted from Ref. [106].*

To produce references that are suitable for the quantitation of partially hydrolyzed gluten, (e.g., in sourdough, starch syrup, malt extracts, and beer), the prolamin fractions of wheat, rye, and barley were digested with pepsin and trypsin or with pepsin and chymotrypsin [108]. The six different digests were compared by reversed-phase high-performance liquid chromatography (RP-HPLC) and SDS-polyacrylamide gel electrophoresis (PAGE), which showed that intact proteins were no longer present in the digests. The crude peptide content ($N \times 5.7$), important as a base parameter for calibration, varied between 65.7% and 96.0%, depending on the cereal species. The analysis of fermented beverages demonstrated that the combination of the enzymatic digests with a competitive ELISA (see Section 4.3.1) was an adequate system for the quantitation of gluten peptides in fermented products.

In conclusion, the structure and composition of the reference should be as similar as possible to that of the target analyte. The prolamin content has to be determined using a prolamin calibrator; and the gluten content, using an appropriate mixture of prolamins and glutelins. In some cases, it is advisable to use special references (e.g., a hordein preparation for barley contaminations or partially hydrolyzed references for fermented products). The calibration curve should always be based on the protein/peptide content and not on the amount of substance. Altogether, the development of a commonly accepted reference material not only for prolamins but also for glutelins and gluten peptides is essential because it would provide a common platform to evaluate, validate, and compare results from various gluten quantitation techniques.

4.3 Immunochemical Methods

To date, immunochemical assays are the methods of choice for gluten analysis [95] and are recommended by Codex Stan 118–1979 and Codex Stan 234–1999 (see Section 3.1). Immunoassays are based on the specific reaction of an antibody (immunoglobulin) with an antigen, which is the substance to be determined. Antibody-containing antisera are produced by immunization of animals (e.g., rabbits or mice) by injection with the corresponding antigen. The antiserum obtained is then tested for its specificity and purified to remove undesirable specificities. The polyclonal antibodies (pAbs) obtained react with different binding sites (epitopes) of the antigen. In the case of gluten quantitation, the results obtained after analysis with pAbs are less influenced by variation of cereal species and cultivar. However, a disadvantage of this method is the high risk of cross-reactions with proteins from nontoxic cereals; in addition, pAbs cannot be produced with a reproducible composition and specificity. More specific mAbs are produced, after immunization, by the fusion of isolated splenocytes with murine myeloma cells to produce hybrid cells, so-called hybridomas. These hybridomas, positive for antibodies against the antigens, are then cloned and grown in a cell culture medium. The resulting mAb preparation can be purified by precipitation and/or affinity chromatography. The advantages of mAbs include absolute reproducibility of specificity and the ability to produce almost unlimited quantities.

A central point of immunoassays is the quantitation of the antibody/antigen complex. Previously, the formation of precipitates or labeling with markers (e.g., luminescent or fluorescent dyes, stable radicals, radioisotopes) was used for measurements. Nowadays, ELISAs are the most frequently used technique, and usually are applied in the immunochemical quantitation of gluten. More recently, immunosensors have been developed.

4.3.1 ELISA

ELISAs are relatively easy to perform, often cheaper than other techniques, and provide rapid results. The most common indicator enzymes used are horseradish peroxidase (substrate 2,2′-azinobis(3-ethylbenzothiazoline-6-sulfonic acid)), alkaline phosphatase (substrate 4-nitrophenylphosphate), and β-D-galactosidase (substrate 4-nitrophenyl-β-galactoside). These enzymes are linked to the antigen by covalent bonds (e.g., by reaction with glutaraldehyde or carbodiimide). Two ELISA systems have been applied most frequently for gluten analysis: sandwich ELISA and competitive ELISA [95]. The principle of the sandwich ELISA is shown in Figure 4.9(A). In sandwich ELISA, mAbs or pAbs are immobilized onto the wells of a microtiter plate. Aliquots of the

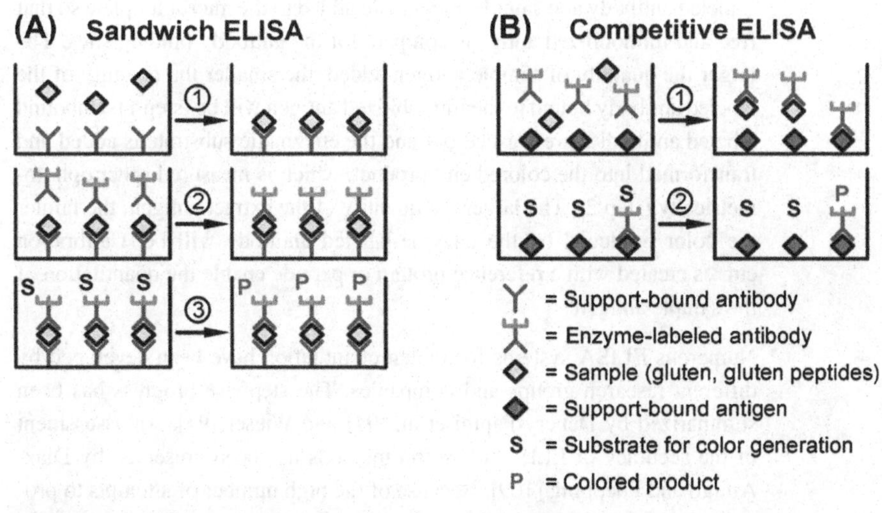

■ **FIGURE 4.9** Different ELISA formats: (A) sandwich ELISA; (B) competitive ELISA. (Please see color plate at the back of the book.) *Adapted from Ref. [95].*

extract containing the antigen to be determined are added and incubated in the microtiter plate, resulting in the formation of the antibody/antigen complex (step 1). After washing, mAbs or pAbs labeled with an indicator enzyme are added and bound to a second binding site of the antigen during a subsequent incubation step (step 2). Thus, the antigen is "sandwiched" between the support-bound unlabeled antibodies and enzyme-labeled antibodies. After the unbound enzyme-labeled antibodies are washed out, the substrate for the enzyme is added, transformed into a colored end product, and measured spectrophotometrically (step 3). The absorbance measured is directly proportional to the antigen concentration in the extract, which can be calculated using a reference protein and a calibration curve. The sandwich ELISA is suitable only for large antigens (proteins) because the antigen must have at least two binding epitopes that are spatially separated to bind both support-bound antibody and enzyme-labeled antibody. In the case of gluten analysis, the sandwich ELISA is inappropriate when partially hydrolyzed (fermented) products such as sourdough products, malt extracts, or beer have to be analyzed, because the gluten peptides may have only one binding site left.

The competitive ELISA is suitable not only for intact proteins but also for small-sized antigens (peptides) with only one antigenic epitope. The assay is composed of three components (Figure 4.9(B)) [95]:

1. the antigen immobilized onto the microtiter plate;
2. a limited and constant quantity of the enzyme-labeled antibody;
3. the antigen from the extract.

Labeled antibody and sample antigen are added to the microtiter plate so that free and immobilized antigens compete for the antibody binding sites. The larger the quantity of sample antigen added, the smaller the quantity of the labeled antibody bound to the immobilized antigen will be (step 1). Unbound labeled antibodies are washed out and the enzymatic substrate is added and transformed into the colored end product, which is measured spectrophotometrically (step 2). The larger the quantity of the extract antigen, the fainter the color produced by the enzyme-labeled antibody will be. Calibration curves created with a reference protein or peptide enable the quantitation of the sample antigen.

Numerous ELISA systems for gluten quantitation have been developed by different research groups and companies. The stepwise progress has been summarized by Denery-Papini et al. [94] and Wieser [95]. An assessment of the accuracy of ELISA detection methods has been presented by Diaz-Amigo and Poepping [109]. Because of the high number of attempts to produce an appropriate immunoassay, only the principles of ELISA kits that currently are commercially available are described here (Table 4.2). The

Table 4.2 List of Commercially Available ELISA Kits for Gluten Detection

Company	Name	Type	Antibody
Abnova	Gluten/Gliadin ELISA Kit	Sandwich	pAb
Astori Tecnica	Gluten ELISA Kit	Competitive	pAb
Biomedal Diagnostics	GlutenTox ELISA Sandwich	Sandwich	G12 mAb
	GlutenTox ELISA competitive	Competitive	G12 mAb
	GlutenTox Sticks	Dipstick	G12 mAb
Biocontrol	Transia Plate Prolamins	Sandwich	R5 mAb
BioCheck (UK)	Gluten-Check ELISA kit	Sandwich	401.21 mAb
Diagnostic Automation	DAI Gliadin/Gluten ELISA	Sandwich	pAb
ELISA Systems	ELISA Systems Gliadin assay	Sandwich	401.21 mAb
ELISA Technologies	Gluten Aller-Tek	Sandwich	401.21 mAb
	EZ gluten®	Dipstick	401.21 mAb
EuroProxima	Gluten-Tec® ELISA	Competitive	α20 mAb
Imutest	Gluten-Check ELISA Kit	Sandwich	401.21 mAb
	Gluten-in-Food Test	Screening test	401.21 mAb
Ingenasa	Ingezim Gluten®	Sandwich	R5 mAb
	Ingezim Gluten® SemiQ	Sandwich	R5 mAb
	Ingezim Gluten® Hidrolizado	Direct	R5 mAb
Morinaga Institute	Wheat Protein ELISA Kit	Sandwich	pAb
Neogen	Alert for Gliadin	Screening test	401.21 mAb
	Alert for Gliadin R5	Screening test	R5 mAb
	BioKits Gluten Assay Kit	Sandwich	401.21 mAb
	Veratox® for Gliadin	Sandwich	401.21 mAb
	Veratox® for Gliadin R5	Sandwich	R5 mAb
	Reveal 3-D for Gluten	Dipstick	401.21 mAb
	Reveal 3-D for Gliadin R5	Dipstick	R5 mAb
R-Biopharm	Ridascreen® Gliadin	Sandwich	R5 mAb
	Ridascreen® Fast Gliadin	Sandwich	R5 mAb
	Ridascreen® Gliadin competitive	Competitive	R5 mAb
	Rida®Quick Gliadin	Dipstick	R5 mAb
Romer Labs	AgraQuant® ELISA Gluten G12	Sandwich	G12 mAb
	AgraStrip® LFD Gluten G12	Dipstick	G12 mAb
Zeulab	Proteon Gluten Express	Dipstick	G12 mAb

oldest immunoassay on the market was developed by Skerritt and Hill in 1990 [99]. This sandwich ELISA uses mAbs (401.21) against heat-stable ω-gliadins. This test has been suggested as suitable for quantitating gluten in all types of uncooked and heat-treated foods. A gliadin preparation extracted with 40% ethanol from the Australian wheat cultivar Timgalen is provided as reference protein. The assay has been successfully evaluated in collaborative studies, validated by the Association of Official Analytical Chemists (AOAC International), and patented and marketed by several companies. The manufacturer-indicated sensitivity of the different test kits ranges from 20 mg to 160 mg of gluten/kg. Major disadvantages of the assay are that it recognizes barley and oat prolamins very poorly and that the results are strongly cultivar-dependent due to the different proportions of ω-gliadins that can range from around 7% to 20% of total gliadins [97]. A second rapid test kit, which is suitable for home use or in process quality control, has been developed to provide rapid qualitative or semiquantitative results and to improve compliance with GFD in CD patients [110].

The Mendez group in Madrid developed a sandwich ELISA based on mAbs (R5) raised against ω-secalins and directed against epitopes such as QQPFP, QQQFP, LQPFP, and QLPFP occurring in CD-toxic sequences of prolamins [111]. The R5 antibody shows very limited reactions with glutelins and no reaction with oat proteins. First data indicated that the R5 ELISA recognizes prolamins from wheat, rye, and barley to the same degree [111]. Recent data suggests that R5 mAbs have a higher reactivity toward secalins and hordeins compared to gliadins, and, therefore, their contents are overestimated when a gliadin reference is used for calibration [108,112]. Within hordeins, the response of two sandwich ELISA kits varied considerably, depending on the hordein fraction, which was enriched either in B-, γ-, D-, or C-hordeins [113]. Several different test kits using R5 mAbs are now on the market, and most systems are adapted to the reference gliadin (PWG-gliadin) described by van Eckert et al. [107]. Two extraction methods are proposed, either with 60% ethanol or with the cocktail (see Section 4.1). The sandwich R5 ELISA was evaluated successfully in collaborative studies [114,115], endorsed as a type I method by the Codex Committee of Methods of Analysis and Sampling (CCMAS) in 2005, recommended by Codex Stan 118–1979 and Codex Stan 234–1999, and approved as AACCI Approved Method 38–50.01 (see Section 3.1). The assay guarantees a limit of detection (LOD) of 1.5 mg gliadin/kg and a limit of quantitation (LOQ) of 2.5 mg gliadin/kg. To simplify and speed up testing, a kit including a stick, in which the R5 mAbs are immobilized, has been developed [116]. The stick is dipped into the diluted sample extract and a red line appears, if the sample contains the corresponding prolamins. The assay has a sensitivity of around 10 mg gluten/kg product. It is particularly suited as a swab method for checking the environment, such as tables and machines, for gluten contamination.

In 2012, a competitive ELISA using R5 mAbs was developed [117]. This test needs only one epitope for binding and also detects small peptides derived from partially hydrolyzed prolamins, for example, those present in fermented cereal foodstuffs, such as sourdough products, malt extracts, and beer. In addition, the competitive system is cheaper and faster than the sandwich system, given that only one antibody is used, and the incubation of the sample and the conjugated antibody is performed in one step within the assay. The calibrator of the first-generation ELISA was a synthetic peptide with the sequence QQPFP and that of the second generation ELISA was a mixture of peptic-tryptic hydrolyzates from wheat, rye, and barley prolamins. The LOD is 1.4 mg prolamin/kg. The combination of the competitive R5 ELISA with prolamin hydrolyzates as reference was shown to be suitable for the quantitation of small amounts of prolamin peptides in fermented products [108]. A successful collaborative study allowed the method to be approved as AACCI Approved Method 38–55.01 [118]. A disadvantage of the competitive R5 ELISA is that it is compatible only with ethanol but not with the cocktail. However, Mena et al. demonstrated that the competitive ELISA can be used in combination with the extractant solvent UPEX for the analysis of any kind of food samples [104] (see Section 4.1).

Two mAbs, named G12 and A1, were raised against the 33-mer peptide of α2-gliadin (see Chapter 2, Section 3.5) and used for the development of a sandwich and a competitive ELISA [119,120]. The affinity of G12 to the 33-mer peptide was shown to be superior to A1, although the sensitivity for gluten detection was higher for A1. The sandwich ELISA contains G12 as the enzyme-labeled antibody and A1 as the support-bound antibody; the competitive ELISA contains only G12. The assays provide an extraction solvent containing a reducing agent so that analysis of both unheated and heat-processed products is possible. Gluten and PWG-gliadin serve as reference proteins for calibration. Both sandwich and competitive ELISAs show a LOD of 2 mg gluten/kg and a LOQ of 4 mg gluten/kg for wheat, rye, and barley prolamins. The detection limit for oat prolamins is much higher. No cross-reactivity to proteins of nontoxic cereals has been observed. A collaborative study of the G12/A1 sandwich ELISA has been carried out recently and the method is expected to be endorsed by the AACCI as Approved Method 38-52.01 in 2014.

In cooperation with EuroProxima (Arnheim, The Netherlands), the Leiden University Medical Center (Leiden, The Netherlands) has developed a competitive ELISA, named Gluten-Tec®, based on a monoclonal antibody that detects an epitope of α20-gliadin including the sequence RPQQPY [121]. The assay uses 60% ethanol and an extraction solvent containing dithiothreitol as reducing agent, such that the extraction of unheated and heat-processed foods is possible. The α20-antibody shows comparable reactivity to wheat and rye prolamins but slightly reduced reactivity to barley prolamins. The antibody has a much lower sensitivity for oats and does not cross-react with proteins from rice, corn, and other nontoxic cereals. The Gluten-Tec® ELISA is calibrated against the synthetic peptide GPFRPQQPYPB. The obtained results in ng peptide/kg food must be converted to mg prolamin and mg gluten/kg food, respectively. A collaborative study revealed a reproducibility similar to that obtained with the sandwich R5 ELISA [122]. The conversion factor of 100 from ng peptide/g to ng gliadin/g was determined experimentally by the analysis of a corn bread sample spiked with wheat flour. The average LOD was 0.41 ng peptide/ml (ethanol extraction) and 0.46 ng peptide/ml (dithiothreitol extraction), respectively. The peptide concentration (ng/ml) is converted to the peptide concentration in a sample (ng/g) by multiplying with a factor of 100. Based on the correlation between amount of peptide and gliadin content, the conversion factor from ng peptide/g to ng gliadin/g is 100. The resultant LOD is 2.5 mg gliadin/kg. Future experiments have to demonstrate that the conversion factor between peptide and gluten can be transferred to samples with different matrices.

4.3.2 Immunosensors

The immunosensor developed by Nassef et al. [123] is based on an antibody raised against the immunodominant CD epitope α56–75 and a chemical surface that uses dithiol compounds for anchoring the capture antibody. The method based on this immunosensor was shown to be highly sensitive and reproducible. Applied to the analysis of commercial gluten-free and gluten-containing raw and processed foodstuffs, an excellent correlation was achieved when compared to a previously developed ELISA based on an anti-gliadin pAb. An electrochemical, magneto immunosensor for the quantitation of gliadin or small gliadin fragments in natural and pretreated food samples has been described by Laube et al. [124]. The immunological reaction was performed on magnetic beads as solid support by the oriented covalent immobilization of the gliadin antigen on tosyl-activated beads. Excellent detection limits were achieved according to the legislation for gluten-free products, and the assay was successfully evaluated using spiked gluten-free foodstuffs.

4.4 **Nonimmunochemical Methods**

4.4.1 Polymerase Chain Reaction

The polymerase chain reaction (PCR) is based on the determination of specific deoxyribonucleic acid (DNA) fragments. DNA analysis is more sensitive by several orders of magnitude than protein analysis. A few molecules of any DNA sequence can be amplified by a factor of 10^6 to 10^8 in a very short time. PCR can be applied for both unheated and heat-treated products because DNA is considerably more heat-stable than proteins. PCR enables the amplification of a specific DNA fragment flanked by two oligonucleotides that act as primers in the amplification reaction catalyzed by DNA polymerase. The amplified product is visualized after gel electrophoresis by a fluorescent dye, by capillary electrophoresis, or by Southern blotting (qualitative PCR). For quantitative PCR, oligodeoxynucleotides labeled with fluorescent or enzyme markers are used, and quantitation is performed by measuring the intensity of fluorescence or color ("real-time" PCR).

The group of Allmann in Berne was the first to apply PCR for gluten analysis. A highly repetitive and specific genomic wheat DNA segment was applied for wheat detection [125]. This qualitative assay was tested with 35 different food samples, ranging from bakery additives to heated and processed products. Wheat starch even with low gliadin contents strongly reacted positive, whereas wheat gluten used as an additive could not be detected. PCR and a sandwich ELISA were compared by the analysis of oat samples spiked with wheat [126]. The results demonstrated that PCR was about 10 times more sensitive than the ELISA system.

A quantitative, competitive PCR system was developed to detect wheat, rye, and barley contaminations using a specific primer pair (WBR11/WBR13) [127]. An internal DNA standard was constructed by adding 20 base-pairs to the original PCR product. The PCR system was applied to 15 commercially available products labeled gluten-free and compared with a sandwich ELISA. Both methods yielded identical results for most samples and were proposed to support each other in testing gluten-free products. The primer pair also was used in a quantitative PCR system to detect traces of gluten in four samples of flours and 13 samples of biscuits designated gluten-free [128]. Real-time PCR using melting curve analysis was established specifically to discriminate wheat, rye, barley, and oat contamination in food samples [129]. Simultaneous PCR and sandwich ELISA analyses gave good correlations. The advantage of using melting curve analysis over gel electrophoresis was that the analysis could be performed in the same closed capillary used for amplification. Thus, the risk of cross-contamination of samples could be eliminated. A one-step, real-time immuno-PCR was introduced for gliadin detection by Henterich et al. [130]. For this technique, R5 monoclonal antibodies were conjugated with an oligonucleotide. The sensitivity of gliadin analysis was increased more than 30-fold above the level reached by ELISA. Three different real-time PCR systems for measuring wheat, rye, and barley DNA were developed by the group of Mujico [131,132]. The combination of these systems allowed both the discrimination of the type of cereal and the determination of the proportion of wheat, rye, and barley in contaminated oat samples. The comparison of PCR and R5 ELISA used for the analysis of corn flour and unheated food samples revealed a good linear correlation [133]. The practical applicability of the real-time PCR method was tested by the analysis of 49 food samples. Three out of 49 samples were found positive for gluten by both PCR and ELISA, and one sample was found positive only by PCR [134]. Real-time PCR assays including homologous target sequences encoding HMW-GS were used to detect different wheat species (common wheat, spelt, kamut), barley, and rye [135]. The sensitivity of the system was dependent on the matrix and ranged from 2.5 mg wheat/kg (vegetable matrix) to 5.0 mg/kg (meat matrix). Oat- and barley-specific systems resulted in a sensitivity of 10 mg/kg. A highly sensitive real-time PCR system for the quantitation of wheat contaminations in gluten free-food was developed and optimized by Mujico and coworkers [136]. The analyses of different products indicated a better sensitivity in the PCR technique compared to R5 ELISA.

In summary, the developed quantitative PCR systems can be recommended as highly sensitive screening tools for the presence of wheat, rye, and barley. It can be regarded as complementary to immunological methods; however, that PCR detects DNA and not protein has to be kept in mind. Samples positive in PCR screening experiments for wheat, rye, and barley have to be reanalyzed by an analytical method targeting gluten proteins. PCR is also unsuitable for the detection and quantitation of gluten in partially hydrolyzed products such as beer, syrups, and malt extracts and of vital wheat gluten used as additive.

4.4.2 Electrophoresis

The separation of proteins by electrophoresis is based on different mobilities in an electric field caused by differences in the number of charged amino acid residues. The application of electrophoresis within the field of cereals has focused on proteins (not peptides) and qualitative characterization (not quantitation). Electrophoresis of cereal proteins began with the use of moving boundary electrophoresis, mainly on starch gels; this then was replaced by PAGE, providing much better separations. Different detection methods after separation have been developed with Coomassie blue and silver being the most commonly applied stain. An important electrophoretic principle is acid (A–) PAGE. It is based on differences in protein charge density at low pH and is used mainly for fingerprinting, especially of prolamins in studies on cultivar differentiation and identification. According to increasing mobility on the gels, gliadins were classified into ω-, γ-, β-, and α-gliadins, and secalins into ω- and γ-secalins. Later studies on amino acid sequences, however, indicated that the classification based on electrophoretic mobility does not always agree with the "true" classification based on amino acid sequences. For example, based on sequence analysis, α- and β-gliadins fall into one group.

Classical capillary electrophoresis separates proteins according to differences in charge and size. The analytes move in the interior of a small capillary filled with a conductive medium owing to an electric field and can be detected by UV absorbance or laser-induced fluorescence after elution. The principle of

SDS-PAGE is based on the covering of proteins with a surplus of negatively charged dodecylsulfate anions such that they are separated in the electric field, dependent only on molecular size (mass). Some cereal proteins have been named according to SDS-PAGE mobility, such as D-, C-, B-, and A-hordeins or HMW-GS and LMW-GS, as well as single HMW-GS (e.g., nos. 1–12). It should be mentioned here that apparent molecular masses upon SDS-PAGE are estimated to be much higher (+10% and more) than the true masses derived from amino acid sequences.

Proteins that are separated by A-PAGE or SDS-PAGE can be detected specifically by reaction with antibodies. Proteins are transferred from the polyacrylamide gels onto a membrane made of nitrocellulose or polyvinylidene difluoride using an electric current (so-called Western blotting). Afterward, protein-specific antibodies that contain a detectable label (e.g., a reporter enzyme similar to the ELISA technique) are added. Reactions between the label and a suitable substrate generate visible products.

The technique of isoelectric focusing (IEF) is based on the different isoelectric points of proteins, such that they can be separated in an immobilized pH gradient gel. IEF (first dimension) is used frequently in combination with SDS-PAGE (second dimension) for 2-dimensional (2D-) gel electrophoresis. 2D-electrophoresis is one of the most effective separation methods for proteins. For example, wheat flour proteins can be separated into hundreds of spots (Figure 2.3). In the field of proteomics, proteins separated by 2D-gel electrophoresis can be identified after tryptic digestion by mass spectrometry (MS) peptide mapping and database search algorithms. Proteomics is used with increasing frequency in CD research, for example, to identify protein expression specific to intestinal tissue, to determine the diagnostic biomarkers in body fluids, or to produce fingerprints of the end products of cellular processes [137,138].

4.4.3 Column Chromatography

Column chromatography has been widely used to characterize, separate, and quantitate cereal proteins. In particular, gel permeation (GP-) liquid chromatography (separates on the basis of molecular weight and size) and reversed-phase (RP-) liquid chromatography (separates on the basis of hydrophobicity) have been applied since the 1980s, whereas cation and anion exchange chromatography have lost importance during the past decades. In special cases, affinity chromatography has been applied, a method based on a highly specific interaction (e.g., between antigen and antibody, enzyme and substrate, or receptor and ligand). The improvement of column materials enabled the application of HPLC, which enhanced separation efficiency and reduced elution time considerably [139]. Detection and quantitation of eluted proteins are carried out by measuring UV absorbance in the range of 200–220 nm. At these wavelengths, the absorbance units are highly correlated with protein quantity independent of the protein type, and the detection limit is around 1–2 μg protein [140]. GP- and RP-HPLC also can be used for the separation and quantitation of peptide mixtures, when appropriate column material is used. An important disadvantage is that the detection technique cannot differentiate between gluten and nongluten proteins and, therefore, is unspecific and not applicable for the analysis of complex foods. In special cases, however, column chromatography can be applied for gluten determination.

Despite this limitation, column chromatography, in particular RP-HPLC, is a highly valuable aid in CD research. For example, it frequently has been used for the characterization of reference materials necessary for gluten analysis, the isolation and identification of proteins and peptides involved in CD pathomechanism, and the follow-up of protein and peptide metabolism. It also is applicable for tracking plant breeding and genetic engineering. Moreover, the combination of liquid chromatography and mass spectrometry (LC-MS) is nowadays an indispensable instrument to identify and quantitate proteins and peptides with high specificity and sensitivity.

GP-HPLC can be applied for both gliadin and gluten determination in wheat starch, which is widely used as base material for gluten-free bread production [22]. Twenty-three starch samples provided by different companies were extracted either by 60% ethanol (gliadins) or 50% 2-propanol plus a reducing agent (gluten). The extracts were concentrated in a vacuum centrifuge and analyzed by GP-HPLC. The results indicated a broad range of gliadin concentrations of between 15 and 574 mg/kg starch. The average coefficient of variation resulting from two determinations was ±2.6%. The correlation coefficient between the contents of gliadins and crude protein ($N \times 5.7$) was $r=0.232$ (Figure 4.2), showing that the crude protein content does not reflect the gliadin content as assumed by the first draft of Codex Alimentarius (see Section 3.1). Considering the ratio of gliadins to glutenins (the latter was calculated by gluten minus gliadins), huge differences were found (0.2–4.9) (Figure 4.10), demonstrating that the general assumption of a prolamin content of gluten of 50% (Codex Stan 118–1979) is not justified. This finding was confirmed by RP-HPLC analyses of prolamins and glutelins from cultivars of different wheat species, rye, barley, and oats [141]. The ratio ranged from 1.4 to 13.9 (Figure 4.10). Thus, the gluten content calculated by multiplying the prolamin content by a factor of 2 is, in part, considerably overestimated. Several other raw materials used for the production of gluten-free products were tested by the GP-HPLC method. Prolamin and gluten determination was, in principle, possible for apple fiber, buckwheat groats, spice mixture, flours of chestnut, millet, and rice, but not for skim milk powder and corn flour [22].

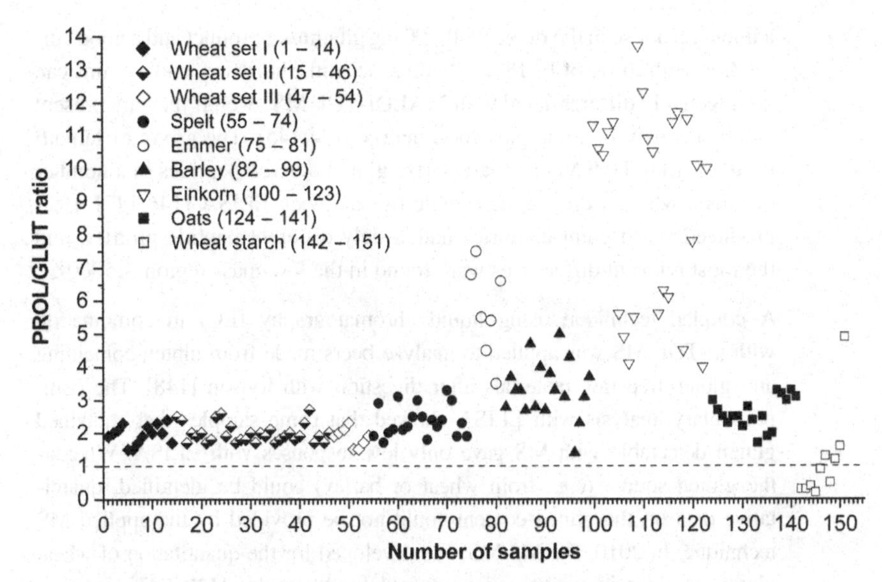

■ **FIGURE 4.10** Ranges of prolamin/glutelin (PROL/GLUT) ratios of flours from different cereal species and of wheat starches. The dotted line represents a ratio of 1 used in the calculation of the gluten content by 2 × PROL [141]. *With kind permission from Springer Science and Business Media.*

4.4.4 Mass Spectrometry

Matrix-assisted laser desorption/ionization time-of-flight mass spectrometry (MALDI-TOF MS) has become an important method to determine the molecular masses of proteins and peptides. The principle of this technique is that ions are generated from the analyte-matrix co-crystallizate in a high vacuum by short laser pulses. The ions released by the laser are accelerated by a short high-voltage impulse into a TOF MS instrument. The heavier ions are slower than the lighter ones, so that the flight time is proportional to the ratio of mass to charge (*m/z*) of the analytes. Calibration is performed with analytes of known masses and the resolution increased by doubling the ion flight path using an electric field as reflector. MALDI-TOF MS allows the simultaneous measurement of masses from around 1000 to 100,000 without chromatographic purification in the low picomol range within a few minutes. Thus, not only intact proteins but also protein hydrolyzates can be analyzed.

The group of Mendez in Madrid was the first to use MALDI-TOF MS for the identification of prolamins from different cereals [142]. Sample preparation was shown to be quite easy and the use of a reducing agent for protein extraction did not deter analysis. Thirty food samples (wheat breads and starches, gluten-free foods) were simultaneously analyzed by MALDI-TOF MS and a laboratory-made sandwich ELISA [143]. The MS results revealed a linear response in the range of 4–100 mg gliadin/kg product and a good correlation with those of ELISA. Gliadins, secalins, hordeins, and avenins can be selectively differentiated with MALDI-TOF MS, even if they are present simultaneously in a complex food matrix [144,145]. The group of Iametti used MALDI-TOF MS to characterize gluten derived peptides in a number of beers, which were not detectable by sandwich ELISA [146,147]. Beer produced in different countries had widely different peptide profiles, and the most relevant differences were found in the low-mass region (<5000).

A coupled technique using liquid chromatography (LC) in combination with Q-TOF MS was applied to analyze beers made from gluten-containing and gluten-free raw materials after digestion with trypsin [148]. The complimentary analysis with ELISA showed that some samples that contained gluten detectable with MS gave only low responses with ELISA. Whereas the gluten source (e.g., from wheat or barley) could be identified, quantitative data on the gluten content could not be provided by the applied MS technique. In 2010, LC-MS/MS was developed for the quantitation of wheat gluten peptides in native and processed food samples [149]. The samples were digested with pepsin, trypsin, and chymotrypsin and then analyzed by LC-MS/MS based on six immunogenic gluten marker peptides. The method detected these marker peptides in the range of 0.01–100 mg peptide/kg product. However, very different ratios of the six marker peptides were found in different foods, and any calculation of the gluten content appeared impossible and was not attempted. Similarly, only relative values expressed as a percentage of the average hordein content of 60 beers could be calculated after LC-MS analyses of peptides without and with tryptic digest. At least two peptides per protein were selected as markers and quantitated in the multiple reaction monitoring (MRM) mode, allowing the detection of hordeins in beer [150].

Altogether, mass spectrometry is a highly valuable nonimmunological approach for the detection of gluten proteins and peptides. However, the conversion of the obtained data into mg gluten/kg product as required by the Codex Alimentarius and other regulations is not possible yet. Moreover, the expensive equipment and expertise it requires will limit the usage of this technique to specialized service laboratories and large food manufacturers.

REFERENCES

[1] Hallert C, Grant C, Grehn S, Granno C, Hulten S, Midhagen G, et al. Evidence of poor vitamin status in coeliac patients on a gluten-free diet for 10 years. Aliment Pharmacol Ther 2002;16:1333–9.

[2] Thompson T, Dennis M, Higgins LA, Lee AR, Sharrett MK. Gluten-free diet survey: are Americans with coeliac disease consuming recommended amounts of fibre, iron, calcium and grain foods? J Hum Nutr Diet 2005;18:163–9.

[3] Alvarez-Jubete L, Arendt EK, Gallagher E. Nutritive value of pseudocereals and their increasing use as functional gluten-free ingredients. Trends Food Sci Technol 2010;21:106–13.
[4] Huettner EK, Arendt EK. Recent advances in gluten-free baking and the current status of oats. Trends Food Sci Technol 2010;21:303–12.
[5] Pawlowska P, Diowksz A, Kordialik-Bogacka E. State-of-the-art incorporation of oats into a gluten-free diet. Food Rev Int 2012;28:330–42.
[6] Zannini E, Miller-Jones J, Renzetti S, Arendt EK. Functional replacements for gluten. Annu Rev Food Sci Technol 2012;3:227–45.
[7] Omary MB, Fong C, Rothschild J, Finney P. Effects of germination on the nutritional profile of gluten-free cereals and pseudocereals: a review. Cereal Chem 2012;89:1–14.
[8] Zannini E, Pontonio E, Waters DB, Arendt EK. Applications of microbial fermentations for production of gluten-free products and perspectives. Appl Microbiol Biotechnol 2012;93:473–85.
[9] Hager AS, Axel C, Arendt EK. Status of carbohydrates and dietary fiber in gluten-free diets. Cereal Foods World 2011;56:109–14.
[10] Gallagher E. Formulation and nutritional aspects of gluten-free cereal products and infant foods. In: Arendt EK, dal Bello F, editors. Gluten-free cereal products and beverages. New York (USA): Academic Press; 2008. pp. 321–46.
[11] Arendt EK, Morrissey A, Moore MM, dal Bello F. Gluten-free breads. In: Arendt EK, dal Bello F, editors. Gluten-free cereal products and beverages. New York (USA): Academic Press; 2008. pp. 289–319.
[12] Engleson J, Atwell B. Gluten-free product development. Cereal Foods World 2008;53:160–84.
[13] Houben A, Hoechstaetter A, Becker T. Possibilities to increase the quality in gluten-free bread production: an overview. Eur Food Res Technol 2012;235:195–208.
[14] Zandonadi RP, Botelho RBA, Araujo WMC. Psyllium as a substitute for gluten in bread. J Am Diet Assoc 2009;109:1781–4.
[15] Cappa C, Lucisano M, Mariotti M. Influence of Psyllium, sugar beet fibre and water on gluten-free dough properties and bread quality. Carbohydr Polym 2013;98: 1657–66.
[16] Hernando A, Garcia E, Llorente M, Mujico JR, Lombardia M, Maeki M, et al. Measurements of hydrolysed gliadins in malts, breakfast cereals, heated/hydrolysed foods, whiskies and beers by means of a new competitive R5 ELISA. In: Stern M, editor. Proceedings of the 19th meeting of the working group on prolamin analysis and toxicity. Zwickau (Germany): Verlag Wissenschaftliche Scripten; 2005. pp. 31–7.
[17] Nic Phiarais BP, Arendt EK. Malting and brewing with gluten-free cereals. In: Arendt EK, dal Bello F, editors. Gluten-free cereal products and beverages. New York (USA): Academic Press; 2008. pp. 347–72.
[18] Comino I, Real A, Gil-Humanes J, Piston F, de Lorenzo L, de Lourdes-Moreno M, et al. Significant differences in coeliac immunotoxicity of barley varieties. Mol Nutr Food Res 2012;56:1697–707.
[19] Codex document ALINORM 08/31/26. Appendix iii. Draft revised codex standard for foods for special dietary use for persons intolerant to gluten. Rome: Codex Alimentarius Commisson WHO; 2008.
[20] Codex Standard 118–1979. In: Codex standards for gluten-free foods. Joint FAO/WHO food standards program. Rome: Codex Alimentarius Commission, WHO; 1981.

[21] Kasarda DD, Dupont FM, Vensel WH, Altenbach SB, Lopez R, Tanaka CK, et al. Surface-associated proteins of wheat starch granules: suitability of wheat starch for celiac patients. J Agric Food Chem 2008;56:10292–302.
[22] Wieser H, Seilmeier W. Determination of gliadin and gluten in wheat starch by means of alcohol extraction and gel permeation chromatography. In: Stern M, editor. Proceedings of the 17th meeting on prolamin analysis and toxicity. Zwickau (Germany): Verlag Wissenschaftliche Scripten; 2003. pp. 53–7.
[23] Peraeaho M, Kaukinen K, Paasikivi K, Sievaenen H, Lohiniemi S, Maeki M, et al. Wheat-starch-based gluten-free products in the treatment of newly detected coeliac disease: prospective and randomized study. Aliment Pharmacol Ther 2003;17: 587–94.
[24] Kaukinen K, Salmi T, Collin P, Huhtala H, Kaerjae-Lahdensuu T, Maeki M. Clinical trial: gluten microchallenge with wheat-based starch hydrolysates in coeliac disease patients – a randomized, double-blind, placebo-controlled study to evaluate safety. Aliment Pharmacol Ther 2008;28:1240–8.
[25] Wieser H, Koehler P. Detoxification of gluten by means of enzymatic treatment. J AOAC Int 2012;95:356–63.
[26] di Cagno R, de Angelis M, Lavermicocca P, de Vincenzi M, Giovannini C, Faccia M, et al. Proteolysis by sourdough lactic acid bacteria: effects on wheat flour protein fractions and gliadin peptides involved in human cereal intolerance. Appl Environ Microbiol 2002;68:623–33.
[27] di Cagno R, de Angelis M, Auricchio S, Greco L, Clarke C, de Vincenzi M, et al. Sourdough bread made from wheat and nontoxic flours and started with selected lactobacilli is tolerated in celiac sprue patients. Appl Environ Microbiol 2004;70: 1088–96.
[28] de Angelis M, Rizzello CG, Fasano A, Clemente MG, de Simone C, Silano M, et al. VSL#3 probiotic preparation has the capacity to hydrolyze gliadin polypeptides responsible for celiac sprue. Biochim Biophys Acta 2006;1762:80–93.
[29] di Cagno R, de Angelis M, Alfonsi G, de Vincenzi M, Silano M, Vincentini O, et al. Pasta made from durum wheat semolina fermented with selected lactobacilli as a tool for a potential decrease of the gluten intolerance. J Agric Food Chem 2005;53:4393–402.
[30] de Angelis M, Cassone A, Rizzello CG, Gagliardi F, Minervini F, Calasso M, et al. Mechanism of degradation of immunogenic gluten epitopes from *Triticum turgidum L. var.* durum by sourdough lactobacilli and fungal proteases. Appl Environ Microbiol 2010;76:508–18.
[31] de Angelis M, Coda R, Silano M, Minervini F, Rizzello CG, di Cagno R, et al. Fermentation by selected sourdough lactic acid bacteria to decrease coeliac intolerance to rye flour. J Cereal Sci 2006;43:301–14.
[32] Rizzello CG, de Angelis M, di Cagno R, Camarca A, Silano M, Losito I, et al. Highly efficient gluten degradation by lactobacilli and fungal proteases during food processing: new perspectives for celiac disease. Appl Environ Microbiol 2007;73:4499–507.
[33] Greco L, Gobbetti M, Auricchio R, di Mase R, Landolfo F, Paparo F, et al. Safety for patients with celiac disease of baked goods made of wheat flour hydrolyzed during food processing. Clin Gastroenterol Hepatol 2011;9:24–9.
[34] di Cagno R, Barbato M, di Camillo C, Rizzello CG, de Angelis M, Giuliani G, et al. Gluten-free sourdough wheat baked goods appear safe for young celiac patients: a pilot study. J Pediatr Gastroenterol Nutr 2010;51:777–83.

[35] Loponen J, Sontag-Strohm T, Venaelaeinen J, Salovaara H. Prolamin hydrolysis in wheat sourdoughs with differing proteolytic activities. J Agric Food Chem 2007;55:978–84.

[36] Koehler P, Wieser H. Peptidases for degradation of gluten and possible use in dietary therapy. In: Stern M, editor. Proceeding of the 24th meeting of the working group on prolamin analysis and toxicity. Zwickau (Germany): Verlag Wissenschaftliche Scripten; 2011. pp. 95–8.

[37] Marx S, Otterbach-Noae J, Langer O, Zotzel J. International patent 2008 WO 2008090126 A1 20080731.

[38] Gianfrani C, Siciliano RA, Facchiano AM, Camarca A, Mazzeo MF, Costantini S, et al. Transamidation of wheat flour inhibits the response to gliadin of intestinal T cells in celiac disease. Gastroenterology 2007;133:780–9.

[39] Mazzarella G, Salvati VM, Iaquinto G, Stefanile R, Capobianco F, Luongo D, et al. Reintroduction of gluten following flour transamidation in adult celiac patients: a randomized, controlled clinical study. Clin Dev Immunol 2012;2012:329150.

[40] Metakovsky EV, Branlard GP, Graybosch RA. Gliadins of common wheat: polymorphism and genetics. In: Wrigley C, Bekes F, Bushuk W, editors. Gliadin and glutenin – the unique balance of wheat quality. St. Paul (USA): AACC International; 2006. pp. 35–84.

[41] Shewry PR, Halford NG, Lafiandra D. The high-molecular-weight subunits of glutenin. In: Wrigley C, Bekes F, Bushuk W, editors. Gliadin and glutenin – the unique balance of wheat quality. St. Paul (USA): AACC International; 2006. pp. 143–69.

[42] Juhasz A, Gianibelli MC. Low-molecular-weight glutenin subunits: insights into this abundant subunit group present in glutenin polymers. In: Wrigley C, Bekes F, Bushuk W, editors. Gliadin and glutenin – the unique balance of wheat quality. St. Paul (USA): AACC International; 2006. pp. 171–212.

[43] Kasarda DD, Qualset CO, Mecham DK, Goodenberger DM, Strober W. A test of toxicity of bread made from wheat lacking α-gliadins coded for by the 6A chromosome. In: McCarthy CF, Fottrell PE, editors. Perspectives in coeliac disease. Lancaster (UK): MTP Press; 1978. pp. 55–61.

[44] Ciclitira PJ, Hunter JO, Lennox ES. Clinical testing of bread made from nullisomic 6A wheats in coeliac patients. Lancet 1980;2:234–6.

[45] Shewry PR, Tatham AS, Kasarda DD. Cereal proteins and coeliac disease. In: Marsh MN, editor. Coeliac disease. Oxford (UK): Blackwell Scientific Publications; 1992. pp. 305–48.

[46] Frisoni M, Corazza GR, Lafiandra D, de Ambrogio E, Filipponi C, Bonvicini F, et al. Wheat deficient in gliadins: promising tool for treatment of coeliac disease. Gut 1995;36:375–8.

[47] Spaenij-Dekking L, Kooy-Winkelaar Y, van Veelen P, Drijfhout JW, Jonker H, van Soest L, et al. Natural variation in toxicity of wheat: potential for selection of nontoxic varieties for celiac disease patients. Gastroenterology 2005;129:797–806.

[48] Molberg O, Uhlen AK, Jensen T, Solheim-Flaete N, Fleckenstein B, Arentz-Hansen H, et al. Mapping of gluten T-cell epitopes in the bread wheat ancestors: implications for celiac disease. Gastroenterology 2005;128:393–401.

[49] van den Broeck HC, van Herpen TWJM, Schult C, Salentijn EMJ, Dekking L, Bosch D, et al. Removing celiac disease-related gluten proteins from bread wheat while retaining technological properties: a study with Chinese Spring deletion lines. BMC Plant Biol 2009;9.

[50] van den Broeck HC, Gilissen LJWJ, Smulders MJM, van der Meer IM, Hamer RJ. Dough qualtiy of bread wheat lacking α-gliadins with celiac disease epitopes and addition of celiac-safe avenins to improve dough quality. J Cereal Sci 2011;53:206–16.
[51] van den Broeck H, Hongbing C, Lacaze X, Dusautoir JC, Gilissen L, Smulders M, et al. In search of tetraploid wheat accessions reduced in celiac disease-related gluten epitopes. Mol Biosyst 2010;6:2206–13.
[52] van den Broeck HC, de Jong HC, Salentijin EMJ, Dekking L, Bosch D, Hamer RJ, et al. Presence of celiac disease epitopes in modern and old hexaploid wheat varieties: wheat breeding may have contributed in increased prevalence of celiac disease. Theor Appl Genet 2010;121:1527–39.
[53] Vincentini O, Maialetti F, Gazza L, Silano M, Dessi M, de Vincenzi M, et al. Environmental factors of celiac disease: cytotoxicity of hulled wheat species *Triticum monococcum*, *T. turgidum* ssp. *dicoccum* and *T. aestivum* ssp. *spelta*. J Gastroenterol Hepatol 2007;22:1816–22.
[54] Carroccio A, di Prima L, Noto D, Fayer F, Ambrosiano G, Villanacci V, et al. Searching for wheat plants with low toxicity in celiac disease: between direct toxicity and immunologic activation. Dig Liver Dis 2011;43:34–9.
[55] van Herpen TWHM, Goryunova SV, van der Schoot J, Mitreva M, Salentijn E, Vorst O, et al. Alpha-gliadin genes from the A, B, and D genomes of wheat contain different sets of celiac disease epitopes. BMC Genomics 2006;7.
[56] Mitea C, Salentijn EMJ, van Veelen P, Goryunova SV, van der Meer IM, van den Broeck HC, et al. A universal approach to eliminate antigenic properties of α-gliadin peptides in celiac disease. PloS One 2010;5:e15637.
[57] Fire A, Xu SQ, Montgomery MK, Kostas SA, Driver SE, Mello CC. Potent and specific genetic interference by double-stranded RNA in caenorhabditis elegans. Nature 1998;391:806–11.
[58] Becker D, Wieser H, Koehler P, Folck A, Muehling KH, Zoerb C. Protein composition and techno-functional properties of transgenic wheat with reduced α-gliadin content obtained by RNA interference. J Appl Bot Food Qual 2012;85:23–33.
[59] van Herpen TWJM, Riley M, Sparks C, Jones HD, Gritsch C, Dekking EH, et al. Detailed analysis of the expression of an alpha-gliadin promoter and the deposition of alpha-gliadin protein during wheat grain development. Ann Bot 2008;102:331–42.
[60] Gil-Humanes J, Piston F, Hernando A, Alvarez JB, Shewry PR, Barro F. Silencing of γ-gliadins by RNA interference (RNAi) in bread wheat. J Cereal Sci 2008;48:565–8.
[61] Gil-Humanes J, Piston F, Tollefson S, Sollid LM, Barro F. Effective shutdown in the expression of celiac disease-related wheat gliadin T-cell epitopes by RNA interference. Proc Natl Acad Sci USA 2010:17023–8.
[62] Stoven S, Murray JA, Marietta EV. Latest in vitro and in vivo models of celiac disease. Expert Opin Drug Discov 2013;8:445–57.
[63] Rashtak S, Murray JA. Review article: coeliac disease, new approaches to therapy. Aliment Pharmacol Ther 2012;35:768–81.
[64] Gilissen LJWD, van der Meer JM, Smulders MJM. Beyond coeliac disease toxicity. In: Fasano A, Troncone R, Branski D, editors. Frontiers in celiac disease. Basel (Switzerland): Karger; 2008. pp. 139–47.
[65] Tanner GJ, Howitt CA, Forrester RI, Campbell PM, Tye-Din JA, Anderson RP. Dissecting the T-cell response to hordeins in coeliac disease can develop barley with reduced immunotoxicity. Aliment Pharmacol Ther 2010;32:1184–91.

[66] CODEX STAN 1–1985. General standard for the labelling of prepackaged foods. Codex Alimentarius Commission; 2010. Amendment 7.
[67] CODEX STAN 118–1979. Codex standard for gluten-free foods. Codex Alimentarius Commission; 1983. Amendment 1.
[68] CODEX STAN 118–1979. Codex standard for foods for special dietary use for persons intolerant to gluten. Codex Alimentarius Commission; 2008. Revision 1.
[69] CODEX STAN 146–1985. General standard for the labelling of and claims for prepackaged foods for special dietary uses. Codex Alimentarius Commission; 1985.
[70] CODEX STAN 234–1999. Recommended methods of analysis and sampling. Codex Alimentarius Commission; 2011.
[71] CODEX STAN 163–1987. Standard for wheat protein products including wheat gluten. Codex Alimentarius Commission; 2001. Revision 1.
[72] CAC/GL 45–2003. Guideline for the conduct of food safety assessment of foods derived from recombinant-DNA plants. Codex Alimentarius Commission; 2008. Amendment 1.
[73] Commission Regulation (EC) No 41/2009 of 21 January 2009. Off J Eur Union 2009;16(3).
[74] Regulation of the European Parliament and of the Council (EU) No 609/2013 of 12 June 2013. Off J Eur Union 2013;181(35).
[75] Regulation of the European Parliament and of the Council (EU) No 1169/2011 of 25 October 2011. Off J Eur Union 2011;304(18).
[76] Government of Canada: Food and drug regulations C.R.C., c.870, Curr 25 August 2013.
[77] Health Canada. Health Canada's position on gluten-free claims, http://www.hc-sc.gc.ca; June 2012 [accessed 05.09.13].
[78] United States Government: United States Code, Title 21, Chapter 9, Subchapter IV, Section 343, January 05, 2009.
[79] Food Allergen Labeling and Consumer Protection Act of 2004. Public Law 108-282, Title II, August 02, 2004.
[80] United States Food and Drug Administration: Code of federal regulations, title 21, Chapter I, Subchapter B, Part 101, Subpart F, Section 101.91.
[81] Food labeling; gluten-free labeling of foods. Fed Regist August 05, 2013;78(150): 47154–79.
[82] Alcohol and Tobacco Tax and Trade Bureau. Use of "Gluten-Free" on TTB-regulated alcohol beverages. TTB Announcement. http://www.ttb.gov; August 22, 2013 [accessed 05.09.13].
[83] Alcohol and Tobacco Tax and Trade Bureau. Interim policy on gluten content statements in the labeling and advertising of wines, distilled spirits, and malt beverages. TTB Ruling. http://www.ttb.gov; May 24, 2012 [accessed 05.09.13].
[84] Australia New Zealand Food Standards Code: Standard 1.2.7 – nutrition, health and related claims. Federal Register Legislative Instruments F2013L00054 January, 07, 2013.
[85] Australia New Zealand Food Standards Code: Standard 2.9.5 – food for special medical purposes. Federal Register Legislative Instruments F2013C00147, February 21, 2013.
[86] Submission on behalf of the Coeliac Society of Australia by Mr Graham Price http://www.pc.gov.au/__data/assets/pdf_file/0008/82286/sub046.pdf [accessed 05.09.13].
[87] Licensing the Crossed Grain Symbol. http://www.coeliac.org.uk.
[88] European Licensing System. http://www.aoecs.org.

[89] Celiac Sprue Association. http://www.csaceliacs.info.
[90] Gluten-Free Certification Organization of the Gluten Intolerance Group. http://www.gfco.org.
[91] Gluten-Free Certification Program of the Canadian Celiac Association. http://www.glutenfreecertification.ca.
[92] Gluten-Free Certification Program of the National Foundation for Celiac Awareness. http://www.gf-cert.org.
[93] E-mail and telephone correspondence with organizations [88–92].
[94] Denery-Papini S, Nicolas Y, Popineau Y. Efficiency and limitations of immunochemical assays for the testing of gluten-free foods. J Cereal Sci 1999;30:121–31.
[95] Wieser H. Detection of gluten. In: Arendt EK, dal Bello F, editors. Gluten-free cereal products and beverages. Amsterdam (The Netherlands): Academic Press; 2008. pp. 47–80.
[96] Haraszi R, Chassaigne H, Maguet A, Ulberth F. Analytical methods for detection of gluten in food - method developments in support of food labeling legislation. J AOAC Int 2011;94:1006–25.
[97] Wieser H, Seilmeier W, Belitz HD. Quantitative determination of gliadin subgroups from different wheat cultivars. J Cereal Sci 1994;19:149–55.
[98] Wieser H. Investigations on the extractability of gluten proteins from wheat bread in comparison with flour. Z fuer Lebenm – Forschung 1998;207:128–32.
[99] Skerritt JH, Hill AS. Monoclonal antibody sandwich enzyme immunoassays for determination of gluten in foods. J Agric Food Chem 1990;38:1771–8.
[100] Denery-Papini S, Boucherie B, Larre C, Pineau F, Popineau Y, Gueguen J, et al. Measurement of raw, heated and modified gluten after limited hydrolysis. In: Stern M, editor. Proceedings of the 16th meeting of the working group on prolamin analysis and toxicity. Zwickau (Germany): Verlag Wissenschaftliche Scripten; 2002. pp. 71–3.
[101] van den Broeck HC, America AHP, Smulders MJM, Bosch D, Hamer RJ, Gilissen LJWJ, et al. A modified extraction protocol enables detection and quantification of celiac disease-related gluten proteins from wheat. J Chromatogr B 2009;877:975–82.
[102] Garcia E, Llorente M, Hernando A, Kieffer R, Wieser H, Mendez E. Development of a general procedure for complete extraction of gliadins from heat processed and unheated foods. Eur J Gastroenterol Hepatol 2005;17:529–39.
[103] Gessendorfer B, Wieser H, Koehler P. Optimisation of a solvent for the complete extraction of prolamins from heated foods. J Cereal Sci 2010;52:331–2.
[104] Mena MC, Lombardia M, Hernando A, Mendez E, Albar JP. Comprehensive analysis of gluten in processed foods using a new extraction method and a competitive ELISA based on the R5 antibody. Talanta 2012;91:33–40.
[105] van Eckert R, Scharf M, Wald T, Pfannhauser W. Determination of proteins with ELISA-methods: doubtful quantitative results? In: Amado R, Battaglia R, editors. Authenticity and adulteration of food – the analytical approach. Proceedings of the 9th European conference on food chemisty, FECS Event No. 220, Vol. I. Swiss Society of Food and Environmental Chemistry; 1997. pp. 263–8.
[106] Schwalb T, Wieser H, Koehler P. Comparison of different protein references and ELISA kits for the detection of gluten in foods. In: Stern M, editor. Proceedings of the 24th workshop on prolamin analysis and toxicity. Zwickau (Germany): Verlag Wissenschaftliche Scripten; 2011. pp. 23–9.

[107] van Eckert R, Berghofer E, Ciclitira PJ, Chirdo F, Denery-Papini S, Ellis HJ, et al. Towards a new gliadin reference material – isolation and characterisation. J Cereal Sci 2006;43:331–41.
[108] Gessendorfer B, Koehler P, Wieser H. Preparation and characterization of enzymatically hydrolyzed prolamins from wheat, rye, and barley as references for the immunochemical quantitation of partially hydrolyzed gluten. Anal Bioanal Chem 2009;395:1721–8.
[109] Diaz-Amigo C, Poepping B. Accuracy of ELISA detection methods for gluten and reference materials: a realistic assessment. J Agric Food Chem 2013;61:5681–8.
[110] Skerritt JH, Hill AS. Self-management of dietary compliance in coeliac disease by means of ELISA "home test" to detect gluten. Lancet 1991;337:379–82.
[111] Valdes I, Garcia E, Llorente M, Mendez E. Innovative approach to low-level gluten determination in foods using a novel sandwich enzyme-linked immunosorbent assay protocol. Eur J Gastroenterol Hepatol 2003;15:465–74.
[112] Kanerva PM, Sontag-Strohm TS, Ryoeppy PH, Alho-Lehto P, Salovaara HO. Analysis of barley contamination in oats using R5 and ω-gliadin antibodies. J Cereal Sci 2006;44:347–52.
[113] Tanner GJ, Blundell MJ, Colgrave ML, Howitt CA. Quantification of hordeins by ELISA: the correct standard makes a magnitude of difference. PLoS One 2013;8:e56456.
[114] Mendez E, Vela C, Immer U, Janssen FW. Report of a collaborative trial to investigate the performance of the R5 enzyme linked immunoassay to determine gliadin in gluten-free food. Eur J Gastroenterol Hepatol 2005;17:1053–63.
[115] Koehler P, Schwalb T, Immer U, Lacorn M, Wehling P, Don C. AACCI approved methods technical committee report: collaborative study on the immunochemical determination of intact gluten using an R5 sandwich ELISA. Cereal Foods World 2013;58:36–40.
[116] Garcia E, Hernando A, Toribio T, Genzor C, Mendez E. Test immunochromatographic rapid assay: a rapid, highly-sensitive and semi-quantitative test for the detection of gluten in foodstuffs. In: Stern M, editor. Proceeding of the 16th meeting of the working group on prolamin analysis and toxicity. Zwickau (Germany): Verlag Wissenschaftliche Scripten; 2002. pp. 55–64.
[117] Haas-Lauterbach S, Immer U, Richter M, Koehler P. Gluten fragment detection with a competitive ELISA. J AOAC Int 2012;95:377–81.
[118] Koehler P, Schwalb T, Immer U, Lacorn M, Wehling P, Don C. AACCI approved methods technical committee report: collaborative study on the immunochemical determination of partially hydrolyzed gluten using an R5 competitive ELISA. Cereal Foods World 2013;58:154–8.
[119] Moron B, Cebolla A, Manyani H, Alvarez-Maqueda M, Megias M, del Carmen TM, et al. Sensitive detection of cereal fractions that are toxic to celiac disease patients by using monoclonal antibodies to a main immunogenic wheat peptide. Am J Clin Nutr 2008;87:405–14.
[120] Moron B, Bethune MT, Comino I, Manyani H, Ferragud M, Lopez MC, et al. Towards the assessment of food toxicity for celiac patients: characterization of monoclonal antibodies to a main immunogenic gluten peptide. PloS One 2008;3:e2294.
[121] Mitea C, Kooy-Winkelaar Y, van Veelen P, de Ru A, Drijfhout JW, Koning F, et al. Fine specificity of monoclonal antibodies against celiac disease-inducing peptides in the gluteom. Am J Clin Nutr 2008;88:1057–66.

[122] Mujico JR, Dekking L, Kooy-Winkelaar Y, Verheijen R, van Wichen P, Streppel L, et al. Validation of a new enzyme-linked immunosorbent assay to detect the triggering proteins and peptides for celiac disease: interlaboratory study. J AOAC Int 2012;95:206–15.

[123] Nassef HM, Bermudo-Redondo MC, Ciclitira PJ, Ellis HJ, Fragoso A, O'Sullivan CK. Electrochemical immunosensor for detection of celiac disease toxic gliadin in foodstuff. Anal Chem 2008;80:9265–71.

[124] Laube T, Kergaravat SV, Fabiano SN, Hernandez SR, Alegret S, Pividori MI. Magneto immunosensor for gliadin detection in gluten-free foodstuff: towards food safety for celiac patients. Biosens Bioelectron 2011;27:46–52.

[125] Allmann M, Candrian U, Hoefelein C, Luethy J. Polymerase chain-reaction (PCR): a possible alternative to immunochemical methods assuring safety and quality of food. Detection of wheat contamination in nonwheat food products. Z fuer Lebensm – Forschung 1993;196:248–51.

[126] Koeppel E, Stadler M, Luethy J, Huebner P. Detection of wheat contamination in oats by polymerase chain reaction (PCR) and enzyme-linked immunosorbent assay (ELISA). Z fuer Lebensm – Forschung 1998;206:399–403.

[127] Dahinden I, von Bueren M, Luethy J. A quantitative competitive PCR system to detect contamination of wheat, barley or rye in gluten-free food for coeliac patients. Eur Food Res Technol 2001;212:228–33.

[128] Olexova L, Dovicovicova L, Svec M, Siekel P, Kuchta T. Detection of gluten-containing cereals in flours and "gluten-free" bakery products by polymerase chain reaction. Food Control 2005;17:234–7.

[129] Sandberg M, Lundberg L, Ferm M, Malmheden Y. Real time PCR for the detection and discrimination of cereal contamination in gluten free foods. Eur Food Res Technol 2003;217:344–9.

[130] Henterich N, Osman AA, Mendez E, Mothes T. Assay of gliadin by real-time immunopolymerase chain reaction. Nahrung 2003;47:345–8.

[131] Mujico JR, Lombardia M, Mendez E. Detection of wheat DNA in foods by a quantitative real-time PCR system: can the measurement of wheat DNA be used as a non-immunological and complementary tool in gluten technology? In: Stern M, editor. Proceedings of the 18th meeting of the working group on prolamin analysis and toxicity. Zwickau (Germany): Verlag Wissenschaftliche Scripten; 2004. pp. 91–8.

[132] Mujico JR, Hernando A, Lombardia M, Benavides A, Silio V, Maeki M, et al. Quantification of wheat, barley and rye contamination in oat samples by real-time PCR. In: Stern M, editor. Proceedings of the 19th meeting of the working group on prolamin analysis and toxicity. Zwickau (Germany): Verlag Wissenschaftliche Scripten; 2006. pp. 87–94.

[133] Mujico JR, Mendez E. Simultaneous detection/quantification of wheat, barley and rye DNA by a new quantitative real-time PCR system. In: Stern M, editor. Proceedings of the 20th meeting of the working group on prolamin analysis and toxicity. Zwickau (Germany): Verlag Wissenschaftliche Scripten; 2006. pp. 39–45.

[134] Piknova L, Brezna B, Kuchta T. Detection of gluten-containing cereals in food by 5'-nuclease real-time polymerase chain reaction. J Food Nutr Res 2008;47:114–9.

[135] Zeltner D, Glomb MA, Maede D. Real-time PCR systems for the detection of the gluten-containing cereals wheat, spelt, kamut, rye, barley and oat. Eur Food Res Technol 2009;228:321–30.

[136] Mujico JR, Lombardia M, Mena MC, Mendez E, Albar JP. A highly sensitive real-time PCR system for quantification of wheat contamination in gluten-free food for celiac patients. Food Chem 2011;128:795–801.
[137] de Re V, Simula MP, Canzonieri V, Cannizzaro R. Proteomic analyses lead a better understanding of celiac disease: focus on epitope recognition and autoantibodies. Dig Dis Sci 2010;55:3041–6.
[138] Mamone G, Picariello G, Addeo F, Ferranti P. Proteomic analysis in allergy and intolerance to wheat products. Expert Rev Proteomics 2011;8:95–115.
[139] Kruger JE, Bietz JA. HPLC – high-performance liquid chromatography of cereal and legume proteins. St. Paul (USA): AACC International; 1994.
[140] Wieser H, Antes S, Seilmeier W. Quantitative determination of gluten protein types in wheat flour by reversed-phase high-performance liquid chromatography. Cereal Chem 1998;75:644–50.
[141] Wieser H, Koehler P. Is the calculation of the gluten content by multiplying the prolamin content by a factor of 2 valid? Eur Food Res Technol 2009;229:9–13.
[142] Mendez E, Camafeita E, Sebastian JS, Valle I, Solis J, Mayer-Posner FJ, et al. Direct identification of wheat gliadins and related cereal prolamins by matrix-assisted laser desorption/ionization time-of-flight mass spectrometry. J Mass Spectrom 1995;(Spec Issue):S123–8.
[143] Camafeita E, Alfonso P, Mothes T, Mendez E. Matrix-assisted laser desorption/ionization time-of-flight mass spectrometric micro-analysis: the first non-immunological alternative attempt to quantify gluten gliadins in food samples. J Mass Spectrom 1997;32:940–7.
[144] Ferranti P, Mamone G, Picariello G, Addeo F. Mass spectrometry analysis of gliadins in celiac disease. J Mass Spectrom 2007;42:1531–48.
[145] Camafeita E, Solis J, Alfonso P, Lopez JA, Sorell L, Mendez E. Selective identification by matrix-assisted laser desorption/ionization time-of-flight mass spectrometry of different types of gluten in foods made with cereal mixtures. J Chromatogr 1998;A823:299–306.
[146] Iametti S, Bonomi F, Ferranti P, Picariello G, Gabrovska D. Characterization of gliadin content in beer by using different approaches. In: Stern M, editor. Proceeding of the 19th meeting of the working group on prolamin analysis and toxicity. Zwickau (Germany): Verlag Wissenschaftliche Scripten; 2005. pp. 73–8.
[147] Iametti S, Bonomi F, Ferranti P, de Martino A, Picariello G. Characterization of peptides and proteins in beer by different approaches. In: Stern M, editor. Proceeding of the 20th meeting of the working group on prolamin analysis and toxicity. Zwickau (Germany): Verlag Wissenschaftliche Scripten; 2006. pp. 47–52.
[148] Weber D, Cleroux C, Godefroy SB. Emerging analytical methods to determine gluten markers in processed foods – method development in support of standard setting. Anal Bioanal Chem 2009;395:111–7.
[149] Sealey-Voyksner JA, Khosla C, Voyksner RD, Jorgenson JW. Novel aspects of quantitation of immunogenic wheat gluten peptides by liquid chromatography-mass spectrometry/mass spectrometry. J Chromatogr A 2010;1217:4167–83.
[150] Tanner GJ, Colgrave ML, Blundell MJ, Goswami HP, Howitt CA. Measuring hordein (gluten) in beer – a comparison of ELISA and mass spectrometry. PLoS One 2013;8:e56452.

Future Tasks

Intensive multidisciplinary research has contributed to substantial progress in understanding the complex features of celiac disease (CD) over the past few decades. However, many questions remain unanswered and need to be addressed by future studies.

DEFINITIONS

Regarding definitions, the scientific literature suffers from a lack of consensus on the use of the terms related to "celiac disease" and the triggering factor "gluten proteins". To ensure that every person involved in CD uses the same terms, it would be desirable to continue corresponding efforts such as the "Oslo definitions" and the "NICE guidance". Depending on the perspective, CD is partly perceived as a food hypersensitivity disorder and partly as an autoimmune condition. As a compromise encompassing both aspects, CD might be defined as an immune-mediated food intolerance with an autoimmune component.

CHAPTER 1

Epidemiology

Although numerous epidemiological studies on CD prevalence have been published, they are often difficult to compare due to different diagnostic tools and number of participants. In some cases, the two terms prevalence and incidence, which have entirely different definitions, are even intermingled or used interchangeably. A standardization of criteria for prevalence determination and a differentiation into cases of active, silent, and potential CD would be helpful to establish a more precise epidemiological picture. Due to lack of awareness and low suspicion of CD, the prevalence of CD is most likely underestimated in developing countries. Prospective studies on prevalence, clinical course, efficacy of treatment, patient compliance, and disease complications are needed along with better education of physicians, screening in at-risk groups, and improving the availability of gluten-free products in developing countries. Studies in areas with a high level of consanguinity may help find genotype-phenotype correlations in CD, identify specific genetic markers, and clarify associations of CD with other autoimmune diseases.

Genetics and Environmental Factors

The strong association between human leukocyte antigen (HLA) class II alleles DQ2/8 and CD development has been proven conclusively. However, these alleles explain only about 40% of the genetic susceptibility to CD, so that non-HLA genes related to CD still await their identification. Furthermore, the response to gluten peptides in DQ2/8-positive individuals without CD needs to be studied in order to elucidate which factors prevent the disease. Susceptibility variants have been determined by advances in genotyping, but the functional consequences of these variants and their respective contributions to disease pathogenesis are still unknown. The role of epigenetics (e.g., methylation, histone modification) has been understudied in CD even though these heritable changes may play an important part in CD susceptibility. The occurrence of unknown genetic defects in CD due to its association with other genetic diseases such as Down's or Turner's syndrome has not been explored enough yet. Finally, the applicability of genetic discoveries in clinical practice needs to be assessed.

In addition to genetic factors, environmental factors such as infections, birth by cesarean section, effects of breastfeeding on infants, timing of gluten introduction into the infants' diet, and standards of hygiene are under discussion as potential contributors to triggering CD. The strength of these associations needs to be studied and recommendations for a possible prevention of CD should be offered. Whether alterations of commensal and pathogenic microorganisms are at least partially a cause or rather a consequence of CD remains controversial. A resolution of this conundrum is important before possible ways to modulate the microbiome can be explored. In particular, the role of viruses and fungi has not received enough attention so far. Little is known on the complex interplay between genetic and environmental factors leading to CD development, and it will be a major area of research to understand their respective contributions and develop possible prevention strategies.

Clinical Features

Nowadays, many CD patients present with predominantly extraintestinal symptoms and nonspecific findings, or are asymptomatic. This poses considerable challenges for correct diagnosis that can be overcome only by raising awareness and improving the education of physicians. A minor number of CD patients also show neurological or psychiatric symptoms that cannot be explained by malabsorption alone. Yet, the precise mechanism underlying these associated neurological disorders and the relationships between CD and schizophrenia or autism are not known. Recent advances have been made in elucidating the pathogenesis of refractory celiac disease (RCD) I and II, but more research is needed to develop new targeted strategies for cures and prevention of overt lymphoma.

Further studies are required to allow a better diagnostic differentiation between CD, non-celiac gluten sensitivity (NCGS), and irritable bowel syndrome (IBS), because the symptoms and nonspecific findings may be similar in patients. The possible advantages of routine HLA-genotyping for IBS patients should be evaluated, because the patients suffer from a comparatively poor health-related quality of life. At the moment, little is known in the field of NCGS, except that the prevalence in the general population is estimated to be much higher than that of CD. Currently, there are no serologic markers or biomarkers for NCGS, and a diagnosis is mainly made by excluding CD, wheat allergy, and IBS and by monitoring an improvement of symptoms after eliminating gluten from the diet. The grain components triggering NCGS have yet to be identified, as have the pathomechanism, potential genetic and environmental factors, and alternative treatment options.

As a disease with an autoimmune component (transglutaminase [TG] 2), CD may be accompanied by other autoimmune diseases and vice versa. Some shared genetic loci have been identified, but more studies are needed for a better risk assessment. The effect of the gluten-free diet (GFD) on the reduction of the risk for developing another autoimmune disease remains controversial. An improved understanding of the association of different autoimmune diseases will enable the development of prevention strategies.

In CD, an exogenous factor (gluten) can lead to the induction of autoimmune features such as autoantibodies and tissue destruction. The adaptive immune response in any autoimmune disease may consequently not need to be directed toward the antigens that are the target of the autoimmune process. That is why it may be possible that exogenous factors are drivers for other autoimmune diseases. Using CD as a model, the existence of these surmised exogenous factors needs to be verified and their relative contribution to driving other autoimmune processes assessed.

Diagnosis

The requirements for clinical enzyme-linked immunosorbent assay (ELISA) kits for IgA/IgG TGA, IgA/IgG DGPA, IgG AGA, and IgA EMA assays are maximal sensitivity and specificity. This cannot be achieved with one single test, so the best combination of tests needs to be determined to rule out as many false negatives and false positives as possible. Laboratory tests often vary in their performance because of different qualities of antigens and cutoff values. Collaborative studies would be useful to evaluate the accuracy of the results measured with different test kits. Performance criteria of specificity, sensitivity, handling, time, and cost of analysis should also be established for the assessment of new diagnostic kits. In the same way, it will be necessary to judge the reliability of recently developed immunosensors.

The most recent ESPGHAN guidelines suggest that the intestinal biopsy can be omitted in children at the physician's discretion, if IgA TGA titers are above 10 times the upper limit of normal. The implications of this recommendation including the titer level need to be monitored in the future. Further studies should focus on determining the cases in which the duodenal biopsy may be expendable. Reducing interobserver variability through template pathology reporting and communication between pathologists, gastroenterologists, and clinicians will enable improved recognition of milder degrees of mucosal injury and the full spectrum of histopathologic changes, including atypical presentation of CD. The use of video capsule endoscopy (VCE) as a relatively noninvasive and safe procedure is currently limited by its inability to obtain biopsies, the possibility that areas of interest may be missed, and the subjective, labor-intensive analysis of VCE images. Therefore, computerized quantitative image processing could be a powerful tool to analyze VCE recordings. Other noninvasive methodologies to detect, quantify, and monitor the activity of CD will need to be developed.

Pathomechanism

The high amounts of proline and glutamine residues make gluten proteins and peptides fairly resistant to cleavage by gastric, pancreatic, and brush border enzymes. After oral intake of wheat, rye, barley, or oat products, gluten proteins are proteolysed in the gastrointestinal tract, but there is no information available about the actual structures and quantities of gluten peptides arriving at the intestinal brushborder. Then, the passage of peptides across the epithelial barrier follows either the trans- or the paracellular pathway, but the respective contribution of either pathway needs to be clarified. The transcellular pathway seems to be predominant, but very few studies have addressed the rate of peptide degradation in the endosomal/lysosomal compartments. Whereas the barrier function of tight junctions is intact in healthy individuals, patients with active CD show increased intestinal permeability due to upregulation of zonulin. This is the reason why gluten peptides may reach the lamina propria unmodified. However, it is still not clear whether this higher permeability is a cause of CD or rather a consequence of villous atrophy and secretion of inflammatory cytokines.

Regarding the adaptive immune response, the cascade, which leads to secretion of TG2 into the extracellular environment, has not been identified, and the question of whether TG2 activity or inflammation comes first will need to be settled. CD-specific antibodies are important markers for the disease and useful for serologic testing, but their role within CD pathogenesis has yet to be clarified.

Regarding the innate immune response, the mode of action of toxic peptides needs to be elucidated. So far, no receptor for gluten peptides has been identified on intestinal epithelial cells. Furthermore, the role of TCR$\gamma\delta^+$ intraepithelial lymphocytes (IELs) in the epithelium of CD patients is under discussion, because their levels remain high even after years on a GFD. More studies are also necessary to assess the respective contributions of genetic and environmental factors, especially gluten peptides or other cereal constituents like amylase trypsin inhibitors (ATIs), in the initiation of the innate immune response.

Both adaptive and innate immune responses are involved in CD, but their mutual interdependence is largely unknown. While the role of gluten peptides in the adaptive immune response is well characterized, much less is known regarding the innate immune response. Elucidating the mechanism of the innate immune response will contribute to a better understanding of CD pathomechanism, of the interaction with the adaptive immune response in CD, and of inflammatory and tissue destructive reactions in general. This will open up new possibilities to design preventive strategies and develop alternative treatments.

CHAPTER 2
Cereal Proteins

The storage proteins of cereals are composed of a very complex mixture of single proteins. Numerous total amino acid sequences of these storage proteins were translated from DNA and RNA by sequencing techniques and entered into databases. However, many entries are either unreviewed or incomplete or the evidence for the existence of the protein is uncertain, predicted, or inferred from homology. Only a minor part of entries have evidence for the existence of the protein at transcript level or at the actual protein level. Therefore, more work needs to be done to complete the amino acid sequences of storage proteins. Database entries also have to be reviewed and the existence of proteins proven at protein level. DNA-derived amino acid sequences contain the signaling peptide. It should also be kept in mind that signaling peptides of gluten proteins have different lengths to avoid confusion on sequence numbering.

Celiac Disease Toxicity

Prior to the actual toxicity tests, the material to be used for testing should be carefully characterized and analyzed for purity, protein/peptide content, and composition. In vivo testing is usually considered the "gold standard" for assessing CD toxicity of cereal proteins, but because of the high sample amounts needed and the burden on CD patients, it has been largely replaced by in vitro testing. In vitro testing may be done with organ culture of intestinal tissue of CD patients or with very frequently used T-cell proliferation assays. Gluten-sensitive T-cell assays are used to compare the level of immunogenic effects, but immunogenicity measured by T-cell tests does not necessarily correspond to toxicity revealed by in vivo or organ culture tests. This is the reason why it would be of interest to test immunogenic agents for toxicity by organ culture as a confirmatory method. An advantage of organ culture is that it is a model for both innate and adaptive immunity and may be used to study their interdependence. Animal models would be valuable to understand new aspects of CD pathomechanism, but at the moment, there is no satisfactory animal model available. Some promising attempts were made using transgenic mice, but a model encompassing all aspects of the disease still needs to be found.

One hypothesis is that ancient strains of diploid or tetraploid wheat may harbor fewer CD stimulatory epitopes because of the absence of the D-genome. However, there is no experimental proof for different levels of CD toxicity within cereal species. Regarding oats, there may be differences in immunogenicity due to variability among cultivars in the content of the two known immunogenic avenin epitopes. The likelihood of finding oat cultivars devoid of these epitopes has been debated controversially, but a completely safe oat cultivar may exist. Long-term assessments of oats in the GFD are still needed as well as stringent quality criteria guaranteeing the absence of gluten contamination in oats consumed by CD patients. A recent in silico analysis of a peptic-tryptic digest of corn zein yielded a few immunoreactive α-zein peptides that might be harmful for a very limited subgroup of CD patients. Comprehensive in vivo and in vitro studies on immunogenicity and toxicity are missing, and caution should be exercised before the safety of corn for CD patients is questioned.

Similarly to that of cereal species, the level of CD toxicity of different prolamin or glutelin fractions and of different protein types is nearly impossible to compare. The majority of investigations was carried out with gliadins, but data on other protein fractions and types, especially from rye and barley, are missing. Likewise, studies on the CD toxicity of gluten peptides were almost exclusively focused on peptides derived from α-gliadins. Corresponding sequences from γ- and ω-gliadins, glutenins, secalins, and hordeins have not been tested yet by organ culture or in vivo challenge. In cases where ω-gliadins were investigated, no differentiation was made between ω5- and ω1,2-gliadins in most cases, although they vary greatly in their glutamine and proline contents.

CHAPTER 3

Conventional Therapy

The GFD is generally associated with a decreased risk of mortality and malignancy in CD patients, but more long-term monitoring is required, because some studies have found contradictory results. A comprehensive, long-term assessment of the risk for mortality, malignancy, osteoporosis, and other conditions in cases of undiagnosed CD is also not available. Currently, a GFD is recommended for silent CD, but not for potential CD, and inconsistent recommendations are given for asymptomatic CD detected by screening in at-risk groups. More long-term studies that carefully weigh the risks and benefits are needed to re-evaluate these recommendations.

Patients following a GFD are advised to ingest less than 20 mg gluten per day, but the true safe exposure threshold of gluten in the diet relative to CD still needs to be defined in the future. After diagnosis, there is no standard guidance for follow-up management to prevent complications. It would be beneficial to define time periods after which another biopsy should be taken and to define whether this repeated biopsy may be omitted and monitoring done solely based on serology. Better communication of the importance of dietary adherence to the GFD to reduce existing risks is essential in particular for patients from ethnic minorities, adolescents, and adults diagnosed in childhood whose compliance is low. Noninvasive tools like descriptive patient surveys to assess compliance to the GFD and the identification of factors to improve compliance are required. More investigations on the health-related quality of life (HRQOL) of CD patients on a GFD would also be desirable to identify factors that might improve the HRQOL. Long-term studies should also monitor the effects of a GFD on the overall nutritional status, especially on the status of vitamins and minerals, and provide guidance on whether a supplementation may be necessary.

Alternative Therapies

CD patients have expressed the wish to have access to a vaccine against CD or to a pill that would occasionally allow them to eat gluten-containing food. Such alternative therapies are still in the early stages of development, and they will have to comply with stringent criteria regarding safety and toxicology before any effective substance can come onto the market. Phase II clinical trials are already under way, but phase III trials are impeded by the lack of noninvasive methodologies to monitor the activity of CD and reflect patient-related outcomes. Regarding oral enzyme therapy, the amount of gluten that can be effectively detoxified in vivo will have to be determined experimentally. The important parameters influencing the amount of gluten will be the enzyme dose, the time available for it to act, and the presence of other proteins and further food constituents. The main application will be to detoxify gluten contamination in the GFD and prevent inadvertent gluten intake. Improved dosage schedules and delivery routes could be developed as alternatives to a once-per-meal enzyme delivery via oral capsule. The amount of gluten that could be tolerated without adverse effects after application of the respective treatment option will have to be answered for all novel therapeutic approaches.

CHAPTER 4

Products from Gluten-Free Raw Materials

The market for gluten-free products is rapidly growing, and numerous products have been developed with improved formulations. However, the aroma, taste, and textural quality of gluten-free products is in many cases still inferior to their conventional counterparts. The enhancement of flavor and mouthfeel is an ongoing challenge, especially in the production of gluten-free bread and beer. Further possibilities for improving processes and formulations will have to be explored.

Products Rendered Gluten-Free

Gluten-free wheat starch is used for the production of gluten-free foods in many European countries due to its favorable textural properties. It is generally well accepted in these countries and the dietary response to a wheat-starch based GFD was as good as that to a natural GFD. However, doubts about its safety for CD patients remain, especially in the United States and Canada, and further studies on long-term effects are recommended. Peptidase treatment of gluten-containing foods has been successful at degrading gluten to not-detectable levels. Prior to its application in food production, the functional consequences of this treatment on ingredients need to be addressed and compared to the initial food. The genetic modification of wheat and barley resulting in strains deficient in gluten may render those cereals less CD toxic. However, it is not clear whether this reduction of CD toxicity would be enough to make these strains safe for CD patients. Other unanswered questions are economic efficiency, the quality of products made from such strains, stability of the genetic modification, and consumer acceptance.

Legislation

With worldwide mobility and traveling, it would be easier for CD patients if regulations regarding gluten-free foods were harmonized in all countries on the basis of the Codex Alimentarius. At the moment, stricter thresholds apply for gluten-free products in Australia and New Zealand than in Europe, the United States, and Canada. On top of that, there are many different gluten-free symbols on product labels. Some of these are allocated by credible gluten-free certification organizations, but others are merely eye-catching symbols for marketing purposes, providing no trustworthy information on whether the product is really gluten-free and safe or not. A universal gluten-free logo assigned to manufacturers and products based on uniform criteria would prevent confusion and concerns for the safety of products labeled as gluten-free.

Gluten Analysis

The accurate determination of the gluten content in many supposedly gluten-free foods remains a considerable challenge. Appropriate sample preparation should remove interfering substances and solubilize all gluten proteins or peptides from the matrix independent of prior heat-treatment, hydrolysis, or fermentation. Apart from the PWG-gliadin provided by the Working Group on Prolamin Analysis and Toxicity, a commonly accepted reference material for gluten is not available so far. Providing a gluten reference material will be essential to evaluate, validate, and compare results from different gluten quantitation methods.

Immunological techniques like ELISA are widely used sensitive methods, but have their limitations due to different reference materials, extraction protocols, and antibodies that are only specific for prolamins. New ELISAs should be capable of detecting both prolamins and glutelins from all CD-toxic cereals with comparable sensitivity. Immunosensors may be promising alternatives to conventional ELISAs, but their performance needs to be validated first. Quantitative polymerase chain reaction (PCR) may be used as a highly sensitive, nonimmunological technique complementary to ELISA. Due to the absence of DNA in certain processed cereal products, applicability for the detection of CD-toxic cereals in all foods and additives may be limited in the future. Mass spectrometry is the most promising nonimmunological approach for the highly sensitive and accurate detection of gluten proteins and peptides. Key considerations to be made are the selection of relevant gluten marker peptides, the conversion of peptide content to gluten content, and the establishment of reliable databases covering as many protein sequence variations as possible.

More research will have to focus on the development of reference materials, the compilation of protein databases, the comparison of analytical methods, and the influence of different matrices to generate accurate, reproducible, and generally applicable protocols for gluten quantitation to ensure the safety of gluten-free products for CD patients.

Further Reading

REVIEWS

[1] Armstrong MJ, Hegade VS, Robins G. *Advances in coeliac disease*. Curr Opin Gastroenterol 2012;28:104–12.

[2] Cotton D, Taichman D, Williams S, Crowe SE. *Celiac disease*. Ann Intern Med 2011. ITC5-2–16.

[3] Freeman HJ, Chopra A, Cladinin MT, Thomson ABR. *Recent advances in celiac disease*. World J Gastroenterol 2011;17:2259–72.

[4] Kaukinen K, Lindfors K, Collin P, Koskinen O, Maeki M. *Coeliac disease – a diagnostic and therapeutic challenge*. Clin Chem Lab Med 2010;48:1205–16.

[5] Meresse B, Georgia Malamut G, Cerf-Bensussan N. *Celiac disease: an immunological jigsaw*. Immunity 2012;36:907–19.

[6] Mubarak A, Houwen RHJ, Wolters VM. *Celiac disease: an overview from pathophysiology to treatment*. Minerva Pediatr 2012;64:271–87.

[7] Rubio-Tapia A, Murray JA. *Celiac disease*. Curr Opin Gastroenterol 2010;26:116–22.

[8] Tack GJ, Verbeek WHM, Schreurs MWJ, Mulder CJJ. *The spectrum of celiac disease: epidemiology, clinical aspects and treatment*. Nat Rev Gastroenterol Hepatol 2010;7:204–13.

[9] Wieser H, Konitzer K, Koehler P. *Celiac disease – multidisciplinary approaches*. Cereal Foods World 2012;57:215–24.

DEFINITIONS

[10] Husby S, Koletzko S, Korponay-Szabo IR, Mearin ML, Phillips A, Shamir R, et al. *European Society for Pediatric Gastroenterology, Hepatology, and Nutrition guidelines for the diagnosis of coeliac disease*. J Pediatr Gastroenterol Nutr 2012;54:136–60.

[11] Ludvigsson JF, Leffler DA, Bai JC, Biagi F, Fasano A, Green PH, et al. *The oslo definitions for coeliac disease and related terms*. Gut 2012;62:43–52.

HISTORY

[12] Guandalinis S. *Historical perspective of celiac disease*. In: Fasano A, Troncone R, Branski D, editors. Frontiers in celiac disease. Basel (Switzerland): Karger; 2008. pp. 1–11.

[13] Losowsky MS. *A history of coeliac disease*. Dig Dis 2008;26:112–20.

[14] Tommasini A, Not T, Ventura A. *Ages of celiac disease: from changing environment to improved diagnostic*. World J Gastroenterol 2011;17:3665–71.

EPIDEMIOLOGY

[15] Barada K, Abu Daya H, Rostami K, Catassi C. *Celiac disease in the developing world*. Gastrointest Endosc Clin N Am 2012;22:773–96.

[16] Ludvigsson JF, Green PH. *Clinical management of coeliac disease*. J Intern Med 2011;269:560–71.

GENETICS

[17] Abadie V, Sollid LM, Barreiro LB, Jabri B. *Integration of genetic and immunological insights into a model of celiac disease pathogenesis*. Annu Rev Immunol 2011;29:493–525.

[18] Hrdlickova B, Westra H-J, Franke L, Wijmenga C. *Celiac disease: moving from genetic associations to causal variants*. Clin Genet 2011;80:203–13.

[19] Kumar V, Wijmenga C, Withoff S. *From genome-wide association studies to disease mechanisms: celiac disease as a model for autoimmune diseases*. Semin Immunopathol 2012;34:567–80.

[20] Trynka G, Wijmenga C, van Heel DA. *A genetic perspective on coeliac disease*. Trends Mol Med 2010;16:537–50.

CLINICAL FEATURES

[21] Bao F, Green PHR, Bhagat G. *An update on celiac disease histopathology and the road ahead*. Arch Pathol Lab Med 2012;136:735–45.

[22] Ensari A. *Gluten-sensitive enteropathy (celiac disease). Controversies in diagnosis and classification*. Arch Pathol Lab Med 2010;134:826–36.

[23] Ludvigsson JF, Green PH. *Clinical management of coeliac disease*. J Intern Med 2011;269:560–71.

[24] Reilly NR, Fasano A. *Presentation of celiac disease*. Gastrointest Endosc Clin N Am 2012;22:613–21.

GLUTEN-ASSOCIATED DISEASES

[25] Aziz I, Sanders DS. *The irritable bowel syndrome-celiac disease connection*. Gastrointest Endosc Clin N Am 2012;22:623–7.

[26] Bolotin D, Petronic-Rosic. *Dermatitis herpetiformis. Part I. Epidemiology, pathogenesis, and clinical presentation*. J Am Acad Dermatol 2011;64:1017–24.

[27] Bolotin D, Petronic-Rosic. *Dermatitis herpetiformis. Part II. Diagnosis, management, and prognosis*. J Am Acad Dermatol 2011;64:1027–33.

[28] Catassi C, Bai JC, Bonaz B, Bouma G, Calabrò A, Carroccio A, et al. *Non-celiac gluten sensitivity: the new frontier of gluten related disorders*. Nutrients 2013;5:3839–53.

[29] Jackson JR, Eaton WW, Cascella NG, Fasano A, Kelly DL. *Neurologic and psychiatric manifestations of celiac disease and gluten sensitivity*. Psychiatr Q 2012;83:91–102.

[30] Pietzak M. *Celiac disease, wheat allergy, and gluten sensitivity: when gluten free is not a fad*. J Parenter Enteral Nutr 2012;36:685–755.

[31] Rubio-Tapia A, Murray JA. *Classification and management of refractory coeliac disease*. Gut 2010;59:547–57.

[32] Sapone A, Bai JC, Ciacci C, Dolinsek J, Green PHR, Hadjivassiliou M, et al. *Spectrum of gluten-related disorders: consensus on new nomenclature and classification*. BMC Med 2012;10:13.

DIAGNOSIS

[33] Bao F, Bhagat G. *Histopathology of celiac disease*. Gastrointest Endosc Clin N Am 2012;22:679–94.

[34] Husby S, Koletzko S, Korponay-Szabó IR, Mearin ML, Phillips A, Shamir R, et al. *European Society for Pediatric Gastroenterology, Hepatology, and Nutrition guidelines for the diagnosis of celiac disease*. J Pediatr Gastroenterol Nutr 2012;54:136–60.

[35] Lebwohl B, Rubio-Tapia A, Assiri A, Newland C, Guandalini S. *Diagnosis of celiac disease*. Gastrointest Endosc Clin N Am 2012;22:661–77.

[36] Leffler DA, Schuppan D. *Update on serologic testing in celiac disease*. Am J Gastroenterol 2010;105:2520–4.

[37] Rozenberg O, Lerner A, Pacht A, Grinberg M, Reginashvili D, Henig C, et al. *A novel algorithm for the diagnosis of celiac disease and a comprehensive review of celiac disease diagnostic*. Clin Rev Allergy Immunol 2012;42:331–41.

[38] Rubio-Tapia A, Hill ID, Kelly CP, Calderwood AH, Murray JA. *ACG clinical guidelines: diagnosis and management of celiac disease*. Am J Gastroenterol 2013;108:656–76.

[39] Volta U, Villanacci V. *Celiac disease: diagnostic criteria in progress*. Cell Mol Immunol 2011;8:96–102.

PATHOMECHANISM

[40] Di Sabatino A, Vanoli A, Giuffrida P, Luinetti O, Solcia E, Corazza GR. *The function of tissue transglutaminase in celiac disease*. Autoimmun Rev 2012;11:746–53.

[41] Fasano A. *Zonulin and its regulation of intestinal barrier function: the biological door to inflammation, autoimmunity, and cancer*. Physiol Rev 2011;91:151–75.

[42] Heyman M, Abed H, Lebreton C, Cerf-Bensussan N. *Intestinal permeability in coeliac disease: insight into mechanisms and relevance to pathogenesis*. Gut 2012;61:1355–64.

[43] Meresse B, Malamut G, Amar S, Cerf-Bensussan N. *Innate immunity and celiac disease*. In: Fasano A, Troncone R, Branski D, editors. Frontiers in celiac disease. Basel (Switzerland): Karger; 2008. pp. 66–81.

[44] Meresse B, Cerf-Bensussan N. *Innate T cell response in human gut*. Semin Immunol 2009;21:121–9.

[45] Qiao SW, Iversen R, Raki M, Sollid LM. *The adaptive immune response in celiac disease*. Semin Immunopathol 2012;34:523–40.

[46] Sollid LM, Jabri B. *Triggers and drivers of autoimmunity: lessons from coeliac disease*. Nat Rev Immunol 2013;13:294–302.

[47] Wang Z, Griffin M. *TG2 a novel extracellular protein with multiple functions*. Amino Acids 2012;42:539–49.

CEREALS

[48] Koehler P, Wieser H. *Chemistry of cereal grains*. In: Gobetti M, Gaenzle M, editors. Handbook of sourdough biotechnology. New York (USA): Springer; 2013. pp. 11–45.

[49] Leszczynska J. *Wheat (Triticum aestivum) allergens*. Chem Biolo Prop Food Allergens 2010:293–318.

[50] Mamone G, Picariello G, Addeo F, Ferranti P. *Proteomic analysis in allergy and intolerance to wheat products*. Expert Rev Proteomics 2011;8:95–115.

[51] Pawlowska P, Diowksz A, Kordialik-Bogacka E. *State-of-the-art incorporation of oats into a gluten-free diet*. Food Rev Int 2012;28:330–42.

CEREAL PROTEINS AND PEPTIDES

[52] Camarca A, Del Mastro A, Gianfrani C. *Repertoire of gluten peptides active in celiac disease patients: perspectives for translational therapeutic applications*. Endocr Metab Immune Disord Drug Targets 2012;12:207–19.

[53] Koehler P, Wieser H. *Chemistry of cereal grains*. In: Gobetti M, Gaenzle M, editors. Handbook of sourdough biotechnology. New York (USA): Springer; 2013. pp. 11–45.

[54] Shewry PR, Halford NG. *Cereal seed storage proteins: structures, properties and role in grain utilization*. J Exp Bot 2002;53:947–58.

[55] Tatham AS, Gilbert SM, Fido RJ, Shewry PR. *Extraction, separation, and purification of wheat gluten proteins and related proteins of barley, rye, and oats*. Methods Mol Med 2000;41:55–73.

TESTING TOXICITY

[56] Lindfors K, Rauhavirta T, Stenman S, Maeki M, Kaukinen K. *In vitro models for gluten toxicity: relevance for celiac disease pathogenesis and development of novel treatment options*. Exp Biol Med 2012;237:119–25.

[57] Marietta EV, Murray JA. *Animal models to study gluten sensitivity*. Semin Immunopathol 2012;34:497–511.

[58] Stoven S, Murray JA, Marietta EV. *Latest in vitro and in vivo models of celiac disease*. Expert Opin Drug Discov 2013:445–57.

GLUTEN-FREE DIET

[59] Dorn SD, Heinandez L, Minaya MT, Morris CB, Hu Y, Leserman J, et al. *The development and validation of a new coeliac disease quality of life survey (CD-QOL)*. Aliment Pharmacol Ther 2010;31:666–75.

[60] Garcia-Manzanares A, Lucendo AJ. *Nutritional and dietary aspects of celiac disease*. Nutr Clin Pract 2011;26:163–73.

[61] Hager AS, Axel C, Arendt EK. *Status of carbohydrates and dietary fiber in gluten-free diets*. Cereal Foods World 2011;56:109–14.

[62] Saturni L, Ferreti G, Bacchetti T. *The gluten free diet: safety and nutritional quality*. Nutrients 2010;2:16–34.

[63] Simpson S, Thompson T. *Nutrition assessment in celiac disease*. Gastrointest Endosc Clin N Am 2012;22:797–809.

[64] Ukkola A, Maeki M, Kurppa K, Collin P, Huhtala H, Kekkonen L, et al. *Patients' experiences and perceptions of living with coeliac disease – implications for optimal care*. J Gastrointest Liver Dis 2012;21:17–22.

ALTERNATIVE THERAPIES

[65] Bethune MT, Khosla C. *Oral enzyme therapy for celiac sprue*. Methods Enzym 2012;502:241–71.

[66] Lindfors K, Laehdeaho ML, Kalliokoski S, Kurppa K, Collin P, Maeki M, et al. *Future treatment strategies for celiac disease*. Expert Opin Ther Targets 2012;16:665–75.

[67] McAllister CS, Kagnoff MF. *The immunopathogenesis of celiac disease reveals possible therapies beyond the gluten-free diet.* Semin Immunopathol 2012;34:581–600.

[68] Osorio C, Wen N, Gemini R, Zemetra R, von Wettstein D, Rustgi S. *Targeted modification of wheat grain protein to reduce the content of celiac causing epitopes.* Funct Integr Genomics 2012;12:417–38.

[69] Perez LC, de Villasante GC, Ruiz AC, Leon F. *Non-dietary therapeutic clinical trials in coeliac disease.* Eur J Intern Med 2012;23:9–14.

[70] Rashtak S, Murray JA. *Review article: coeliac disease, new approaches to therapy.* Aliment Pharmacol Ther 2012;35:768–81.

[71] Sollid LM, Khosla C. *Novel therapies for coeliac disease.* J Intern Med 2011;269:604–13.

[72] Wieser H, Koehler P. *Detoxification of gluten by means of enzymatic treatment.* J AOAC Int 2012;95:356–63.

GLUTEN ANALYSIS

[73] Diaz-Amigo C, Popping B. *Accuracy of ELISA detection methods for gluten and reference materials: a realistic assessment.* J Agric Food Chem 2013;61:5681–8.

[74] Haraszi R, Chassaigne H, Maquet A, Ulberth F. *Analytical methods for detection of gluten in food – method developments in support of food labeling legislation.* J AOAC Int 2011;94:1006–25.

[75] Wieser H. *Detection of gluten.* In: Arendt EK, dal Bello F, editors. Gluten-free cereal products and beverages. Amsterdam (The Netherlands): Academic Press; 2008. pp. 47–80.

DIETETIC PRODUCTS

[76] Arendt E, dal Bello F. Gluten-free cereals products and beverages. Elsevier Academic Press; 2008.

[77] Caputo I, Lepretti M, Martucciello S, Esposito C. *Enzymatic strategies to detoxify gluten: implications for celiac disease.* Enzyme Res 2010:e174354.

[78] Houben A, Höchstätter A, Becker T. *Possibilities to increase the quality in gluten-free bread production: an overview.* Eur Food Res Technol 2012;235:195–208.

[79] Zannini E, Jones JM, Renzetti S, Arendt EK. *Functional replacements for gluten.* Annu Rev Food Sci Technol 2012;3:227–45.

Index

Note: Page numbers followed by f indicate figures; t, tables.

Color Plates

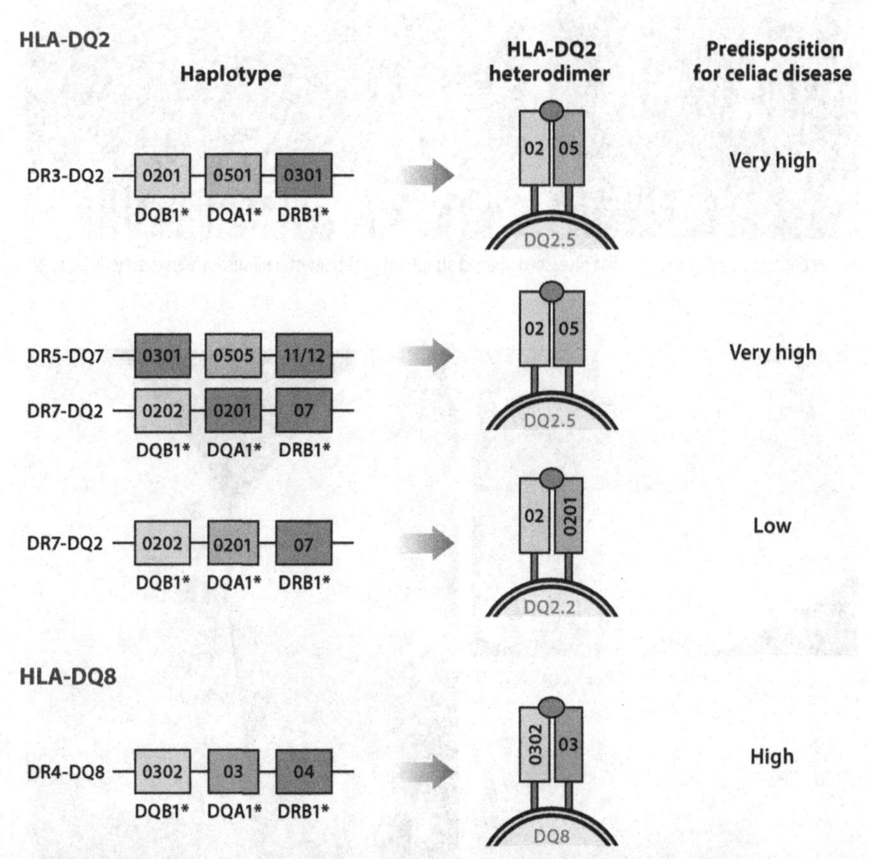

■ **FIGURE 1.4** Human leukocyte antigen (HLA) associations in celiac disease (CD). The great majority of CD patients express the HLA-DQ2.5 heterodimer, which is more strongly associated with CD than are the DQ8 and DQ2.2 heterodimers. *From Abadie et al. [30], with permission.*

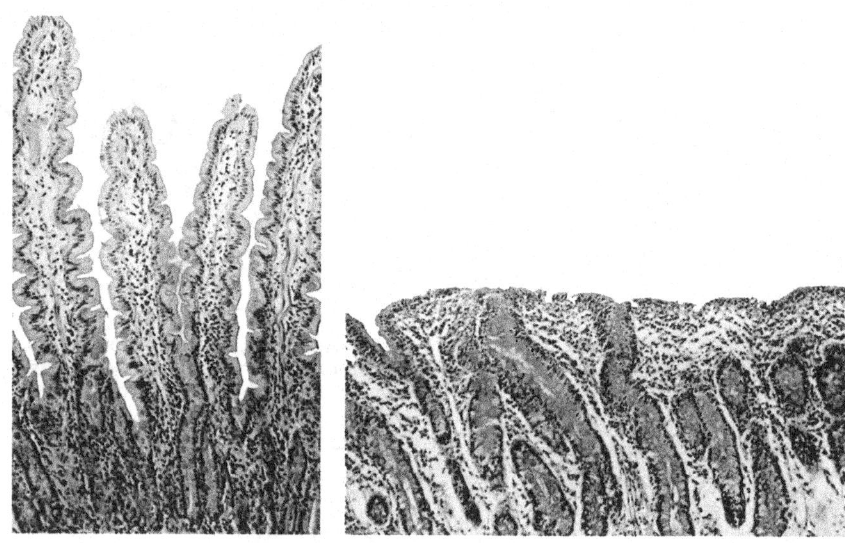

■ **FIGURE 1.6** Cross-section of normal (left) and celiac disease-damaged atrophical (right) intestinal mucosa. *Reprinted with permission from the German Celiac Society.*

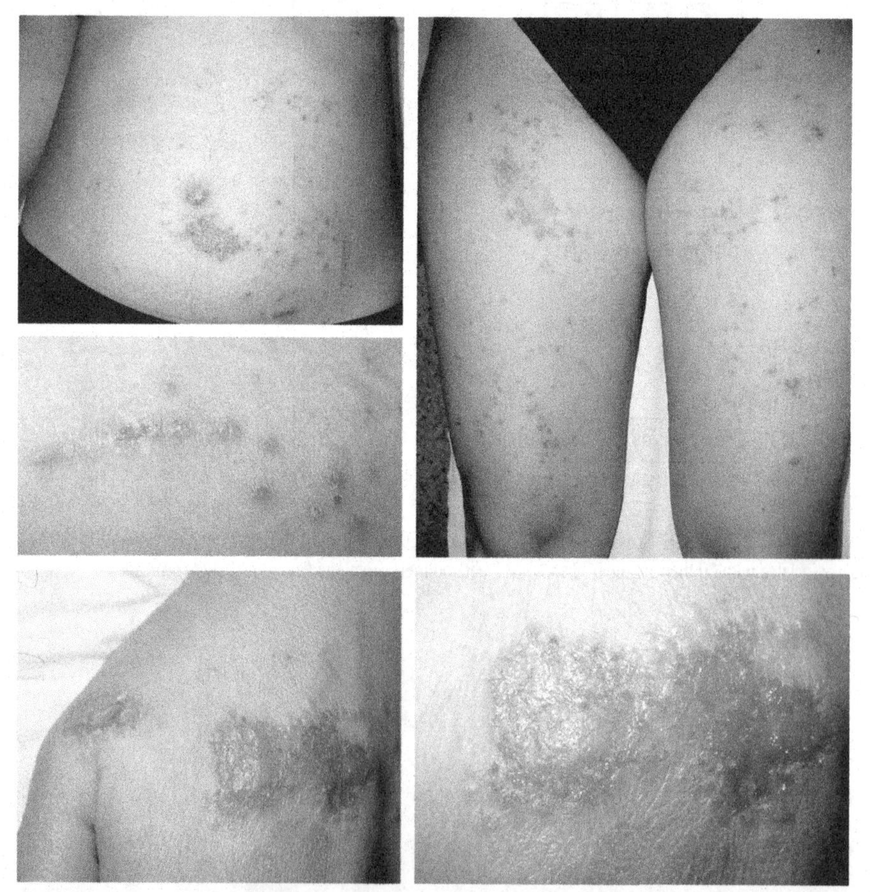

■ **FIGURE 1.7** Erythematous, papular, and vesiculous lesions in a patient with dermatitis herpetiformis. *From Caproni et al. [144].*

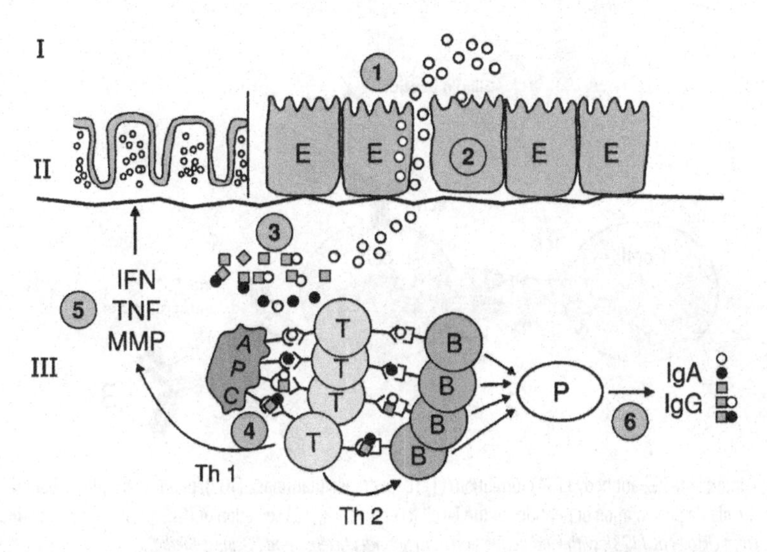

■ **FIGURE 1.10** Schematical representation of the adaptive immune response in the intestinal lymphatic tissue and destruction of enterocytes in the pathogenesis of celiac disease. I = intestinal lumen; II = epithelium; III = lamina propria; APC = antigen-presenting cell; B = B cell; E = enterocyte; IFN = interferon-γ; Ig = immunoglobulin; MMP = matrix metalloproteinase; P = plasma cell; T = CD4+ T cell; TG2 = tissue transglutaminase; Th = T helper; TNF = tumor necrosis factor. For steps 1–6, see text.

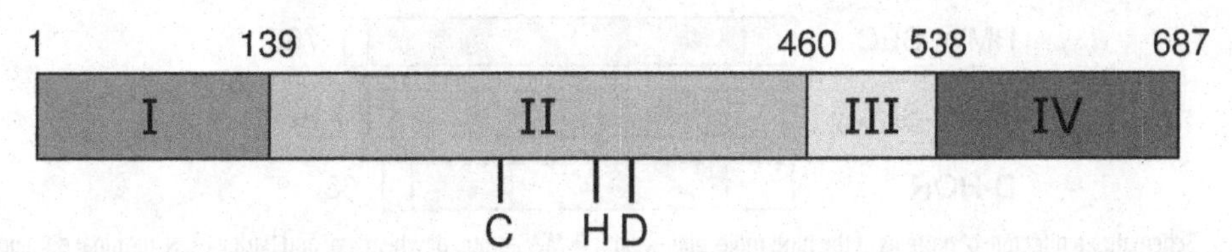

■ **FIGURE 1.13** Different domains of tissue transglutaminase (TG2): I = β-sandwich; II = α/β catalytic core with cysteine (C) 277, histidine (H) 335, and aspartic acid (D) 358 of the active site; III = β-barrel-1; IV = β-barrel-2. *Adapted from Ref. [305].*

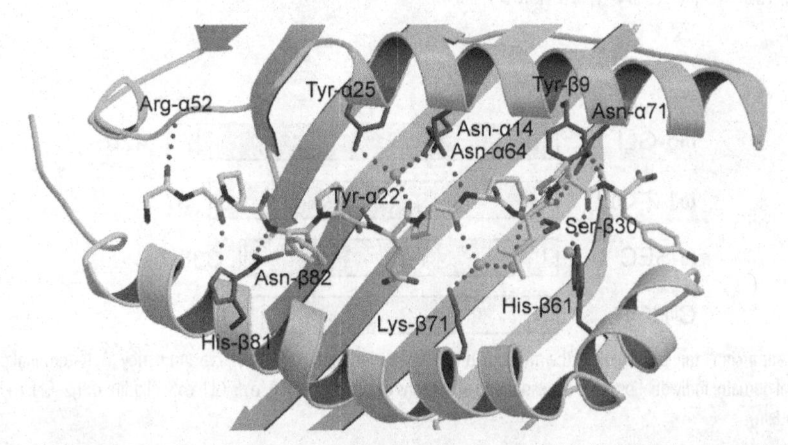

■ **FIGURE 1.15** Putative hydrogen-bonding network in the DQ2.5/peptide complex (shown as red dashes). Peptide α57–68/E65 is shown in yellow, α-chain in green, and β-chain in blue. *According to Ref. [320], copyright 2004 National Academy of Sciences, USA).*

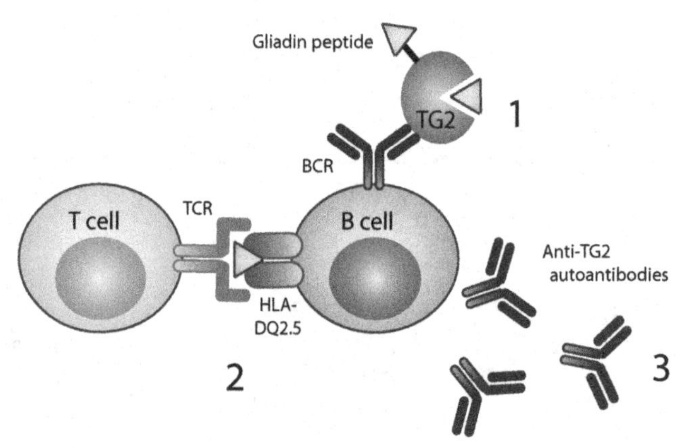

■ **FIGURE 1.20** Model explaining anti-TG2 antibody (TGA) formation. (1) Tissue transglutaminase (TG2)/peptide complex is bound to TG2-specific B-cell receptors (BCR); (2) help from T cells via presentation of peptides to the T-cell receptor (TCR); (3) secretion of TG2-specific autoantibodies after B-cell differentiation into plasma cells. *From Qiao et al. [123], with kind permission from Springer Science and Business Media.*

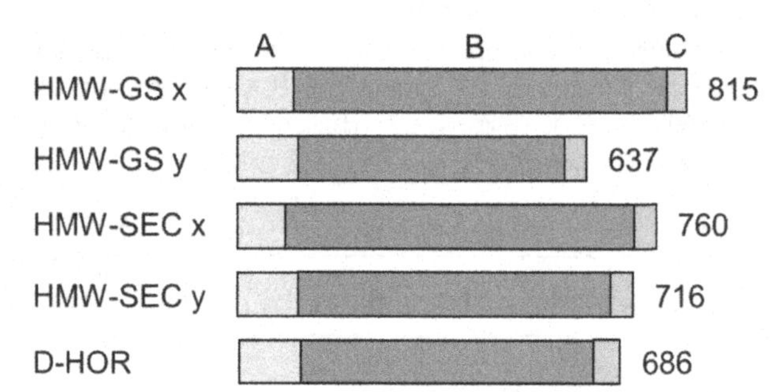

■ **FIGURE 2.6** Schematic architecture of proteins of the high molecular-weight (HMW) group of wheat, rye and barley (A, N-terminal domain; B, repetitive domain; C, C-terminal domain; individual proteins correspond to accessions given in Table 2.5; HMW-GSx, wheat high-molecular-weight glutenin subunit x-type; HMW-GSy, wheat high-molecular-weight glutenin subunit y-type; HMW-SECx, rye high-molecular-weight secalin x-type; HMW-SECy, rye high-molecular-weight secalin y-type; D-HOR, D-hordein).

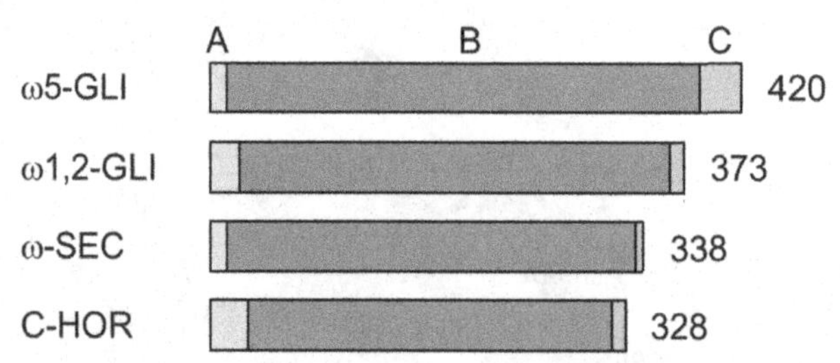

■ **FIGURE 2.7** Schematic architecture of proteins of the medium-molecular-weight group of wheat, rye and barley (A, N-terminal domain; B, repetitive domain; C, C-terminal domain; individual proteins correspond to accessions given in Table 2.6; ω5-GLI, ω5-gliadin; ω1,2-GLI, ω1,2-gliadin; ω-SEC, ω-secalin; C-HOR, C-hordein).

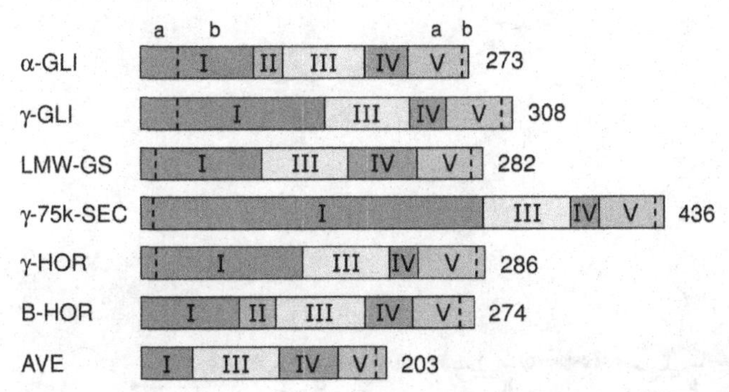

■ **FIGURE 2.8** Schematic architecture of proteins of the LMW-group of wheat, rye, barley and oats (sections I–II, N-terminal domain; sections III–V, C-terminal domain; individual proteins correspond to accessions given in Table 2.7; α-GLI, α-gliadin; γ-GLI, γ-gliadin; LMW-GS, wheat low-molecular-weight glutenin subunits; γ-75k-SEC, γ-75k-secalin; γ-HOR, γ-hordein; B-HOR, B-hordein; AVE, avenin).

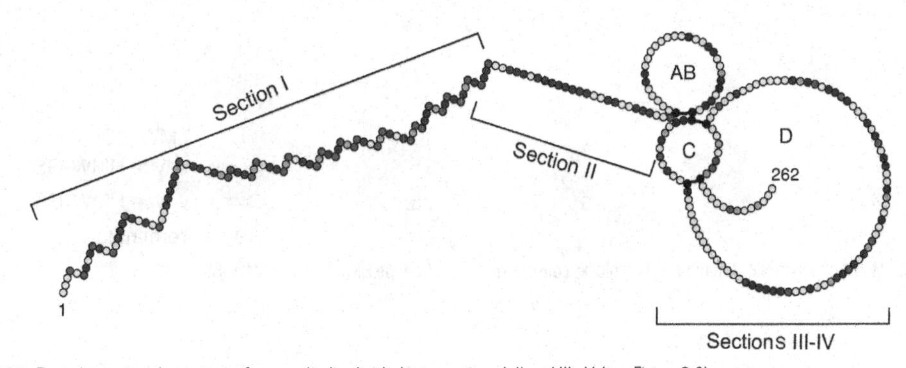

■ **FIGURE 2.11** Two-dimensional structure of an α-gliadin divided into sections I, II and III–V (see Figure 2.8).

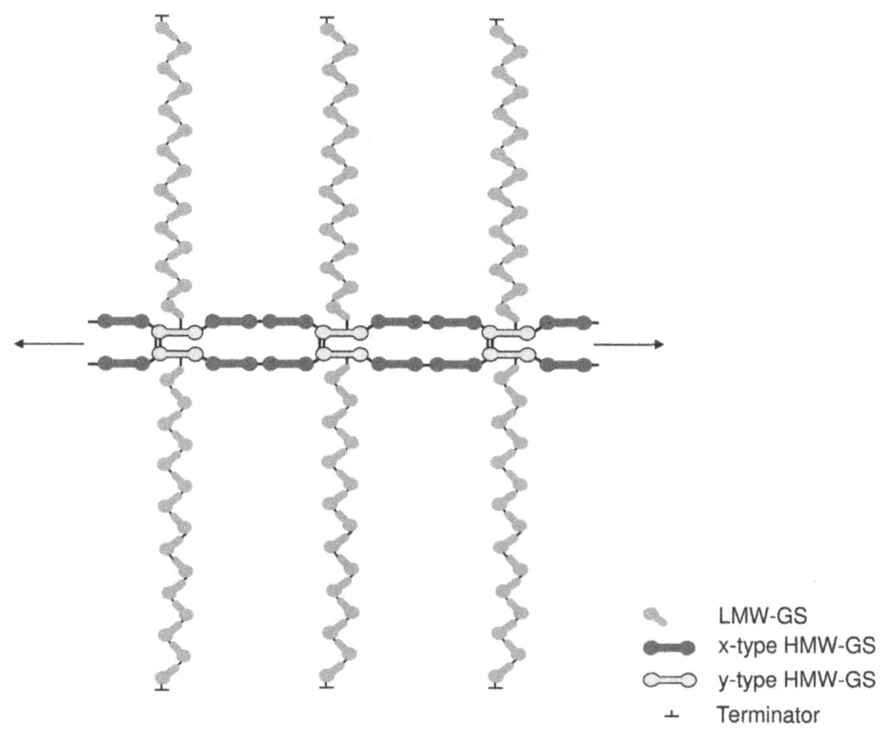

FIGURE 2.12 Model of polymeric glutenin building blocks consisting of x- and y-type HMW-GS and LMW-GS.

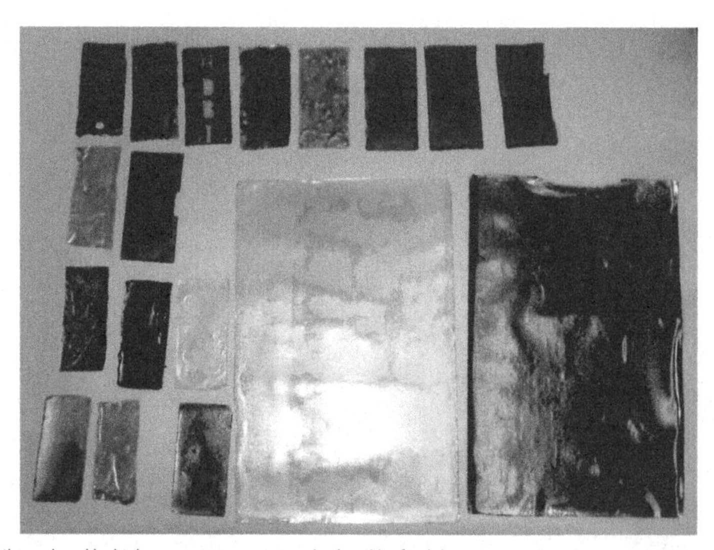

FIGURE 2.13 Gluten foils produced by high-pressure treatment and colored by food dyes.

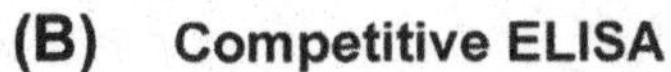

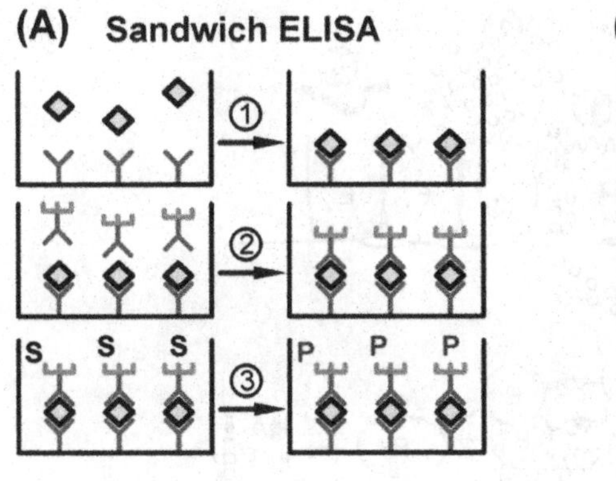

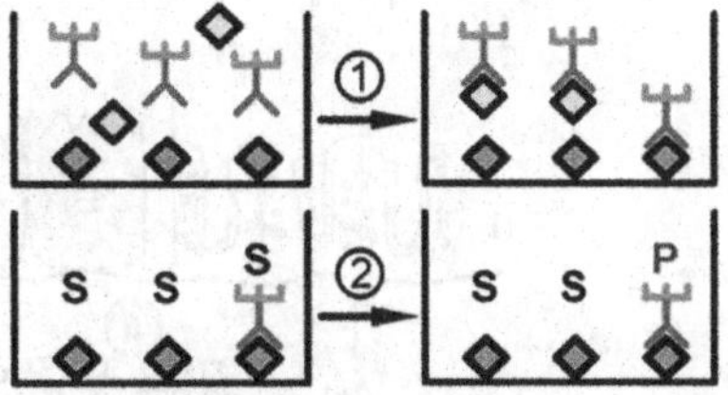

FIGURE 4.9 Different ELISA formats: (A) sandwich ELISA; (B) competitive ELISA. *Adapted from Ref. [95].*

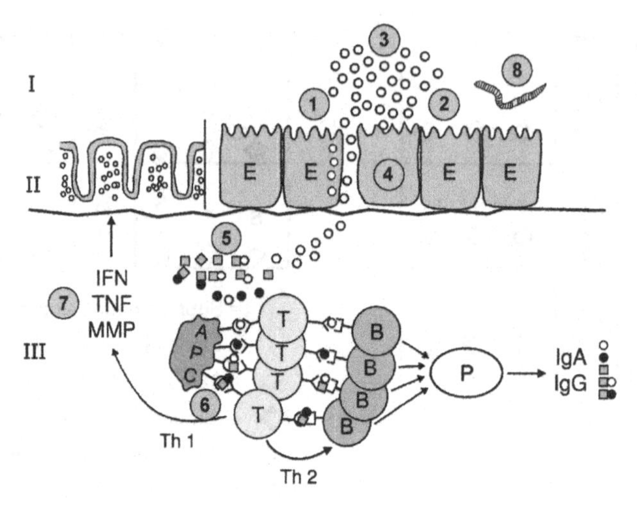

FIGURE 3.1 Scheme of the immune response in the pathomechanism of celiac disease (CD) and indication of possible future treatments of CD. (1) Oral enzyme therapy; (2) gluten-sequestering polymers; (3) probiotic bacteria; (4) permeability inhibitors; (5) inhibition of transglutaminase 2 (TG2); (6) human leukocyte antigen (HLA)-DQ blocking; (7) modulation of inflammation; and (8) hookworm therapy.

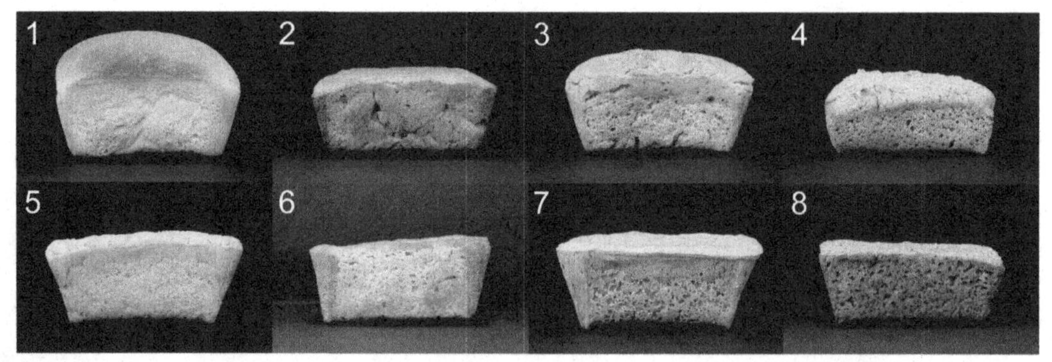

FIGURE 4.1 Appearance of breads from different cereal flours baked under standardized conditions (1, wheat; 2, rye; 3, barley; 4, oats; 5, rice; 6, corn; 7, buckwheat; 8, sorghum).

Printed in the United States
By Bookmasters

Printed in the United States
By Bookmasters